Clinical Trials in Cardiology

Edited by

Bertram Pitt
Professor of Internal Medicine, Division of Cardiology, University of Michigan School of Medicine, Ann Arbor, MI, USA

Desmond Julian
Emeritus Professor of Cardiology, University of Newcastle upon Tyne; Formerly Medical Director of the British Heart Foundation, London, UK

Stuart Pocock
Professor of Medical Statistics, Department of Epidemiology and Population Health, London School of Hygiene and Tropical Medicine, London, UK

W. B. Saunders Company Ltd
London ● Philadelphia ● Toronto ● Sydney ● Tokyo

W. B. Saunders Company Ltd 24–28 Oval Road
London NW1 7DX, UK

The Curtis Center
Independence Square West
Philadelphia, PA 19106-3399, USA

Harcourt Brace & Company
55 Horner Avenue
Toronto, Ontario M8Z 4X6, Canada

Harcourt Brace & Company, Australia
30–52 Smidmore Street
Marrickville, NSW 2204, Australia

Harcourt Brace & Company, Japan
Ichibancho Central Building, 22-1 Ichibancho
Chiyoda-ku, Tokyo 102, Japan

A catalogue record for this book is available from the British Library

ISBN 0-7020-2156-3

Typeset by Paston Press Ltd, Loddon, Norfolk
Printed in Great Britain by The University Press, Cambridge

Contents

Contributors

Stephen G. Ball
Professor of Cardiology, Institute for Cardiovascular Research, University of Leeds, Leeds, UK

Jean-Pierre Boissel
Professor and Head of Department, Clinical Pharmacology, Claude Bernard University, Lyon, France

Steven Borzak
Director, Cardiac Intensive Care Unit, Division of Cardiovascular Medicine, Henry Ford Hospital, Detroit, MI, USA

John G. F. Cleland
Honorary Consultant Cardiologist, Western Infirmary, Glasgow, UK; British Heart Foundation Senior Research Fellow, MRC Clinical Research Initiative in Heart Failure, University of Glasgow West Medical Building, Glasgow, UK

Julian Collinson
Clinical Research Fellow, Clinical Trials and Evaluation Unit, Royal Brompton Hospital, Sydney Street, London, UK

Pim J. de Feyter
Catheterization Laboratory, University Hospital Dijkzigt, Rotterdam, The Netherlands

Marcus Flather
Director, Clinical Trials and Evaluation Unit, Royal Brompton Hospital, Sydney Street, London, UK

Sidney Goldstein
Division Head Emeritus, Division of Cardiovascular Medicine, Henry Ford Hospital, Detroit, MI, Professor of Medicine, Case Western University, Cleveland, OH, USA

Alistair S. Hall
Senior Lecturer in Cardiology, Institute for Cardiovascular Research, University of Leeds, Leeds, UK

Robert A. Henderson
Consultant Cardiologist, Division of Cardiovascular Medicine, University Hospital, Queens Medical Centre, Nottingham, UK

Desmond G. Julian
Emeritus Professor of Cardiology, University of Newcastle upon Tyne; Formerly Medical Director of the British Heart Foundation, London, UK

Thomas Killip
Professor of Medicine, Department of Medicine, Albert Einstein College of Medicine, Executive Vice President, Beth Israel Medical Center, 16th First Avenue, New York, USA

Alain Leizorovicz
Director of Research INSERM, Clinical Pharmacology, Claude Bernard University, Lyon, France

Gordon D. Murray
Robertson Centre for Biostatistics, University of Glasgow, UK

Michael F. Oliver
Professor Emeritus, National Heart & Lung Institute, Imperial College School of Medicine, London, UK

Bertram Pitt
Professor and Associate Chairman, Department of Internal Medicine, Division of Cardiology, University of Michigan School of Medicine, Ann Arbor, USA

Stuart J. Pocock
Professor, Department of Epidemiology & Population Health, Medical Statistics Unit, London School of Hygiene and Tropical Medicine, UK

Elliot Rapaport
Professor of Medicine, William Watt Kerr Professor of Clinical Medicine, Associate Dean for San Francisco General Hospital School of Medicine, Department of Medicine, San Francisco General Hospital and Department of Medicine & Cardiovascular Research Institute, University of California, San Francisco, USA

Kumar Ravi
Fellow in Cardiology, Department of Medicine, Beth Israel Medical Center, New York, USA

J. Ian S. Robertson
Formerly visiting Professor of Medicine, Prince of Wales Hospital, Chinese University, Hong Kong

Jacques E. Rossouw
Visiting Scientist, Office of Disease Prevention, The National Institutes of Health, Bethesda, MD, USA

Freek W. A. Verheugt
Professor of Cardiology, Chairman, Division of Cardiology, Academisch Ziekenhuis Nijmegen, Nijmegen, The Netherlands

Robert West
Reader in Epidemiology, University of Wales College of Medicine, Heath Park, Cardiff, UK

Harvey D. White
Director of Coronary Care & Cardiovascular Research, Green Lane Hospital, Auckland, New Zealand

Lars Wilhelmsen
Professor, Department of Medicine, Östra University Hospital, Göteborg S-416 85, Sweden

Preface

Clinical trials now form the essential basis for much of cardiological practice. Over the last few years, the design, conduct and reporting of clinical trials has improved greatly so that more trials now are well-designed and sufficiently powered to answer the clinical questions addressed. Nonetheless, there are still too many trials that do not measure up to acceptable standards, and the interpretation of trials is far from an exact science. In creating this book, therefore, we have invited distinguished experts in the field to review the published cardiovascular trials critically, and we have also considered the standards by which such trials should be evaluated. We hope this approach will prove more valuable than the uncritical tabulations of trial results that are increasingly available.

In producing this book, we would like to thank the authors who contributed so willingly. We would wish to express our appreciation of the help and advice of Linda Clark and Miranda Bromage of W. B. Saunders Company Ltd.

SECTION I

Basic Principles

1

Introduction

Bertram Pitt, Desmond Julian and Stuart J. Pocock

In recent years there have been many exciting developments across a wide range of therapeutic practices in cardiology, and we can anticipate substantial further advances in the future. However, it is increasingly recognized that, while there is a plethora of potential treatment innovations, only a minority of such ideas turn out to be of real patient benefit, and occasionally an apparently promising therapeutic initiative may actually be harmful to patient welfare.

Hence it is essential that any potential new treatment in cardiology be subjected to the most rigorous testing. Of crucial importance is that such evaluation be objective and fair, with every attempt being made to avoid bias in patient selection, management, follow-up, and outcome assessment. The randomized controlled clinical trial is the only reliable means of achieving such high standards of clinical investigation. Many early phase, small-scale clinical trials are undertaken to evaluate short-term physiological responses to potential new treatments and, while these can give valuable supportive evidence as to which treatments might be of genuine patient benefit, they cannot in themselves give definitive evidence as to which treatments have important (often longer term) influence on patient survival and avoidance of major clinical events (e.g. myocardial infarction).

This book is dedicated to reviewing the information from major randomized clinical trials with an emphasis on those trials and clinical areas for which there is evidence of an effect on morbidity and/or mortality. Each of the authors has been asked critically to review the major clinical trials in their area of expertise and to give their opinion as to what we have learned from these trials, point out deficiencies in the accumulated data, and, where possible, suggest areas for further clinical investigation.

While an individual clinical trial may have a major impact on clinical practice, it is more likely that it is the accumulated information from several clinical trials that is necessary to place the information in proper perspective, to alter clinical decision-making and practice based upon evidence rather than our own experience or intuition.

The introductory chapters are meant to provide the clinician and clinical investigator with the elements of a well-designed clinical trial, an understanding of the clinical trial process, as well as information on how to interpret clinical trials and implement their results in clinical decision-making. In view of the increasing importance of randomized clinical trials for the development of treatment guidelines, it is essential that the trials adhere as closely as possible to these principles. Subsequent chapters then apply these principles to relevant clinical indications. The specific clinical topics covered are described briefly below.

3

The use of lipid-lowering agents was one of the most contentious issues in medicine until the results of the major clinical trials were presented. Now, their great benefits and low risks, at least for the statins, have been amply demonstrated, but questions remain as to the selection of patients and as to the lipid levels that justify treatment.

Hypertension has been the subject of numerous trials over several decades, but many of these were too small, or poorly designed. Interpretation has, therefore, been difficult, and there are still uncertainties about the choice of agent and about the severity of hypertension that warrants therapy. Nonetheless, trials have effectively proved the value of antihypertensive agents in preventing stroke and heart failure. It is less clear how successful they are at reducing mortality from ischemic heart disease.

The past decade has seen many advances in the treatment of the ischemic syndromes, but there have been remarkably few major studies on the prognosis of stable angina, the commonest of them all. By contrast, there have been many good studies of unstable angina, although the rival merits of anticoagulants and the antiplatelet agents have still not been clarified. Nor do we yet know the exact role of beta-blockers, nitrates, and calcium antagonists. Furthermore, the place of angioplasty after unstable angina is only now being subjected to major study.

Studies done more than a decade ago demonstrated the superiority of coronary bypass surgery over medical treatment in improving prognosis in certain categories of patient with stable angina, but can we apply the results of these studies to contemporary practice, when both surgical techniques and medical management have been transformed? More recently, trials have compared surgery with coronary angioplasty in patients with angina. These have helped to clarify the risks of the two procedures and have provided an indication of the relative benefits in the first few years, but longer term follow-up is necessary before one can draw definitive conclusions. Furthermore, the development of stents is promising, and recent trials have given some indication of their potential, but more trials are needed before their ultimate place is established.

Nowhere in medicine has the value of large randomized trials been better demonstrated than in showing the beneficial effects of thrombolysis in myocardial infarction. Their role in the management of this condition is clear, and the size of the trials, particularly when examined by meta-analysis, has helped to define the categories of patient that can be best helped by this treatment, and those most at hazard. The effectiveness of aspirin has also been shown, but trials have yet to demonstrate convincingly the benefits and harm of anticoagulants in this context.

Angiotensin converting enzyme (ACE) inhibitors have been established as essential elements in the treatment of heart failure, and also after myocardial infarction complicated by heart failure or poor left ventricular function. They have also been shown to reduce mortality when administered on the first day of a heart attack, but controversy continues as to whether they should be given to all patients (for whom there are no contra-indications) at this time, or whether they should be reserved for those most likely to benefit.

Large and well-designed studies have established the value of beta-blockers in the postinfarction patient, although the precise indications and contraindications are not universally agreed. By contrast, trials of calcium antagonists have been much less impressive and, indeed, these agents can be hazardous. However, it may be that the benefits and risks of individual calcium antagonists depend upon their pharmacological characteristics, and further information is required before the issue can be considered resolved.

At one time, antiarrhythmic therapy seemed a promising way of managing patients after myocardial infarction who were at high risk because of 'warning' arrhythmias. This approach appeared particularly attractive when it was shown that certain drugs could virtually eliminate these arrhythmias. The trials have provided a sobering experience, for it appeared that agents that seemed to be most effective in treating the surrogate outcome of 'warning arrhythmias' were those most likely to increase mortality. These trials dramatically illustrate the dangers of relying on small trials and surrogate end-points.

Heart failure is a dangerous disorder which is becoming more frequent with the aging population. The numerous trials in this area have been rewarded with both success and disaster. In spite of the significant advances in treatment, the mortality remains high, and will be the subject of many new trials of a variety of therapeutic approaches. Cardiac rehabilitation is a very practical area of patient management which is difficult to study because of confounding factors and the frequency of noncompliance. Furthermore, it is not easy to define because of the various physical and psychological modalities that may be incorporated. Nonetheless, several major trials have been conducted, and it is appropriate that this book concludes with a chapter devoted to their critical assessment.

Clinical trials now form the most solid basis for the practice of cardiology. It is important that cardiologists and others concerned with both patient management and research in cardiology are not only cognisant of the best available evidence, but also that they can weigh up the merits and deficiencies of the increasing number of trials that are being undertaken. This book has been planned to combine a clear account of clinical trial principles with a detailed consideration of the major trials in cardiology. We hope that our efforts will prove of value.

2

Trial Design and Conduct

Jean-Pierre Boissel and Alain Leizorovicz

Introduction

Are Clinical Trials in Cardiology Specific?

Clinical trials represent a fundamental advance in the history of the development and evaluation of effective therapies. They are scientific experiments and, because of this, they can be universally understood and their results applied, provided they are designed and conducted according to now well-codified principles. These principles have been described in numerous papers and textbooks, and are reiterated in the following sections of this chapter.

The concept of a clinical trial is essentially the same for any medical domain. It applies to the evaluation of drugs as well as of surgical procedures, physical therapies and psychotherapies. It can be extended to the evaluation of diagnostic tests. Ultimately, clinical trials can, and will increasingly be, used to evaluate medical strategies. Strategies consist of a set of interventions, possibly in combination with different diagnostic procedures. Examples of the evaluation of strategies in cardiology have been published; for example, invasive versus conservative attitude to acute myocardial infarction (MI), and pre-hospital versus hospital thrombolysis in acute MI. Given the above, what factors could be identified as being specific to trials in cardiology?

The prevalence of cardiac disease is so high in developed countries that despite a risk of fatal complications that is probably lower than for cancers and acquired immune deficiency syndrome (AIDS) (two other domains where therapeutic research is particularly active), the mortality and morbidity due to cardiac disease still rank number one in the adult population. Given this, the definition of relevant therapeutic objectives for cardiac patients, and therefore for clinical trials in cardiology, is straightforward, i.e. to reduce mortality and major cardiac complications (MI, severe heart failure). These clinically relevant outcomes are relatively few in cardiology, and they are quite simple to assess.

There is also usually little dilemma about the individual benefit of prolongation of life, which may be philosophically and ethically disputable in other types of disease such as severely disabling stroke or end-stage metastic cancer. Cardiovascular mortality or total mortality has, therefore, been chosen as the main endpoint in many trials.

7

Large, Simple Trials and Small but Definite Benefit

The relatively low hazard rates associated with outcomes of clinical treatment in cardiac disease and, in particular, the low death rate, necessitate that large to very large numbers of patients be enrolled in clinical trials and/or a follow-up period of several years is used in order to observe a sufficient number of outcomes. The usefulness and, as importantly, the feasibility of performing powerful large-scale trials in cardiology was demonstrated in the late 1970s by Peto and coworkers.[1,2] The proposed concept was much more than a mere statistical theory. It postulated that a small but definite relative improvement in mortality from diseases as common as MI might lead, when applied to the whole population, to the saving of hundreds of thousands of lives per year. The only way to demonstrate such benefits and to convince prescribers that they are real and certain (narrow confidence intervals) is to use a large sample size. The consequence is that such trials, requiring as they do hundreds or thousands of investigators, should, although rigorous, be simple to perform. In the following years several large to very large scale trials involving tens of thousands of patients were performed successfully by different teams. A review of the clinical trials of the management of acute MI shows that hundreds of thousands of patients have been enrolled in hundreds of trials, the latest and the largest trial involving more than 60 000 patients.[3] However, with very large trials it is possible to demonstrate a very small relative benefit, and an even smaller absolute benefit. Although this is feasible, is it worthwhile? The issue is that, with such small benefit, many patients may be treated for each successful case. All the patients who were treated for nothing will add to the cost of the treatment and the burden of its administration, and, even more worryingly, to the risk of adverse reactions.

Future Issues in Clinical Trials in Cardiology

As described above, we are now able to identify very small individual benefit of treatment, and this in itself poses a serious problem with regard to efficiency. One way to solve the dilemma is to think in terms of a therapy target population.[4] The aim of performing clinical trials in cardiology is no longer merely to prove that a treatment is efficacious, but to focus on (1) estimating the magnitude of the benefit a treatment provides and (2) to whom it is really beneficial.

Because of the high prevalence of cardiac diseases and because of major therapeutic advances obtained owing to the numerous clinical trials done over the past two decades, objective changes in health statistics of cardiovascular morbidity and mortality at the community level have already been observed. Likely further improvement will occur when results of trials are applied to a broader population and when long-term effects of effective primary or secondary prevention are observed. The current availability of treatments that definitely improve the vital prognosis of conditions such as MI, angina pectoris, congestive heart failure, hypertension, and hypercholesterolemia leaves the cardiologist faced with new tasks, i.e. to assess small, but definite, improvements provided by new drugs over already effective treatments. In addition, as some treatments were proven effective before the assessment of newer effective therapies, is there a need to re-evaluate them in combination with the newer agents?

Trials comparing different thrombolytic agents in acute MI require tens of thousands of patients to demonstrate any relative improvement in mortality of the order of 15%. Is there a real need for such new agents and, therefore, is it necessary to perform a very large scale trial each time? The definition of a relevant clinical improvement is not easy and may not be the responsibility only of physicians. Ideally, it is the responsibility of the community, or its elected representatives or health insurers, to set desirable objectives in terms of level of health and to assign corresponding resources for therapeutic research and coverage of care costs.

A reduction in mortality may no longer always be a relevant endpoint when comparing active treatments. Provided survival and major complications are similar, quality of life, symptoms, practicability, and cost may become the predominant factors in the choice of treatment. However, the evaluation of these endpoints raises new clinical and methodological problems. New trial designs have been proposed to test for equivalence or (weighted or nonweighted) combined outcomes. It is not always clear whether these trials answer real new clinical questions, or whether the main objective of their promoters is to decrease the sample size and hence the duration and cost of the trials.

These questions deserve a review of what can be considered as established practice and reflection on the implications of the new challenges for the evaluation of treatments in cardiology. However, the general principles of the methodology and conduct of clinical trials will remain the same. The purpose of this chapter is to review the latter aspects of trials and to look at the major difficulties raised by their practical application. Textbooks on clinical trial methodology are available for a more detailed account.[5–7]

Principles of the Experimental Method

A clinical trial is an experiment in which data are collected. The analysis of the data, according to the trial design, leads to a piece of information that is scientific in nature. As such, a clinical trial should meet the fundamental requirements of scientific investigation. Clinical trial methodology is based on the principles of the experimental method, as laid down in the 19th century.[8] These principles are as follows: (1) The hypothesis to be tested must be proposed and written before the start of data collection; the hypothesis is converted by means of a modification of the investigated system (e.g. the patient, the care providing unit). (2) The investigated system is the experimental unit. (3) The experimental design must be such that testing of the hypothesis relies on the comparison between a group of modified experimental units and a control group of unmodified units; this comparison is the key that provides the researcher with access to the results of the experiment. (4) The number of experimental units must be large enough to smooth any idiosyncratic reactions of the experimental units. (5) In order to establish a causal relationship between the modification of the system and the outcome, the two groups must be alike and managed identically except for the intervention itself, prior to, during and after the intervention that induces the modification, up to the completion of data collection.

Originally, these principles could not be applied directly to field research with full efficiency. Practical refinements of the principles came later, with the discovery of the statistical model and the concept of confounding factors. However, before going on to the modern era of experimental methodology, let us consider some of the consequences on the conduct of clinical trials of the first of the above-mentioned principles.

The Need for a Prior Hypothesis

There should be an hypothesis at the very beginning. A clinical trial is an experiment aimed at testing an hypothesis, which usually concerns the efficacy of a given intervention regarding an event, symptom, or impaired quality of life in patients with a defined condition and a particular profile of eligibility. This hypothesis represents the output of a long and complex process, and is gradually built up around reasoning based on available knowledge, intuition, observed or assumed functional relationships, and careful analysis of the health problem in which the trialist is interested. One aspect of the reasoning is the building of a therapeutic model, and the other is the problem formulation. The two processes are fairly intricate and, although they are interdependent, we will consider them separately.

The word 'model' is used in various contexts. Here, it is used to indicate any representation of reality built up from a mixture of empirical knowledge, scientific facts, assumptions, and hypotheses. Such a model could be merely discursive, or could be more elaborate with functional quantitative links between its components. The latter case is mathematical when the links are quantitative, and logical when no attempts are made to introduce quantities. A functional model can be used to predict a future event in an observational setting or a consequence in an experimental setting. Scientists, philosophers, and writers have admitted that reality can only be approached through models.

All models share common features that convey their inability to describe precisely and fully the reality. Models are reductions of reality, because of the unavoidable lack of knowledge and/or because one wants to make the model simpler than reality for practical or technical reasons. Models are never fully exact, not only because they are a reduction of reality, but also because of the inherent lack of knowledge. Observations or experiments will eventually demonstrate the falsity of a model. For the purposes of this chapter on clinical trial methodology, a model should be viewed as an operational step in knowledge building.

The complex hypothesis that a clinical trial is designed to test is drawn from a therapeutic model. It is merely a predicted consequence of the model, which has been obtained by bringing together a pathophysiological model of the condition and the outcome to be cured or prevented, and a pharmacological model (or any similar model for a nonpharmacological therapy) that describes the assumed mechanism of action of the intervention. The pathophysiological model is a representation of the present knowledge about the mechanism of the disease and the related event to be cured or prevented by the intervention. The therapeutic model integrates the assumed mechanism of action of the intervention into the pathophysiology of the disease, the result of this integration being a likelihood of efficacy of the intervention. Because, like any model, the therapeutic model is very likely to be approximate or even false, its predicted consequences should be tested appropriately.

There are various ways to test a therapeutic model, since one can formulate at least as many hypotheses as there are components in a model, although there is a single ultimate hypothesis, i.e. that the treatment has some effect on the therapeutic objective. The proper test (falsification) of this ultimate hypothesis is the randomized controlled trial with a defined clinical outcome. In fact, what a clinical trial actually tests is not the hypothesis. Rather, it tests one of the consequences of the hypothesis, i.e. the magnitude of the effect of the intervention. The size of the effect is predicted by the model, while the real size can be measured owing to the features of the randomized clinical trial methodology, in particular the comparison. However, the predicted size of the effect might be wrong, e.g. the real effect may be smaller. Hence a negative test does not necessarily mean that the model is false.

The problem formulation stems from other considerations, these being related both to the doctors' professional activity (in particular, how they interact with their patients' problems and on which problems their own interest is focused) and epidemiology and health system prejudices. An important consideration here is the burden of the disease and its related event(s) on individual patients and the community.

The formulation identifies the therapeutic objective, i.e. the event to be prevented (which will become the clinical outcome of the clinical trial), the eligibility criteria for trial participants, the duration of observation for recording the occurrence of the event, and the accepted concomitant therapeutic care. It also fixes the size of the effect that seems clinically relevant, and now increasingly often, the economic constraints.

It can be seen that the problem so formulated stems from the therapeutic model. The therapeutic model is built up because (1) physiopathological and pharmacologic (or similar) models exist beforehand, and (2) there are ill patients who need care. More precisely, therapeutic objectives have been defined on the basis of nosology and epidemiology. Furthermore, the problem is almost directly represented in the hypothesis.

The hypothesis should be fixed before the start of data collection. This is a stringent proviso for the validity of any causal relationship found between the trial outcome and the intervention. It also explains why the results of *post hoc* analyses are a low level of evidence, besides giving rise to difficulties with statistical inference, which will be considered later on.

Confounding Factors, Randomization, and Blinding

Confounding Factors

Several factors can affect the evolution of a patient's condition following the administration of a therapy. The effect of the intervention is just one factor, and it cannot be differentiated from the others merely by observing the patient's course. Other factors at play are regression to the mean value, spontaneous improvement or worsening of the disease, the effects of concomitant therapies, and the placebo effect. The effects of all these factors are correlated with time.

Regression to the mean is seen when a subject is selected on the basis of a high or low value of a physiologic parameter such as blood pressure or blood sugar. It is a purely statistical phenomenon, the extent of which is dependent on the patient recruitment process, i.e. the cut-off level for selection. Because the same parameter is also measured later in the study, this new observed value will, on average, be closer to the population mean. As the patient-eligibility criteria usually require some sort of 'abnormal' value, many subjects entered in a trial are prone to show this phenomenon. The result is that, after a while, the 'abnormal' value has moved towards the mean value of the population from which the subjects were selected. Now, suppose that the patient's disease evolution is assessed using the observed change in the parameter. The purely statistical change could be mistakenly viewed as a change in the disease state.

The spontaneous evolution of many diseases is not predictable with precision, particularly when the time-scale of observation is short compared to the overall duration of the disease. This is true not only on an individual basis, but also on a group basis.

The placebo effect is known to affect, most of the time favorably, the evolution of a patient's disease. It is an inevitable component of all therapies. Even if it is still mysterious, nobody would deny it exists. Its intensity and the weights of its components (patient's trust in the doctor or in the pill, patient's expectation of or faith in cure) are not predictable. Many medicines are supposed to 'work' only through the placebo effect.

Thus, following the administration of a therapy, the observed change in the disease severity, however assessed, is the result of the effect of several factors. This could be represented by the following symbolic equation:

Change in disease state from t_0 to t
= Therapy effect + Placebo effect + Regression to the mean   (2.1)
+ Spontaneous improvement or aggravation + Effect of other confounders

Because the effect of the therapeutic intervention cannot be separated from the effects of the other factors, the latter are called confounding factors. In a clinical trial, the application of the third principle, that of comparison, enables one to separate out the effect of the therapy (and to ensure the conclusion of a causal relationship), because the outcome of the experiment is the difference in the mean changes observed in the 'treated' group and in the 'control' group. Thus, for a clinical trial the above equation becomes:

Difference in changes from t_0 to t =
Change in disease state from t_0 to t in the treated group   (2.2)
− Change in disease state from t_0 to t in the control group

This equation holds true provided that the effects of the various confounding factors are the same in both groups. The comparison condition has two components: (1) the two groups should be identical prior to the administration of the treatment or the control; and (2) the two groups should be kept identical during the data-collection process, except for the administration of treatment to one group. The tool used to achieve the first component is randomization, and that used to meet the second is 'blinding'.

Randomization

The actual randomization process will be described in detail in a later section. Here, let us consider just a few important conceptual points. The allocation of a subject to the control or treatment group should be fully independent of the subsequent treatment/control administration. This independence is best guaranteed by using an 'automatic' process that operates independently of the investigator, the patients, and the environment (nurses, wards, family, etc.), and is totally blind to them. The guarantee of groups being balanced in terms of patient characteristics and the strength of confounding factors is strictly dependent on respecting this process. *Post hoc* exclusion of randomized patients can induce a bias that is impossible to remove. However, the very nature of a random procedure means that it could happen that, just by chance, the two groups are not balanced. Sometimes the imbalance can be demonstrated by comparing the baseline data for the two groups, or can be prevented by stratifying the randomization with regard to one or more key prognostic factors.

Blinding

The highest level of blinding that can be achieved in a trial is double-blindness. However, this can only usually be applied when testing drugs. Surgical treatments or lifestyle interventions, for example, cannot be tested in double-blind trials, although they can be submitted to randomized trials. This limitation might mean that it is not possible to relate with full confidence the observed difference to the effect of the experimental therapy. If possible, the evaluation of patients to determine any occurrence of an outcome should be made by an independent observer who is blind to the treatment group. What can be evaluated without bias is the intention to administer the therapy. For instance, with a surgical procedure, a positive outcome of the randomized trial might be due to the anesthesia, the surgeon 'placebo effect', the postprocedure care, the concomitantly used drugs, or any other component of the action that followed the intention to treat a patient with the surgical procedure. The other advantage of blindness is that it guarantees unbiased data collection and an unbiased assessment of the outcome events. In open (unblinded) trials, one should rely only on 'hard' outcomes, such as death, and an independent, blind, critical event committee (see later) should be employed.

The Size of the Effect

In general, doctors think about the efficacy of a therapy in qualitative terms; i.e. the treatment is either efficacious or not. However, estimating the size of the effect, i.e. the magnitude of the benefit that patients will ultimately obtain from receiving the treatment, is a major component of the assessment of a therapy. The size of the effect is inherent in both the aim of a clinical trial and the hypothesis-testing operation. In addition, it is a key issue in selecting the most appropriate therapy for a given patient.

A prior estimate of the size of the effect, or at least a guess at the smallest size that is either likely given the therapeutic model, or therapeutically relevant, is required to compute the number of patients to recruit in a trial (see later section). On the other hand, the decision to undertake a trial to test a hypothesis is made only if a sizeable efficacy could reasonably be expected according to the therapeutic model. The trial itself could be viewed as a tool for measuring the size of the effect of a treatment through the difference in the changes observed in the two groups.

Even at this stage, when no data on the efficacy of a treatment are available, one could predict that the size of the effect will depend on the type of patients selected. This can be inferred from the therapeutic model, and also (and at the very least) from purely arithmetic considerations. If the benefit when expressed as the relative risk is constant over the range of untreated risks, the absolute benefit (the difference in, say, the rates of events in untreated and treated patients) will vary. If, however, the absolute benefit is constant, the relative risk will vary. With an effect model intermediate between a multiplicative one (constant relative risk) and an additive one (constant absolute benefit), both efficacy indices will vary according to the untreated risk, as they will if the effect model is nonlinear. Besides this arithmetic interaction, there is a second type of interaction that leads the size of the effect to depend on characteristics of the patients other than those merely correlated with the untreated risk. Variations in the genotype and the environment of the patients could decrease or increase the size of the treatment effect. These interactions may be called 'biologic'. In fact, the difference between arithmetic and biologic interactions is not so clear-cut because: (1) the cause of the arithmetic interaction is the spontaneous variation in the untreated risk across populations and subgroups, which obviously has strong biologic components, genetic as well as environmental; and (2) biologic interaction could add to the arithmetic interaction.[9]

Thus, the size of the effect is a key component of the therapeutic model, the hypothesis, and the design of the clinical trial. The process of evaluating a new therapy has both qualitative and quantitative outcomes, the former depending on the latter. It is concluded that a therapy is effective (qualitative interpretation of the outcome) when the observed size of the effect is sufficiently large in comparison to the precision of its estimate (quantitative interpretation of the outcome). However, the most important part of the outcome for the clinician and the patient is the quantitative one.

Application of the Statistical Model

A major advance was made with the introduction of statistics to the evaluation of therapies. The aim of applying the statistical model is to solve three related issues: the variability between one observation and another, either in the same patient at two different times (intrapatient variability) or in different patients at the same time (between-patient variability); the chance variation in the results of the same experiment repeated several times; and the prediction of future events based on prior observed series or data. The two statistical tools that provide a solution to these issues are the test of significance, and the point estimate and its confidence limits.

The Test of Significance

The test of significance provides arbitrary, but reasonable, rules for deciding whether the trial outcome, i.e. the observed difference between the changes in the two groups, is due to chance or could be accepted as corresponding to a real difference. The principle consists of setting a null hypothesis, i.e. that the value of a real difference in the changes is zero, and computing the probability (P value) of the observed difference given the null hypothesis. If the P value is high, the experiment was not able to demonstrate a difference, either because no difference exists or because their were insufficient data. This could be due to either a lower than anticipated size of the effect, or to a greater than expected variability in outcome. In either case, the number of patients included in the trial was too small, which is equivalent to saying that the power of the trial (to detect the effect) was too low. Note that the test of significance cannot differentiate between these two alternatives. If the P value is small, usually less than 0.05, one may conclude that the difference is not likely to be a chance finding. Note that the test itself tells us nothing about any causal relationship between the observed difference and the tested treatment. This issue relies on the lack of bias in the design and execution of a trial.

Multiple Statistical Inferences

The statistical null hypothesis is drawn from the hypothesis that the trial is designed to explore:

One (therapeutic) hypothesis $\Rightarrow$ One (statistical) null hypothesis $\Rightarrow$ One trial $\Rightarrow$
One test of significance   (2.3)

The above equation is an important landmark in statistical science. However, if more than one significance test is performed on the same batch of data, the risk of drawing incorrect conclusions is increased, because the probability of one P value being less than 0.05 if all the null hypotheses are true increases with the number of tests.

Estimation of the Size of the Treatment Effect

Once the difference between the changes in the treated and the control patients has been calculated and tested for statistical significance, the next question for the researchers to consider is the size of the treatment effect, particularly if the P value is small. The answer is obtained through a two-step procedure.

First, one should demonstrate that the difference between the two groups was caused by the intervention, and therefore, that the observed size of the effect is a true value, given the experimental setting. This is achieved by considering to what extent the actual conduct of the trial met the principles of the experimental method, adhered to the intended study protocol, was consistent with the components of the therapeutic model (e.g. whether the observed compliance was within the acceptable range), and was proper for testing the (therapeutic) hypothesis. One thus determines a 'level of evidence' to support the causal relationship. Inevitably, this is a subjective judgement, since no established scale of level of evidence exists. The lack of such a scoring instrument is due to the number of components involved and the difficulty in weighting each one.

Secondly, provided that the first step ended with a satisfactory support of the causal relationship, one would like to know the value of the size of the effect. The statistical theory of estimation shows that the most likely value of the true effect is the observed difference, but that other values, although less likely, are perfectly consistent with the collected data. In order to provide the researcher with a range of such values, one computes a confidence interval; that is, the range of true values that are not significantly different from the observed difference at the $X\%$ level. As X is usually set at 5% significance, this is customarily a 95% confidence interval.

Trial Experimental Design

In the preceding sections we have assumed the simplest experimental design, i.e. two parallel groups of patients, one receiving the test therapy, the other being the control, and patients being randomly assigned to either group. However, a more complex design may sometimes be appropriate. The interested reader is referred to the specialist textbooks for more detail on this subject.[10,11] Here, we only consider briefly two alternative designs that have a good pay-off in assessing the clinical benefit of therapies in cardiology.

More than Two Parallel Groups

When the optimal dose of treatment is unknown, one will need several treatment groups, each receiving a different dose. Thus, referring to Equation (2.3), there is more than one hypothesis because of the additional component, the dose. At the end of the trial more than one statistical test could be made, depending on the approach used to explore the dose–effect relationship. Alternatively, more than one concurrent therapy could be tested in a single trial against the same control. Clearly, in such a case there is more than one (therapeutic) hypothesis and more than one statistical test, which are not independent. However, the corresponding therapeutic models do share common features, e.g. the same control treatment and often a part of the mechanism of action is the same for all the tested therapies. Great attention should be paid to the multiple statistical inference issue.

Factorial Design

If, instead of several competing therapies, there is more than one therapy to be tested that have dissimilar therapeutic models and act through different noninteractive mechanisms, one should consider the factorial design. The principle is quite simple: instead of one question per trial, a single trial is conducted to address two or more questions. The only common features of the various hypotheses are the patients and the outcome. In addition, one should assume that there is no interaction between the two (or more) treatments with regard to the size of the effect, i.e. one assumes that the effects are purely additive.[2] In principle, the number of subjects required is the same as for a trial addressing just one of the two (or more) hypotheses. The price to pay in such a trial is that results are limited to the no-interaction assumption; this requires a little more work in the preparation and setting up of the trial, and a common set of eligibility criteria, unless one accepts a rather complex inclusion procedure.[12] With two treatments and their controls, there will be four subgroups, or 'cells'. Randomization is used to allocate patients to one of the four combinations.

A Tool for Measuring an Effect

As stated above, a clinical trial is a tool that has been developed to measure the effect of an intervention through a comparison with another intervention, called the control or reference intervention. The nature of the effect is defined by the outcomes set for the trial, the outcomes being derived directly from the objectives, which, in turn, were derived from the hypothesis. When setting the objectives of a trial a thorough reflection should be made by the clinicians and the statisticians, because the design and analysis of the trials should be adapted to the question.

The Effect of What?

This question was alluded to earlier in this chapter, when we introduced the concept of intention to treat. In pragmatic-type trials, with clinical outcomes, the effect to be measured is the one of the intention to treat with the tested treatment. Besides the nature of the specific treatments themselves (tested treatment and control), there are other differences between the groups, even in totally blind trials. Side-effects can lead to treatment withdrawal more often in one group than in the other. Even if the rates of withdrawal are similar in the two groups, the reasons for stopping treatment or for patients not continuing the treatment may be different. Compliance could be unevenly distributed for reasons other than side-effects. In addition, the anticipated effects of the treaments might influence the duration of their administration. If one wants to measure the (pharmacological) effects of the chemical species that constitute a medicine, one should set up a more explicative-type trial, in which the patients are highly selected, have a homogenous profile, and, if possible, will provide high compliance with the test therapy. These are usually preliminary studies, with intermediate outcomes being given preference over clinical outcomes.

Definition of the Eligible Population

Physicians are interested to know whether, for patients having a predefined disease type, risk, personal characteristics, and no current contraindications, whether treament with a new therapy will improve the patient's risk compared to a reference treatment. Of interest is the overall effect, which actually includes the true treatment effect, compliance with the prescribed treatment, and unwanted treatment-related events.

As it is impossible to predict the precise effect of treatment at an individual level, the observation of a group of patients enrolled in a clinical trial serves to provide an estimate of the average effect. To be relevant to future clinical practice, the study population should be defined to be as close as possible to the type of patients the physician has to manage. However, although the goal of having an eligible population identical to the therapist's target population is highly commendable, it is never reached. Furthermore, the population that is actually enrolled in a clinical trial will differ from the overall eligible population.[13]

Of utmost importance is the setting of the time of randomization. Study patients should be randomized at the time at which the physician wants to initiate treatment. Once a patient has been randomized to a group, treatment should be given immediately. However, if for any reason the treatment needs to be modified or discontinued at a later point in the trial, the outcome should still be measured and taken into account in the analysis of the original treatment group according to the intention-to-treat principle.

The first reported large-scale placebo-controlled trials on the treatment of acute MI by fibrinolysis were criticised by some cardiologists because a number of the patients enrolled (10–12%) did not have a confirmed MI. It was suggested that the results for these patients be removed from the analysis. It took time to make these physicians realize that the question addressed in these trials was the value of early treatment in patients with suspected MI. A delay in initiating treatment in order to confirm the diagnosis by measuring enzymes and observing significant Q waves on the electrocardiogram (ECG) would have led to the selection of true MI patients. Furthermore, a delay may have reduced the effect of treatment on the very same patients because an interaction between time to treatment and effect was in fact observed. If the data on patients without confirmed MI had been removed from the analysis, a different question from the intended one would have been answered. Also, it would most likely have introduced a bias into the comparison, because active treatment may prevent the completion of MI in some patients treated very early. Patients who die very early during treatment (on the first day) may not have an accurate diagnosis based on enzymes and the ECG, and there is an imbalance in favor of more deaths occurring during day one in patients receiving fibrinolysis. In addition, fibrinolytics interfere with the time of release of enzymes.

Thus, for similar reasons, removing data on poor compliers or noncompliers, or of patients experiencing adverse events, even when these are labeled 'unrelated to the treatment', can often lead to major biases in the data and distortions from the initial objectives of the trial.

The Power of a Trial

The power of a trial is its ability to provide evidence in support of the hypothesis of primary interest, i.e. to sort out the effect it is aimed at measuring if that effect exists. This property is of utmost importance. A trial with low power is useless because it will have very little chance of achieving the investigator's goal. Such a trial is also a waste of resources, although one could say that, even if the results obtained are inconclusive, a trial provides information that could be in the future entered in a meta-analysis. In order that a trial has the best chance of detecting the expected effect of a treatment, it should have sufficient statistical power as well as sufficient pharmacological power (i.e. the appropriate dose should be given) and design power (i.e. the proper design). The power linked with the conduct of the trial (i.e. the quality of the completed trial) is considered later.

When one talks of the power of a trial, one is usually referring to its statistical power. If β is the risk of not concluding that there was a statistically significant effect when the effect exists in reality, also called type II error, then the statistical power ω is:

$$\omega = 1 - \beta \tag{2.4}$$

Thus, the statistical power of a trial is a probability, which indicates the chance that the expected difference could be detected at a prespecified level of statistical significance. It can be set, when designing a trial, not to be inferior to a prespecified level. The higher the set level of power the higher are the chances that the expected (minimum) difference between the treatment groups will be demonstrated. In most cases it is not reasonable to set the power below 0.80. The level of the power has a direct impact on the required sample size: the higher the intended power, the larger the sample size needed.

The choice of the statistical power for a trial goes well beyond mere statistical considerations. At the end of a trial a statistical test is performed to assess how much the observed difference corresponds to a real difference. The only conclusion of classical statistical tests is to reject or accept the null hypothesis with a given level of risk of a false-positive conclusion (α or type I error), usually 0.05. If the null hypothesis cannot be rejected because the computed P value is greater than the prespecified level of significance, this does not mean that a difference does not exist and that the effect of the tested treatment is nill. One cannot say either that the two compared treatments are equivalent or that the therapeutic model is refuted in a qualitative (i.e. the treatment has an effect) or even quantitative (i.e. the anticipated size of the effect) sense.

Consequences for Placebo-Controlled Studies

If the trial is placebo (or no treatment) controlled, one conclusion based on a lack of statistical evidence (i.e. a nonsignificant result) would be to not recommend the use of the new 'active' treatment. However, the clinician interpreting the results would be much more confident that a clinically relevant difference had not been missed if the power, and hence the sample size, was large. If a treatment is actually effective but, because of lack of power, the results of trials are not clearly significant, it will not be widely used and many patients who could have benefited from the treatment will not receive it. Physicians have a moral, ethical, and (in some countries) legal obligation to offer to their patients state of the art management. If the true positive effect of an existing treatment is not established because of lack of significant evidence from underpowered trials, physicians cannot be expected to offer the best available treatments to their patients. Thus, that trials have sufficient statistical power is not only a methodological requirement, but also an ethical issue. However, many published trials are still underpowered.[14]

Fibrinolytics were discovered in the mid-1940s. The hypothesis that they could be effective in acute MI was made shortly after. The first randomized controlled trial of fibrinolytics in acute MI was published in 1959.[15] Over the next 30 years, about 30 trials were performed. Almost all these trials had a limited sample size and their results could not demonstrate a definite and statistically significant beneficial effect of the treatment on mortality. In the mid-1980s, several groups performed large-scale trials, all of which confirmed beyond any doubt that fibrinolytics could decrease by about 20% the risk of 1-month mortality. If these trials had been performed in the 1950s and their results applied at that time, given an incidence of one million MI per year in developed countries and a 1-month mortality of 15–17% (it was actually higher 10 years ago), it is easy to estimate that the lives of about a million patients could have been prolonged. One should also recall the possible thousands of deaths induced by the precription of class I antiarrhythmics until a sufficiently large study (CAST) was performed and showed a definite excess in mortality in patients receiving the active treatment as compared to placebo.[16]

Consequences for Studies Comparing Active Treatments

Trials looking for differences between treatments. If the results of a study comparing active treatments, usually a reference treatment and a new treatment, show no statistically significant difference, the logical conclusion would be to recommend to continue the use of the reference treatment. However, the temptations for the authors or the physicians to conclude that both treatments can be considered equivalent is not always resisted. The confusion between no statistically significant difference and equivalence is widespread, and is all the more misleading because 'negative' results are more likely to be observed in trials with small sample sizes where true differences between treatments may exist but be missed because of a lack of power. Of course 'negative' results from trials with adequate power to demonstrate reasonable differences are much more informative, because such trials have a narrower confidence interval for the difference.

The availability of effective treatments such as fibrinolytics, aspirin, beta-blockers, and angiotensin converting enzyme inhibitors for MI makes it increasingly difficult to launch new mortality studies because: (1) thanks to the combination of these treatments, the event rate in the control group will be low (typically less than 10%); and (2) any reasonably expected improvement obtained with a new drug when evaluated against one of the above can only be relatively modest (less than 10–15%).

Trials like ISIS 3, GISSI 2, and GUSTO 1 were performed with the objective of detecting small but definite differences in mortality between streptokinase and t-PA, should any such differences exist.[17–19] To do this it was necessary to enrol tens of thousands of patients. The final result was the observation of a significant 10% improvement in mortality in favor of accelerated r-TPA in the latter trial. Since then new fibrinolytic agents have been developed and the question was raised as to whether new very large-scale trials would be needed to evaluate these agents. From a methodological point of view, if a further 10–15% improvement in mortality is deemed clinically relevant, the answer is that about 25 000 patients should be enrolled to assess this objective. Investigators for several good, and some less good, reasons are looking for alternative assumptions and study designs that require smaller sample sizes. Some of these designs involve the use of more frequent events, such as combined outcomes or surrogate outcomes. The problem with surrogacy is that it is doubtful that one could find an appropriate surrogate outcome.[20]

Another attractive way to limit the sample size is to aim at demonstrating rather large differences. For example, instead of a 15% reduction in mortality with a new thrombolytic (from 7% to 6%), the objective would be to look for an at least a 30% reduction (from 7% to 5%). With $\alpha = 0.05$ and $\omega = 95\%$, the required sample size then goes down from 32 000 to 6800. Although this approach is rather unrealistic, it is acceptable in terms of cost/benefit ratio. Given the present mortality rate in patients presenting with acute MI who are treated with a thrombolytic, only a new treatment that further increases by, say, more than 20 per 1000 the number of lives saved would be considered clinically more useful than the currently used fibrinolytics. However, it should be made clear in the protocol and in the publication that failure to reach statistical significance in these conditions means that, whatever the actual results, the new treatment will not be recommended. Another caveat on such a design is the low power for such a trial in assessing safety.

Trials designed to show equivalence between active treatments. Most clinical trials are performed to demonstrate superiority of one kind of treatment over another. As more effective treatments are now available, definite clinically significant improvements on a major clinical outcome are less likely to be obtained from new treatments. Thus the main interest in developing new treatments may not be associated with major clinical events but with gaining improvements in secondary, however important, features, such as side-effects, quality of life, treatment practicability, or cost. However, such criteria can only be considered if the new treatment is at least as effective as the reference treatment with regard to major clinical outcomes. Therefore, it could be envisaged that a trial be designed with the objective of showing 'equal efficacy' on major clinical outcomes and benefit on some other outcomes. As mentioned previously, it is impossible to establish equal efficacy, and a non-statistically-significant result of a clinical trial does not imply equal efficacies of the tested treatments. To overcome this problem it has been proposed to set *a priori* an interval within which the difference between the treatments could be considered not clinically relevant and to evaluate at the end of the study the probability that the observed difference is outside the preset interval. If this probability is low, say less than 5%, the treatments are considered equivalent with regard to the chosen outcomes. This interval and the corresponding statistical test define the equivalence of the treatments. Equivalence trials may, therefore, seem attractive. However, before deciding to embark on such a trial design, one should be aware of the stringent requirements of such an approach.

(1) The choice of the primary outcome of equivalence and of the secondary outcome of superiority. This choice should not allow a possible excess of rare, but severe, adverse events (e.g. hemorrhagic strokes with fibrinolytics) to be missed. If the main criterion (equivalence) is total mortality and the secondary criterion (superiority) is, say, indirect cost, the sample size may be not large enough to detect an excess of rare severe adverse events. Therefore, if, for instance, one is interested in demonstrating that the new intervention is cheaper than the reference one, there should be at least two equivalence criteria: total mortality and severe adverse events.

(2) The choice of the width of the interval of equivalence. The demonstration of the equivalence of the two compared treatments is based on the criterion chosen to define equivalence and the width of the interval of equivalence. Should the interval be mistaken, the relevance of the equivalence, and thus of the whole trial, might be seriously disputed. If the criterion is total mortality, should one choose 10%, 1% or 0.01% as the width of the interval? The narrower the interval, the larger will be the resources needed to carry out the trial. Also, in terms of ethics and public health, these three intervals are extremely different.

(3) The sample size. Perhaps the main problem lies in the large number of patients needed. For example, an investigator wants to evaluate a new fibrinolytic in the treatment of acute MI in order to establish its equivalence to a reference thrombolytic. The investigator might be satisfied if the new treatment is shown not to be worse than the reference treatment. This is an equivalence problem. With the reference treatment resulting in a 6% mortality rate (the GUSTO trial[18]), an accepted relative increase of no more than 5% would require a sample size of 98 000 patients (with one-sided $\alpha = \beta = 0.05$). Even if one accepts that a relative increase in mortality of up to 10% is not clinically relevant, the required sample size is still 25 000. In general, the sample size required to test for equivalence between treatments is usually of the same order as for testing clinically significant efficacy.

Pharmacological Power

Usually, the 'power' of a trial is taken to mean its statistical ability to meet the stated objectives, and refers directly to the sample size. However, when considering the ability of a trial to meet its objectives in a broader sense, there are other important design aspects that deserve careful attention in order to optimize the chances of detecting the expected efficacy. For example, an understanding of the mechanism of action of the treatments, the choice of drug regimen in both the reference and the new-treatment group, and the optimal length of follow-up are crucial issues.

An obvious requirement is to use in the control group (when the reference treatment is not a placebo) the best established, or at least the most commonly established, treatment as the reference, so that the results of the study may be relevant to prescribers, drug agencies and patients. The largest and most clinically relevant effect of a drug would be obtained if the titration and the duration of treatment were optimal according to the corresponding therapeutic model. Attempting to select the optimal regimen is a delicate if not impossible task. If good and relevant phase I and phase II trials have been performed, the optimum daily dose, route of administration, and schedule of dosing of the drug should be known with sufficient validity and precision. These data are essential in choosing the treatment regimen. However, well-designed, informative, and carefully conducted dose-finding studies are the exception rather than the rule. In the name of efficiency and rapidity, in-depth pharmacological studies of the mechanism of action of a drug have not always been completed when phase III trials begin. Thus it is not surprising that the treatment regimen selected for use in a trial may not be adequate, sometimes resulting in an undue excess of side-effects, an apparent inefficacy, or both, whereas another regimen with the same drug could have proven effective. This situation may be termed a lack of 'pharmacological power'. When proper phase II trials are not and cannot be available because of a lack of relevant intermediate outcomes, several dose regimens may be considered in phase III trials.

Increasing the dose of a drug does not always increase its efficacy but it usually increases the number and the severity of adverse effects. An increase in side-effects may also affect compliance to the treatment, and thus further decrease both the pharmacological and statistical power of a trial. For example, an apparently small increase in the dose of heparin given as initial treatment of MI patients, who otherwise received aspirin and fibrinolytics, led to an excess of bleeding events that justified a change in protocol during the course of a large-scale trial.[21] Not surprisingly, no proper dose-finding studies have been undertaken for the use of heparin in the management of MI or similar conditions, and what is usually referred as the 'therapeutic range' has been empirically based on safety data rather than on efficacy data. However, it is more surprising that no sufficiently large dose–effect trials have been done on the use of streptokinase or t-PA in acute MI.

Optimal pharmacological power also requires a relevant administration scheme. The same dose of a fibrinolytic given to the same type of patient would obviously not have the same efficacy if given very early or very late after onset of symptoms. The duration of treatment with a hypolipidemic agent should be long enough to see the effect of the drug, if one assumes that the effect is essentially mediated by a retardation of the progression of atherosclerosis, in contrast to the almost immediate protection that could be expected from antithrombotic drugs in the same type of patient. Hence, the treatment regimen is dependent on the therapeutic model, which is the basis of the hypothesis that the trial is aimed at testing. Thus the pharmacological power is dependent on the relevance of the therapeutic model.

In the past, there has been confusion between pharmacological power and statistical power. The example of the use of aspirin in the secondary prevention of MI is typical. The first large controlled study was published in 1974.[22] The study compared aspirin 300 mg to placebo in 1200 patients. A 20% reduction in mortality was observed in favor of aspirin, but the difference was not statistically significant. The medical community believed that the reason for the insufficient efficacy of the drug was too low a dose. Subsequent trials that addressed the same question used doses of aspirin up to 1500 mg. These doses were shown to have a similar efficacy on mortality, but at the price of a higher risk of gastrointestinal disorders. It was about 10 years before it was realized that 300 mg or less of aspirin per day could be recommended for the secondary prevention of MI.

Measuring an Effect of a Therapy

The ultimate goal of a clinical trial is to estimate, through the process outlined in the previous sections, the extent of the beneficial effect of a therapy. There are still a few specific aspects to consider before getting into the practical conduct of a clinical trial.

Clinical Outcome

As the goal is patient benefit, the primary outcome studied should be of clinical relevance. A clinical outcome is anything that represents directly either the quantity or the quality of life. In western cultures, there exists a tacit hierarchy in clinical outcome: (1) death; (2) clinical nonlethal events; (3) disability, painful symptoms, limitated autonomy; and (4) quality of life.

Often, so-called 'surrogate' outcomes are used instead of clinical outcomes in clinical trials, because these are supposed to allow trials to be just as informative but to be of shorter duration and smaller sample size, and hence less expense. This is a mistaken belief and the fallacy of surrogacy has been demonstrated.[20] The conditions that any intermediary outcome criterion (i.e. any variable correlated with the clinical event) needs to meet in order for it to be an informative substitute for clinical-efficacy evaluation are so stringent as to be inapplicable in most, if not all, real situations.

Finally, we should mention the issue of using combined outcomes, e.g. a mix of death, recurrent MI, and the need for angioplasty or coronary bypass. The use of such outcomes is becoming quite common in clinical trials in cardiology. However, no full account of their limitations and the requirements for their relevance is currently available. Caution is recommended.

Indices of Clinical Efficacy

The difference between two groups in the case of a binary clinical outcome such as death or a nonfatal event reduces to a difference in the risk (rate) R of the outcome, $R_c(F) - R_t(F)$, where the subscripts c and t denote the groups, and F denotes control and treatment 'failure' (i.e. the occurrence of the event). This is called the *absolute benefit*. Another way of representing the results is as the *relative risk*, $R_t(F)/R_c(F)$. These two indices share the same information (i.e. the size of the effect), but they are not interpreted in the same way. To understand this, suppose that the relative risk is constant for a given therapy. If $R_c(F)$ varies, which occurs when patients with the illness are at varying risk of the event, the absolute benefit will vary accordingly. *Table 2.1* shows some values of both indices for post-MI patients treated with a beta-blocking agent. The absolute benefit is much smaller for a low-risk patient than for a high-risk patient, when the relative risk is the same for both.

Another useful index of efficacy is the reciprocal of the absolute benefit; that is, the number of patients that must be treated in order to achieve one success (i.e. one disease event or one death prevented). If the absolute benefit is 0.05, then the number of subjects to be treated for one success is $1/0.5 = 20$. *Table 2.1* gives some examples of the number of post-MI patients to be treated with beta-blocking agents during 1 year. With long-term therapies, e.g. in hypertension, this idea could be extended to give the number of patient-years of treatment required for one success.

Table 2.1 Comparison of absolute benefit and relative risk[a]

Relative risk	$R_c(F)$	$R_t(F)$	Absolute benefit	NST
0.750	0.050	0.038	0.013	80
	0.100	0.075	0.025	40
	0.150	0.113	0.038	27
	0.200	0.150	0.050	20
	0.250	0.188	0.063	16
0.375	0.050	0.019	0.031	32
	0.100	0.038	0.063	16
	0.150	0.056	0.094	11
	0.200	0.075	0.125	8
	0.250	0.094	0.156	6
0.188	0.050	0.009	0.041	25
	0.100	0.019	0.081	12
	0.150	0.028	0.122	8
	0.200	0.038	0.163	6
	0.250	0.047	0.203	5

[a]Relative risk = $R_t(F)/R_c(F)$. Absolute benefit = $R_c(F) - R_t(F)$. $R_c(F)$, risk for untreated patients; $R_t(F)$, risk for treated patients.
NST, number of patients that must be treated for one success.
NST = 1/Absolute benefit.

Clinical Significance

Consideration of the index of efficacy issue leads to the difficult question of what is a clinically significant efficacy. It is obvious that a very small absolute benefit could be meaningless for patient welfare, taking into account the burden and the cost of therapy. This problem is partly solved by the physician balancing the advantages and the disadvantages of giving the therapy to a patient, once his or her untreated risk has been predicted. Another part of the solution relies on those who evaluate the therapy. With simple, large-scale trials, a very small effect size can be identified. Whether this is a useful endeavor depends on several factors. The absolute benefit might be too small to be useful for patients at average risk in the control group, but worthwhile for those in the high-risk range. This explains why in clinical trials aimed at evaluating clinical benefit it is wise to recruit patients that cover a large range of risk rather than to rely on restrictive eligibility criteria. However, even if the expected effect is limited, it can be unethical to deprive patients of the therapy, especially if the new therapy is the first to show promise for the disease under consideration or if the social burden of the disease is high (e.g. high prevalence, high risk, or high cost for the community). Furthermore, the discovery of an effective therapy could foster further research in the field.

There is no straightforward answer to the question of what is a clinically significant efficacy, essentially because the question of clinical significance is complex and requires further reflection. This has an obvious bearing on the issue of extrapolation, which is now described.

Extrapolation of Clinical Trial Results

Strictly speaking, the results of a clinical trial are valid only for patients that match those in the studied population. However, doctors have to care for patients who differ to varying degrees from the study population. Thus, when a therapy is allowed to be prescribed, the population to which it is disseminated is different from the original study population.[23,24] To what extent can one extrapolate from the trial results? In a preceding section we introduced the concept of interactions between the size of the effect and the patient profile. Extrapolation is feasible if these interactions have been assessed and demonstrated. The means of identifying interactions are outside the scope of this chapter. They are not standardized and require much further work before they are validated. Let us just say that meta-analysis, particularly the meta-analysis of joint individual record databases, is basically the best way available at the present time of exploring these interactions.[25–27] Subgroup analysis is also a useful approach, although it has much less validity. Finally, the maintenance of a clinical-trial log, where all the patients considered for eligibility are registered together with their main characteristics, helps to define the study population as compared to the therapy target population.[26] However, this is rarely done because of the extra workload.

Subgroup Analysis

Subgroup analysis consists of reanalyzing the data on treatment differences using subsamples of patients defined according to subcategories of one or more baseline variables.[28] The categorization can be decided on before the start of the trial (*a priori* subgrouping) or after the trial has been completed (*post hoc* subgrouping). In the former case, the intended subgrouping is stated in the protocol, i.e. before any analysis is undertaken. The level of evidence of the results is somewhat better for *a priori* than *post hoc* subgrouping, but in both cases is still much lower than for the primary analysis, i.e. the one that tests the overall hypothesis. Even worse is data-derived subgrouping. The worst case is *post hoc* subgrouping when the primary analysis does not reach statistical significance. The level of evidence is then particularly weak, even from a generating hypothesis point of view. A fairly good example of the low validity of *post hoc* subgrouping is a review of the trials of beta-blockers in post-MI patients. In 1987, the long-term effect of late intervention with beta-blocker treatment on the survival in these patients had been assessed in nine trials. Attempts were made in most trials to determine whether specific *post hoc* subgroups of patients would benefit more from the treatment than others. These subgroup analyses suggested that certain characteristics are associated with a particular benefit from beta-blockers: anterior location of the infarct, tachycardia, cardiomegaly on chest X-ray, diabetes, electrical and/or mechanical failure, age below 65 years, and age above 60 years (note the inconsistency between the two latter findings). A meta-analysis of subgrouped data explored the validity of these findings across the nine trials and with regard to the pooled data.[27] A fairly good homogeneity of relative risk was found across all the sub-groups, thus dismissing all the previous hypotheses of interaction.

All subgroup analyses share four different drawbacks, the relative weights varying from case to case.

(1) Multiple statistical inference. The same argument mentioned earlier applies here. By increasing the number of tests one cannot interpret conventional levels of statistical significance. The risk of spurious findings is underlined by the wording 'data dredging'.

(2) Risk of unbalanced subgroups. Unless the randomization was stratified according to

predefined subgroups, there is no guarantee that the treated and control patients in the subgroups are similar. As the power of testing for balance between treated and control subgroups is usually very low, such a check, although currently done, is of limited value. On the other hand, stratification is limited by the number of variables that can be managed in practice.

(3) Low power for detecting an interaction. Obviously, subgrouping decreases the statistical power of each statistical test, because the number of statistical units is reduced.

(4) Validity. As subgroup analysis does not explore an *a priori* hypothesis, it does not comply with the first principle of the experimental method, and hence it is not deductive. According to Popper,[29] subgroup analysis cannot be accepted as a refutation test. Of course, this limitation does not hold with *a priori* subgrouping, provided that the corresponding hypothesis is clearly stated and is consistent with the therapeutic model. In such a case, note that the number of statistical tests can be greater than the number of hypotheses, unless the hypotheses have been translated into statistical interaction tests, which they should have been (i.e. do not use subgroup *P* values).

Whatever its limitations, subgroup analysis is common, but should only be done as a secondary analysis.[27] Such an analysis can be done to explore data with the aim of sparking new hypotheses to be investigated in future trials, and is useful for gaining insight about possible interactions that will be explored later in the process of extrapolation to the therapy target population. The overall message is clear: subgroup analysis should only be tackled and interpreted with great caution.

The Conduct of a Clinical Trial

The Need for an Unbiased Database

Clinical trials are scientific experiments with a carefully designed protocol that describes all the conditions of the realization of the experiment. In other scientific domains, if an experiment has been carefully designed, the protocol strictly adhered to, and the data correctly collected, other investigators should be able to reproduce the experiment, and it is highly recommended that they do so to give external validity to the findings of previous researchers. This rule should also apply in therapeutic research, and careful consideration of the ethical concerns of research in human beings strongly argues in favor of repetition of positive or inconclusive clinical trials. However, although theoretically compulsory in clinical research as well, the repetition of trials is rarely done sufficiently to validate the results of a positive clinical trial. The main reason for this is quite obvious: it would not be ethically justified to repeat a study if one tested treatment is known with sufficient evidence to be less effective than the other.

Three factors support the idea that this lack of trial repetition should not apply to the situation where a single trial has led to statistically significant results. First, the intensity of the effect demonstrated might be particular to the studied population.[30] Secondly, despite a high degree of apparent internal validity and a low risk of statistical error, the findings could be spurious. In both these cases, dissemination of the treatment could induce considerable harm in future patients. Finally, the identical duplication of a clinical trial is not feasible, because of the continuously varying patient profiles and environment. Thus, one should realize that the repetition of a clinical trial is not a duplication. Anyway, this ethical concern regarding repetition of clinical trials, together with several other reasons such as the avoidance of additional cost, make it difficult to repeat a positive clinical trial many times. Therefore, a clinical trial should be conducted in such a way that the results may be trusted; because the room for external validation is limited, there is a need to ensure a high degree of internal validity.

Introduction to Quality Control and Quality Assurance

Quality assurance is a primary requirement for clinical trials for scientific, ethical, economic, and legal reasons. The numerous techniques that have been developed for controlling the conduct of trials and assuring their quality fill tens of kilograms of binders making up standard operating manuals and several volumes of the official literature in many countries, not to mention textbooks and articles. In the last decade, new posts have been created for specialist staff in quality assurance departments and audit departments, both in the pharmaceutical industry and in hospital and academic departments and government agencies. Despite, or maybe because of, this expansion, the fundamental bases for such efforts may be overlooked by physicians, and even sometimes by the specialists in charge of quality assurance. The main objective of quality control is to guarantee as much as possible the collection of unbiased data for the analysis. The objectives of quality are met first by preventive measures: a well-planned study, a scientifically sound protocol with a clear description of the study procedures, tested procedures for feasibility including simple unambiguous case report forms, trained and permanently motivated participants, check-lists, reminders for follow-up visits, etc. Secondly, during the study, an ongoing program for the detection/correction of errors on data as well as on procedures should be set up, usually with the combined help of computer programmers and clinical research staff. Finally, periodic descriptive statistics of key indices of quality, such as accrual rates, the completeness of the collection of case-report forms, the data error rate, and the rate of deviations from the protocol, allow all participants to make timely and appropriate decisions regarding the conduct of the study.

Guidance for Quality Assurance

To obtain an unbiased database, three important requirements must be met.

(1) It must be ensured, without any ambiguity, that all randomized patients (and no others) are accounted for in the analysis of their original group. This is the denominator for calculating the event rate in each treatment group. The best randomization procedure that guarantees compliance to the above requirement is centralized randomization: having verified eligibility, the investigator contacts an independent randomization centre (by telephone, computer network, fax), gives basic information on the patient, some form of coded identification, and asks for randomization. In return, within minutes (or within seconds with remote-entry computerized randomization) the treatment identifier allocated to the patient is transmitted to the investigator. Treatment with the study material should begin immediately in order to avoid the risk of any contraindication developing before any treatment is given. The randomization list held by the randomization centre is the only list used to define the study population of the analysis.

(2) All patients must be correctly classified at the end of the study with regard to the occurrence of the main outcome event. This is the numerator for calculating the event rate in each treatment group. Choosing a simple, easy to measure, and universally accepted definition of outcome is the easiest way to fulfil this requirement. For example, in a study population of a few hundred coronary heart disease patients, it is relatively easy to obtain

the vital status for all patients at 6 months, whereas to obtain a coronary angiogram or even a noninvasive test, such as a stress test, for all patients may be very difficult. However, it is crucial for the validity of the trial that the rate of patients lost to follow-up for the main outcome is kept as low as possible. One guideline is that a sensitivity analysis attributing the opposite extreme outcome to patients lost to follow-up in each group should not substantially alter the conclusions of the study. During the study continuing efforts should be made to detect potential losses to follow-up (patients who have missed visits) and to try to obtain information on these patients. In order to obtain a standardized and unbiased classification of measurements or outcome events for the analysis of a trial, a central assessment and validation by a committee or a laboratory blinded to treatment allocation is recommended, if not compulsory, for outcomes that may be interpreted subjectively. All possible events should be notified and the detection of potential events should be declared on the case-report forms. The purpose of this procedure is to minimize the risk of missing any outcome events (i.e. the risk of false-negative results), while accepting at this stage a rather high rate of false-positive results. All relevant documentation is then provided by the investigator for the description of the event. Finally, the outcome validation committee reviews blindly the documentation and classifies the event according to prespecified definitions that meet the objectives of the trial.

(3) It must be ensured that the management of patients during follow-up, including extra protocol diagnostic procedures, concomitant treatments, compliance with study treatment, notification of outcome, and adverse events, is not systematically influenced by the knowledge of the nature of the study treatment. A double-blind design should be planned whenever possible.

Safety and Efficacy Data Monitoring

Continuous Assessment of the Accumulating Data: Ethical versus Methodological Constraints

It is not unusual in trials performed in cardiology that large numbers of patients are required and that studies last several years because of the time necessary to recruit patients and to observe long-term outcomes. Before the planned end of the study it may be possible that the collected data are already sufficient to show the superiority of one treatment over another or to show an unacceptable excess of severe adverse events. For ethical reasons it would not be justified to continue such a trial should clear results against or in favor of the tested treatment already be available. Thus, there is a requirement to look at interim results. The evaluation of interim results serves primarily to protect patients participating in the study, for whom investigators have moral and legal obligations, and also to protect all patients with the same condition who may benefit from the new treatment or, on the contrary, benefit from avoiding a hazardous treatment. Although almost everybody would agree with these principles, their application in practice has generated much uncertainty and debate. For a brief introduction to the issues and problems, the reader is referred to two published papers, one written from a specifically statistical point of view[31] and one written from a broad perspective.[32] In this section, we will raise the most striking points that investigators should be aware of.

The level of evidence needed to discontinue prematurely a trial for efficacy or safety reasons is a matter for discussion; there is no universal answer and discontinuation should be determined in the context of each new trial. The decision depends on the therapeutic model, the efficacy outcome, the anticipated or unexpected adverse events, the overall spontaneous evolution of the disease, the basic risk of the eligible patients, the availability of established, nonconcurrent therapies, and the available data on the intervention, including those from previous as well as ongoing similar clinical trials. This catalog of factors explains why, although the goals are rigorous and scientifically indisputable, the principles and procedures given below should be flexible.

While, for ethical reasons concerning the subjects involved in the trial, it is justified to stop a trial as soon as efficacy or adverse effect differences are clearly observed, the study should not be stopped too prematurely for similar ethical reasons, but concerning present or future patients outside the trial. Assuming that the identified effect is real, and the trial was stopped rightly, a marginal statistical significance may not convince future prescribers and the treatment will remain largely unused. It is not therefore ethical to act on results that may not be accepted as sufficiently convincing. The history of the evaluation of class I antiarrhythmics, mentioned in a previous section, illustrates this dilemma. CAST was stopped prematurely only after a highly significant excess of death had been observed in the treated group.[16]

Finally, one should realize the central statistical issue raised by making several interim evaluations of the data. Each time the data are assessed, the risk of mistakenly rejecting the null hypothesis (i.e. of concluding that the tested treatment is more effective than the control) increases. At the first interim analysis this risk is no longer kept at the *a priori* accepted value (usually 0.05). Hence, one of the problems in designing a procedure for efficacy and safety monitoring is to adjust the threshold value for each interim analysis in such a way that the overall risk is kept at the desired value (say, 0.05), in order to safeguard against stopping the trial on the basis of overoptimistic statistical arguments.

Statistical Considerations

It can be demonstrated[33] that, even in the case of a trial comparing two treatments of identical efficacy, if interim analyses are performed frequently enough, merely by chance some of these analyses will show differences for which a classical statistical test may lead to a P value of less than 0.05. As mentioned above, conventional P values cannot be used directly in interim analysis. Several methods have been proposed for adjusting these levels for interim analyses.[31,34–36]

Some methods are based on the continuous monitoring of differences each time a pair of patients included in each treatment group has reached the follow-up. These methods, which pertain to the sequential design, are of low practical value because of the constraint that one must wait for the achievement of follow-up of the previous pair before including the next one. However, they constitute a valuable model from which the group sequential methods were derived. Instead of looking at a pair of patients, the latter methods consider equal-sized groups of consecutively recruited patients. Each interim analysis is based on the data accumulated so far. The accrual continues without interruption. Similar techniques plan the analysis on the basis of specific numbers of outcome events instead of groups of patients. Finally, other methods focus on the consumption of the desired risk of a false-positive conclusion, and allow the P value to be adjusted according to the overall type I error and the number of prespecified interim analyses, while using conventional statistical tests.

All these techniques are formulated such that early decisions to stop a trial require very stringent levels of significance. Premature discontinuation is therefore unlikely, unless a much larger than expected difference is observed. However, the degree of guarantee against an early mistaken decision varies with the type of method used.

Asymmetric Decision Rules

Decision-making for interim analysis cannot be reduced to an algorithm based on the result of a statistical test. As stressed above, when making such a decision, among other factors, the prior knowledge about the treatments being evaluated should be taken into account. If the trial is a confirmatory trial in which the new treatment has already been shown in another trial or in a meta-analysis to be effective (or detrimental) less stringent evidence may be required than in the first phase III trial of a new drug. Such considerations may lead to the acceptance of a one-sided approach for the final analysis[37] and asymmetrical decision rules for data monitoring.[38] The aim of a placebo-controlled trial is to show that the active treatment is effective, not to demonstrate that it is worse than placebo. Obviously, it would not be reasonable to call for the same level of evidence to stop the trial for efficacy as for lack of efficacy. A one-sided approach or, as an alternative, an asymmetrical two-sided approach, may then be chosen, with a smaller adjusted P value for efficacy (i.e. a difference favoring the new treatment) than for the reverse (i.e. a difference favoring placebo). Finally, there are situations where investigators would be willing to stop a trial early if it appears that, even if the trial were continued to its planned end, an inconclusive result or a smaller than expected effect is likely. This latter attitude is not widely accepted, for the reasons that the estimate of the results obtained in a study involving an adequate sample size is always informative, and that statistical methods or rules are not yet fully validated for such a purpose.

Asymmetrical decision rules have undisputed application in combined efficacy and safety monitoring, where they are most frequently applied. In this case, the rule is asymmetrical in two ways: (1) the number of checks for safety is higher than for efficacy), and (2) the adjusted P value for deciding to stop is higher for safety than for efficacy. The MAST trial was interrupted early thanks to an asymmetrical rule which allowed the decision to stop to be made owing to safety concerns (there was an increase in symptomatic cerebral bleeding in the treated group), with a much lesser level of evidence and at an earlier stage than would have been required for efficacy.[39] Hence, such a rule is more conservative for efficacy than for safety. The consequence is that in incorrect decision to stop a trial prematurely for reasons of safety is more likely than for reasons of efficacy. On the other hand, even a significant excess of side-effects in one active treatment group might not lead to a trial being stopped if the overall clinical benefit is in favor of the treatment. For example, it was deemed acceptable to continue a placebo-controlled trial with fibrinolytics in acute MI despite an excess of severe bleedings and even fatal cerebral hemorrhages, because these events were largely counterbalanced by the overall benefit in terms of total mortality.[2]

Meta-monitoring for Efficacy and Safety

Although it is far from being settled or even precisely formulated, the issue of common monitoring for safety, and, to a lesser extent, for efficacy, has been raised following various recent experiences such as the excess of symptomatic cerebral bleedings in the thrombolyzed groups of placebo-controlled trials of thrombolysis in acute stroke.[39] Three trials were stopped prematurely within 1 year. Had a meta-monitoring procedure been in operation, all three trials, and the two others that were run to completion, would have been stopped even sooner, and fewer patients would have been submitted to a hazardous treatment. The principle is exactly the same as the one underlying the choice of a less stringent rule for safety than for efficacy. Instead of looking at data from each single trial, in terms of deciding whether to stop a trial early it would be more efficient to look at pooled data from all the trials altogether. As the proof of efficacy requires a greater level of evidence, the latter need not necessarily apply to efficacy monitoring.

Implementation of Data Monitoring in a Clinical Trial

It is clear from the above discussions that data monitoring cannot be improvised during the course of a study when investigators suddenly have doubts about the efficacy or safety of the treatments. The whole process should be planned in advance and described in the protocol. The statistical method, the number of analyses, the outcome variables to be monitored, and the level of significance set for each one at each analysis should be stated in the protocol. However, it is unnecessary, and perhaps unwise, to specify the exact decisions that are to be made according to the results of a specific statistical test. A data-monitoring committee is in charge of looking at the interim data analyses, not of making irrevocable decisions. The committee passes recommendations on to the investigators, who will make the decision of whether to proceed or to stop. Members of the data-monitoring committee should be appointed before the start of the study and all must have proven skill, both methodological and practical, in clinical trials. It is also necessary to appoint recognized specialists in the disease and the treatments being evaluated, as well as biostatisticians familiar with the problems of interim analyses. All should be sensible, wise and cool headed, be independent of the sponsor, and have no vested interest in the results of the study. Such personnel are not involved in the trial otherwise. This independence will ensure confidentiality of the interim results, and thus prevent the potential introduction of biases by investigators in the conduct of the study. Confidentiality also prevents early discontinuation of the study by investigators who may be prematurely convinced of the efficacy of a treatment by the early results, the consequence being the impossibility of carrying the trial to its end. For these reasons, even in single-center trials or trials involving a few centers, such a committee is recommended. In some trials interim analyses are performed by an independent statistical centre which is the only unit where the treatment code can be opened for statistical computations before the completion of the trial.

Conclusion

In the past two decades many advances in cardiology have been achieved thanks to proper randomized clinical trials. These advances concern both the care of patients and the knowledge of the mechanisms of cardiac diseases. However, many problems remain that require more trials with a more elaborate methodology. Although the basic principles will not change, new methods are needed to solve such problems as the identification of the interaction between the size of the effect and patient characteristics in order to allow cardiologists to make more relevant decisions as to whether a given therapy is worth prescribing to a given patient. Prescribers should know enough about these problems and the relevant methods in order to handle better the information that is provided by clinical trials.

References

1. Yusuf S, Collins R, Peto R. Why do we need some large, simple randomized trials? *Stat Med* 1984; **3**: 409–20.
2. ISIS-2 (Second International Study of Infarct Survival) Collaborative Group. Randomised trial of intravenous

streptokinase, oral aspirin, both, or neither among 17 187 cases of suspected acute myocardial infarction: ISIS-2. *Lancet* 1988; **ii**: 349–60.

3. ISIS-4 (Fourth International Study of Infarct Survival Collaborative Group). ISIS-4: randomised factorial trial assessing early oral captopril, oral mononitrate, and intravenous magnesium sulphate in 58 050 patients with suspected acute myocardial infarction. *Lancet* 1995; **345**: 669–85.
4. Collet J-P, Boissel J-P, VALIDATA Group. Sick population-treated population: the need for a better definition. *Eur J Clin Pharmacol* 1991; **41**: 489–91.
5. Friedman LM, Furberg CD, DeMets DL. *Fundamentals of Clinical Trials.* Boston: John Wright, 1981.
6. Pocock SJ. *Clinical Trials: A Practical Approach.* Chichester: Wiley, 1990.
7. Schwartz D, Flamant R, Leelough J. *L'essai Thérapeutique Chez l'Homme.* Paris: Flammarion Médecine/Science, 1970.
8. Bernard C. *Introduction à la Médecine Expérimentale.* Paris: Baillière, 1865.
9. Boissel J-P, Gueyffier F, Haugh M. Response to 'Inclusion of Women and Minorities in Clinical Trials and the NIH Revitalization Act of 1993 – The perspective of NIH Clinical Trialists'. *Controlled Clin Trials* 1995; **16**: 286–8.
10. Armitage P. *Statistical Methods in Medical Research.* Oxford: Blackwell, 1971.
11. Cochran WG, Cox GM. *Experimental Designs.* New York: Wiley, 1957.
12. Boissel J-P, Leizorovicz A, Gillet J. Comparison of treatments with different set of eligibility criteria: example of P.RE.COR trial. *Controlled Clin Trials* 1985; **6**: 225–6.
13. Boissel J-P, Leizorovicz A, Picolet H. Ducruet T, and the APSI investigators. Efficacy of Acebutolol after acute myocardial infarction (the APSI Trial). *Am J Cardiol* 1990; **66**: 24C–31C.
14. Freiman JA, Chalmers TC, Smith H, Kuebler RR. The importance of beta, the type II error and sample size in the design and interpretation of the randomized control trial: survey of 71 negative trials. *N Engl J Med* 1978; **299**: 690–4.
15. Fletcher AP, Sherry S, Alkjaersig N, Smyrniots SE, Jick S. The maintenance of a sustained thrombolytic state in man. II. Clinical observations on patients with myocardial infarction and other thrombo-embolic disorders. *J Clin Invest* 1959; **38**: 1111–9.
16. The Cardiac Arrhythmia Suppression Trial (CAST). The cardiac arrhythmia suppression trial (CAST). *N Engl J Med* 1989; **321**: 386–91.
17. Gruppo Italiano per lo Studio della Sopravivenza nell'Infarto Miocardico. GISSI-2: a factorial randomised trial of alteplase versus streptokinase and heparin versus no heparin among 12 490 patients with acute myocardial infarction. *Lancet* 1990; **336**: 65–71.
18. The GUSTO Investigators. An international randomized trial comparing four thrombolytic strategies for acute myocardial infarction. *N Engl J Med* 1993; **329**: 673–82.
19. ISIS-3 (Third International Study of Infarct Survival Collaborative Group). ISIS-3: a randomised comparison of streptokinase vs tissue plasminogen activator vs anistreplase and of aspirin plus heparin vs aspirin alone among 41 299 cases of suspected acute myocardial infarction. *Lancet* 1992; **339**: 753–70.
20. Boissel JP, Collet JP, Moleur P, Haugh M. Surrogate end-points: a basis for a rational approach. *Eur J Clin Pharmacol* 1992; **43**: 235–44.
21. GUSTO-IIa Investigators. Randomized trial of intravenous heparin versus recombinant hirudin for acute coronary syndromes. The Global use of Strategies to Open Occluded Coronary Arteries (GUSTO) IIa Investigators. *Circulation* 1994; **90**: 1631–7.
22. Elwood PC, Cochrane AL, Burr ML, Swetnam PM. A randomized controlled trial of acetyl-salicyclic acid in the secondary prevention of mortality from myocardial infarction. *Br Med J* 1974; **i**: 436–40.
23. Boissel J-P. The impact of clinical trials on the practice of medicine. *Controlled Clin Trials* 1989; **10**: 120S–34S.
24. Boissel J-P, Nemoz C, Gillet J, Salewski B, Biaz N. Groupe de Pharmacologie Clinique et de Thérapeutique de la Société Française de Cardiologie. La prescription médicamenteuse dans le postinfarctus: résultats de l'EPPI (étude de prescription postinfarctus). *Arch Mal Coeur* 1990; **83**: 1777–82.
25. Fibrinolytic Therapy (FTP) Collaborative Group. Indications for fibrinolytic therapy in suspected acute myocardial infarction: collaborative overview of early mortality and major morbidity events from all randomised trials of more than 1000 patients. *Lancet* 1994; **345**: 311–22.
26. Gueyffier F, Boutitie F, Boissel J-P, et al. INDANA: a meta-analysis on individual patients data in hypertension. Protocol and preliminary results. *Thérapie* 1995; **50**: 353–62.
27. The Beta-Blocker Pooling Project Group. The Beta-Blocker Pooling Project (BBPP): subgroup findings from randomized trials in post infarction patients. *Eur Heart J* 1988; **9**: 8–16.
28. Freedman LS, Simon R, Foulkes MA, et al. Inclusion of women and minorities in clinical trials and the NIH Revitalization Act of 1993 – The perspective of NIH clinical trialists. *Controlled Clin Trials* 1995; **16**: 277–85.
29. Popper KR. *The Logic of Scientific Discovery.* London: Hutchinson, 1968.
30. Boissel JP, Collet JP, Lièvre M, Girard P. An effect model for the assessment of drug benefit: example of antirrhythmic drugs in postmyocardial infarction patients. *J Cardiovasc Pharmacol* 1993; **22**: 356–63.
31. Canner PL. Monitoring clinical trial data for evidence of adverse or beneficial treatment. In: Boissel JP, Klimt CR (eds), *Multicenter Controlled Trials: Principles and Problems.* Paris: INSEZRM, 1979; 131–50.
32. Boissel J-P, Boutitie F, Leizorovicz A, Pinzani V. Issues and problems with repeated interim analysis in clinical trials. *J Nephrol* 1994; **7**: 97–101.
33. Armitage P. *Sequential Medical Trials.* Oxford: Blackwell, 1975.
34. Boutitie F, Bellissant E, Blanchard J, et al. Surveillance d'essais cliniques et analyses intermédiaires. 1. Les comités de surveillance. *Thérapie* 1992; **47**: 345–9.

35. Boutitie F, Bellissant E, Blanchard J, *et al.* Surveillance d'essais cliniques et analyses intermédiaires. 2. Métodes statistiques. *Thérapie* 1992; **47**: 351–5.
36. Pocock SJ. Group sequential methods in the design and analysis of clinical trials. *Biometrika* 1977; **64**: 191–9.
37. Boissel J-P. Controlled clinical trials: today's challenges for statisticians and designers. *Controlled Clin Trials* 1981; **1**: 333–7.
38. DeMets DL, Ware JH. Asymetric group sequential boundaries for monitoring clinical trials. *Biometrika* 1982; **69**: 661–3.
39. Hommel M, Boissel J-P, Cornu C, *et al.* Termination of a trial of streptokinase in severe acute ischaemic stroke. *Lancet* 1994; **345**: 57.

3

Interpreting a Trial Report

Desmond G. Julian and Stuart J. Pocock

Introduction

The first consideration when undertaking a clinical trial is to ensure that its design and conduct conform to best practice, but the analysis and reporting of its results are of almost equal importance. As described in Chapter 1, the principles of trial design are now clearly formulated, but less attention has been paid to the way in which trials are presented and extrapolations are made. In this chapter, we will address these issues and provide guidelines by which the quality of a report may be judged. In assessing the usefulness of any clinical-trial report, one has three realms of concern:

(1) *Internal validity.* Was the trial a fair comparison of the specific treatments studied on the specific patients recruited? That is, was the design and conduct reliable and unbiased, was the follow-up and analysis complete and appropriate, and were the conclusions well matched to the results?
(2) *Trial size.* Were enough patients studied, was follow-up sufficient, and were enough clinical outcomes observed to reach a precise comparison (estimate) of any differences between treatments?
(3) *External validity.* Were the trials' findings of direct relevance to determining treatment policy for future patients? That is, were the patients entered, the treatment regimens, and the measures of patient response appropriate for evaluating treatment as intended for patients in normal clinical practice?

Internal Validity

Randomization

(a) Were patients randomly assigned to treatment? This is, of course, an absolutely essential prerequisite for an unbiased study.

(b) Were sufficient details provided of the method of randomization to establish with confidence that it was performed correctly in all patients? There are numerous ways in which the process of randomization can go awry, and hence a trial report's methods section should contain a brief account of how the randomization was prepared and administered.

(c) Was the method of assignment such that no intended treatment allocation was known by patient or investigator (clinician) until after randomization was completed? One must be

particularly careful that the clinician entering the patient cannot know or predict to what group the next patient will be allocated, nor should the clinician be able to withdraw the patient once the allocation is known. In a fully double-blinded trial, this is unlikely to be a problem, but in some trials (especially those involving surgery or angioplasty), the use of a completely fool-proof method of randomization (such as a telephone randomization system) is necessary. Even then, a difficulty may arise if any patient, having given consent, changes his or her mind. This emphasizes the importance of the 'intention-to-treat' principle, but if such behavior is common it may seriously affect the validity of the trial.

(d) Was baseline comparability of treatment groups established? This is crucial information and major baseline variables should be included in the paper. In large trials, baseline incompatabilities are unlikely, but even here such evidence that the 'fair play' of randomization had achieved balanced treatment groups should still be presented.

Masking

(a) Was the randomized treatment received by any individual patient adequately masked? For instance, if appropriate, was the trial double-blinded? Where possible, trials should be double-blind. This cannot always be the case, as with procedures such as cardiac surgery and angioplasty. But there are other circumstances when investigators feel blindness is impractical, e.g. in anticoagulant trials. Less credence can be placed on trials when they are not double-blind, as it is likely that the patients in the different groups will be cared for and evaluated differently in respects other than the randomized treatment under investigation. If the primary outcome is hard, for example death, unmasking may not be so important, but great caution should be exercised if soft endpoints, such as the need for surgery or quality of life issues, are being addressed.

(b) Were the care-givers aware of the treatment allocation? As mentioned above, if the clinical staff involved know or can suspect the treatment allocation this may bias assessment and affect the concomitant therapy given. Difficulty is experienced in trials in which one of the treatments under investigation has common and characteristic side-effects (such as flushing with vasodilator drugs), or requires a specific and complex type of monitoring (as with anticoagulants), but even then attempts at preserving blinding may be only partially successful at reducing the scope for bias.

(c) Were the patients aware of the treatment allocation? In nonblinded trials, it is inevitable that they are. In blinded trials, they usually will not be, but as they should be informed of the potential benefits and adverse effects of the treatment they are to be given, it is often not difficult for them to guess their treatment allocation. Even so, a fairer comparison is more likely to be achieved if patients are not explicitly informed of their allocated treatment.

(d) Were the outcome assessors aware of the treatment allocation? Especially where soft endpoints are concerned, it is highly desirable that those who assign events to prespecified categories should be unaware of the treatment group to which the affected patients belong. This is usually best achieved by having an Endpoint Committee, which views the relevant data blinded to the treatment allocation. This is particularly important when such endpoints as myocardial infarction and sudden (as opposed to nonsudden) death are concerned, because a knowledge of the treatment received might have influenced the diagnostic category chosen.

(e) Were individual patient data entered into the database without awareness of treatment allocation (and was the data analyst masked to treatment allocation!)? It is highly desirable that

those entering data into the database are unaware of the treatment allocation of patients. There is some debate as to whether statisticians analyzing trial data (and the data monitoring committee evaluating interim results) should be blinded as to which treatment is which, but at present most studies do not conform to this practice.

Patient Follow-up

(a) Were there randomized patients who did not receive their randomly allocated treatment? It commonly happens that a few patients in a trial never receive the treatment to which they were allocated. Reasons for this include death or other clinical events before the treatment can be initiated, patient or doctor refusal, and errors in administration. The published report should include information on such patients, and it is usually appropriate to include them in the intention-to-treat analysis. However, intractable problems may arise if there have been errors in the randomization process, so that the patient was assigned no number or the wrong treatment, or the phial containing the medication was destroyed before the first dose. Such problems should be declared and it is a matter of judgement whether such cases should be included in the trial, or whether some compensatory method can be used.

(b) Is it clearly stated how many patients were followed, when assessment visits occurred, and for what period of time clinical events were observed? The proposed duration of the study and the pattern of planned visits for each patient should have been stated in the protocol, e.g. each patient was to be studied for a minimum of x days, months or years, and followed-up for a fixed period or to the calendar date end of the study. It is important that the time period used in the analysis is clearly specified and any deviation from the original protocol intent is justified. In particular, one must not change the duration of the study retrospectively to provide the most statistically significant result.

(c) How many patients did not comply with their intended treatment, transferred to other treatments, or withdrew from follow-up altogether? Each of these items should be clearly indicated in the report. It is important to recognize that, in accordance with the principle of 'intention to treat', the aim is that no patients should be withdrawn from full follow-up and analysis, even though they have withdrawn from the assigned treatment. Losses to follow-up should be kept to a minimum, and also documented in the trial report. Noncompliance in studies is common and may vitiate the results of the study. Methods of detecting noncompliance should be stated. In drug trials, these might include pill counts, but there are much superior methods of verifying compliance, which should be used if practicable.

(d) Are the reasons for such noncompliance, transfers, or withdrawals clearly stated? In particular, if treatment side-effects or lack of patient improvement are substantial contributory reasons for these protocol deviations, they provide important clues on the less beneficial aspects of a randomized treatment, and full documentation of such adverse consequences is essential.

Approaches to Statistical Analysis

(a) Were the predefined primary outcome(s) stated and analyzed clearly? Most trials have several outcome measures of interest, and this can provoke interpretation problems if there are no prespecified priorities of emphasis. In particular, in the absence of any predefined priorities, a manipulative investigator might be prone to emphasize the most impressive

(significant) of the treatment differences observed across multiple outcomes. Hence, it is appropriate usually to predefine a single primary outcome and its intended analysis. In some circumstances, a trial clearly has two (or, rarely, more than two) key outcomes of primary interest.

(b) *Was the intention-to-treat principle used for the primary analysis?* Analysis by intention to treat means that *all* the patients randomized to each treatment group (and *all* their follow-up time) are included in the comparative analysis, regardless of whether individual patients failed to receive all or some of their intended treatment. This analysis principle is considered essential for obtaining a fair (unbiased) comparison of the randomized treatment *policies* as actually implemented. If substantial numbers of patients do deviate from their intended treatment, and especially if this is unevenly distributed across the treatments, then supplementary analyses might usefully explore the outcome in relation to such compliance (e.g. with on-treatment analyses), but still the primary emphasis should be on analysis by intention to treat.

(c) *Was the intended sample size specified and justified?* In linking the published trial results to the intended trial design it is useful to see a documented rationale for the prespecified number of patients required, and how that number matches up to the actual number of patients included in the results. The credibility of reported results is generally enhanced if the numbers of patients are consistent with scientifically justified prior intentions.

(d) *Was the study terminated earlier or later than planned?* There are valid reasons for terminating studies earlier than planned; for example, if the unblinded results show that the benefit or harm from any treatment is so extreme that it would have been unethical to continue. Termination for these reasons is made more credible if it is justified by predefined statistical stopping guidelines. Termination may be justified for a variety of other reasons, including evidence of benefit or harm from sources outside the trial, inability to recruit patients for the trial, and financial considerations. However, it is unacceptable for pharmaceutical companies to terminate trials because they have 'lost interest'.

(e) *Why was the trial reported now?* There are several well-documented cases of trials being reported prematurely, before complete data were available, and this has led to conclusions that have subsequently had to be withdrawn. In some cases, trials have been reported verbally to meetings but not published subsequently or only after inordinate delay. This is not acceptable, as it does not allow for timely peer review. One also needs to recognize that any trial that is stopped and published early because of an impressive treatment difference may well be prone to exaggerate the true effect. This is particularly true if trialists are prompted to time their publication when results are on a 'random high', since if more substantive results on more patients and follow-up were allowed to accrue one would anticipate some 'regression to the truth'.

(f) *Were steps taken to ensure that a sponsor was not able to review the data unblinded during the conduct of the trial?* The role of the sponsor in the trial must be made clear. It is now generally agreed that the sponsor (whether industrial or governmental) should not be aware of the unblinded results with respect to the main outcomes during the conduct of the trial, because their vested interest in the result is so great. Information needs, therefore, to be provided as to how the data were handled, who held the code, and who was unblinded and when.

(g) *Was there an independent data and safety monitoring committee?* It is now usual practice for there to be a small data and safety monitoring committee (DSMC), composed of experts in the clinical situation being studied, together with experienced clinical trialists and statisticians. These individuals should be independent of the investigators and sponsor and be the only persons who have access to unblinded data during the conduct of the trial.

They should undertake the interim analyses and make recommendations with regard to the continuation of or stopping the trial for reasons of efficacy or safety. The report should describe the function and composition of the DSMC.

Results and Conclusions

(a) *Was an appropriate analytic technique employed?* Of course, it is crucial that the analysis of the trial data be performed correctly using appropriate statistical methods. The trial report should present results and define statistical methods in such a way as to instil confidence in the reader that the data have been analyzed and interpreted correctly.

(b) *Were appropriate measures of variability, including confidence intervals, reported?* The statistical objective of any trial is usually to provide estimates of the magnitude of treatment difference for patient outcomes of primary interest (e.g. relative risk of mortality or disease event, mean difference in a quantitative outcome). The degree of uncertainty in these estimates is dependent on the trial's size: the more patients evaluated, the more precise is the estimate. It is good statistical practice if the extent of uncertainty in the estimates of treatment difference is expressed in the results, usually by including confidence intervals around each (point) estimate.

(c) *Were unadjusted summary data on primary outcome measures and important side-effects reported?* Whereas (sometimes complex) statistical techniques are of value in expressing the magnitude and statistical significance of treatment differences, it is important that the reader of a trial report be provided with basic summary data as well. Thus, for disease events, deaths, and side-effects the numbers of patients affected in each group should be tabulated, and for key quantitative measurements appropriate information on variability (mean and standard deviation, or a tabular or graphical display of distributions by treatment group) should be provided.

(d) *Was the actual probability value stated, and was it clear whether the significance testing was one- or two-sided?* Trial reports often oversimplify the findings of statistical tests of significance by declaring $P < 0.05$ (significant) or NS (not significant), whereas it is better statistical practice to declare the actual P value. For instance, the strength of evidence for a treatment difference being greater than could plausibly arise by chance, is contained in the actual P value, i.e. $P = 0.001$ is much more convincing than $P = 0.04$, and $P = 0.06$ is not without interest as regards a possible real treatment difference, whereas $P = 0.5$ means that there is no suggestion of a true difference.

(e) *Was there appropriate interpretation of the statistically (nonsignificant) differences?* Over-dogmatic interpretation of significance tests is a common pitfall in all medical publications. In particular, $P < 0.05$ does not 'prove' that the treatments are different and $P > 0.05$ does not establish that the treatments are equivalent. More correctly, the smaller the P value the stronger the evidence that a true difference may exist, and one should avoid overly dogmatic conclusions based on the achievement (or not) of any particular level of statistical significance.

(f) *Was appropriate emphasis placed on displaying and interpreting the statistical analysis, in particular controlling for unplanned analyses (e.g. subgroups, multiple endpoints, multiple analysis)?* The presentation of results should be consistent with the study's predefined primary objectives, and one should avoid undue *post hoc* emphasis on any particular subsidiary findings that indicate especially large treatment differences. For instance, if a trial's primary results show no evidence of a difference, it is tempting for authors to find some secondary analysis that is statistically significant, e.g. a particular patient subgroup or another measure of patient response or a specific time period of follow-up, and build their unjustifiably positive conclusions on that issue.

(g) *Were the conclusions regarding treatment comparisons wholly compatible with the predefined primary objectives and results presented?* Yusuf et al.,[1] in discussing the analysis and interpretation of treatment effects in subgroups, refer to *proper* and *improper* subgroups. A *proper subgroup* is characterized by a common set of baseline parameters, such as age, gender, and disease characteristics (e.g. previous infarction, infarct location, pretreatment electrocardiogram (ECG) findings). These authors define an *improper subgroup* as a 'group of patients characterized by variable measures after randomization and potentially affected by treatment, e.g. separate examination of patients with a patent coronary artery in a trial of a thrombolytic agent when it is determined after initiating the randomized treatment'. They add 'comparisons of responders to non-responders or compliers to non-compliers based on information collected after randomization are particular egregious forms of improper subgroup analysis because response and adherence may be markers of a good prognosis, not necessarily measures of therapeutic efficacy'.

For statistical reasons, the number of subgroups to be analyzed must be few, even if they have been identified prospectively. As indicated above, any unplanned subgroup analysis is highly suspect, but it is not unreasonable to look at subgroups for which there is sound biological plausibility, particularly if their relevance has been suggested from other studies. In principle, such subgroup analyses should be regarded as hypothesis generating, with a view to confirmation by further trials, but such further trials are seldom feasible. Of course, the fact that subgrouping is questionable statistically does not mean that there are not subgroups that behave differently with regard to treatment effects.

A further issue here is the presentation of results in terms of the absolute rather than the relative benefit achieved. It is, unfortunately, very common that claims are made of a certain percentage reduction in an endpoint. This is of little clinical interest if the risk is low, but even a small relative reduction may become of great interest if the risk is high.

(h) *If it was allowable in the protocol to administer the active trial treatment to the control group if 'clinically indicated', was this allowed for in the conclusions?* Many trials compare the use of the agent being studied in all those recruited into the study with the selective use of the agent for clinical indications. If this leads to administration of the trial drug to many patients in the control group, depending upon the beliefs and practices of the participants, then even in a very large trial one may be unable to draw reliable conclusions about the therapy under investigation.

Trial Size

Number of Patients

Regardless of the statistical (non)significance, is it evident that the study was on too few patients to reach a reliable and generalizable conclusion? In any specific field of cardiovascular clinical research, sufficient experience and common sense has usually been acquired for there to be general agreement on what constitutes an adequate number of patients and length of follow-up in a clinical trial. Sadly, most trials are far too small and readers should be skeptical of their findings whether they be positive, negative, or equivocal in their conclusions.

Statistical Significance

If the trial was small and still reached a statistically significant result, has adequate consideration been given to publication bias, problems of internal validity, and the possibility of an artificially inflated (lucky!) treatment difference? For a small trial to produce a statistically significant treatment difference, the observed magnitude of effect must be large, often implausibly so. Thus, small 'statistically significant' trials are prone to exaggerate the real (possibly nonexistent) effect and should be interpreted with great caution. In particular, small trials are prone to publication bias, e.g. authors do not publish small 'negative' trials, so that the medical literature on small trials is largely biased towards exaggeration of the truth and a high risk of false-positive findings (type I error).

Lack of Statistical Significance

If the trial has not achieved a conventionally significant treatment difference, could this be because insufficient patients were studied? Small trials lack statistical power to detect realistically modest but important treatment differences, and so there is a substantial risk of a false-negative finding (type II error) having occurred. Thus, one needs to guard against conclusions that claim 'no effect' when the trial had little chance of picking up such an effect owing to a lack of sufficient patients. This is particularly important in trials where the objective was to investigate the equivalence of the treatments under comparison, where it is all too easy to slip from the term 'insufficient evidence of a difference' to the unduly dogmatic claim 'no difference exists'.

Use of Confidence Intervals

Was the imprecision of estimates given adequate emphasis in the trial's summary and conclusions? In a small trial the confidence interval for any treatment difference will be very wide, often including implausibly large effects as well as quite modest effects (and of course a zero effect if the difference is not statistically significant). Thus, confidence intervals are a valuable statistical tool in defusing overenthusiastic interpretations of too few data.

External Validity

Patients Studied

(a) *Were the patients included in the trial adequately representative of the patients to be encountered in normal clinical practice? Were the eligibility criteria too narrow or too broad?* Each trial should indicate clearly the inclusion and exclusion criteria. In some trials, the definitions are deliberately imprecise, so as to include all patients presenting who might suffer from the condition under study. Although very successful in recruiting large numbers of patients, such a definition necessarily means that patients with other diagnoses are included. When much tighter criteria are employed, a great proportion of patients will be excluded. Another problem relates to the willingness of investigators to recruit patients of various kinds. Thus, many trials have deliberately excluded women, but may not have made this clear. Likewise, there is undoubtedly a bias against recruiting the elderly, even if they are not excluded by definition. Concern about the risks of the therapy under test may mean that there is a tendency to recruit a relatively low-risk group of patients. Several studies have confirmed this impression in trials of thrombolytic therapy.

(b) Were adequate steps taken to ensure that a high proportion of eligible patients was randomized? In particular, was a log kept of all patients with the appropriate condition, and how do randomized patients compare with those not randomized (both eligible and ineligible)? There is considerable merit in maintaining a log of patients with the condition under study, whether or not they meet the criteria of the study, as a way of determining the proportion and characteristics of the patients recruited. When this has been done, it has been possible not only to determine the percentage of the population recruited, but to find out to what extent those excluded were similar to those included. In many studies, the excluded patients have fared much worse than the placebo or control group in the trial. In general, the mortality of placebo groups in trials is substantially lower than that anticipated. However, logs have a limitation because of the difficulty of defining who should be included. The characteristics of patients included in or excluded from trials can vary greatly from country to country and center to center.

(c) Was the setting of the trial and the manner of patient selection appropriate? Were the eligibility criteria too narrow or too broad? Have the authors inappropriately extrapolated their findings to types of patients that were not adequately represented? It is not uncommon for authors to generalize from the limited types of patients included in their trial to patients with the condition under study as a whole. For instance, one needs to recognize that hospital-based studies do not readily extrapolate to patients in general practice (who may have less severe disease).

Treatments

(a) Were the treatments under comparison, including dose schedule, duration of treatment, noncompliance, and the control group regimens (placebo or standard treatment) appropriate for normal clinical practice and determining future treatment policy in such patients? In evaluating the relevance of any treatment difference (or lack of) one needs to look at the active and control policies as actually implemented in the trial and consider their applicability to normal practice. If the control were placebo, but other active treatments have previously shown evidence of effect, then the trial cannot directly justify the treatment's use over such alternatives. If the duration of treatment was relatively short then extrapolation to longer treatment periods in a chronic condition may be unjustified. If details are lacking on actual drug use (i.e. departures from the intended dose schedule, especially if due to adverse events), then the applicability to future patients will be unclear.

(b) Were all aspects of current good clinical practice (e.g. ancillary care) adequately taken into account? It is important that use of other treatments (drugs on top of the randomized comparison) is clearly specified, both in terms of inclusion/exclusion criteria and the actual numbers of patients receiving such ancillary treatments. The aim is to make clear the role of a new treatment in the context of other existing treatments. In particular if a new drug is seen as a potential supplement to other established drugs, then the possible risk of adverse multidrug interactions needs to have been investigated.

Outcome Measures and Follow-up

(a) Were the outcome measures (endpoints, indicators of patient response) appropriate for reaching overall conclusions about the treatments under investigation? In conditions in which

the mortality is high, mortality may be the only appropriate primary endpoint, but when mortality alone is not a satisfactory endpoint, it may have to be combined with other endpoints. These composite endpoints may pose problems. For example, death may be increased and myocardial infarction reduced. In some heart failure trials, the quality of life has been improved but the mortality increased. The interpretation of such results is clearly a matter more of judgement than of science.

(b) Was too much evidence given to surrogate markers of response (e.g. physiological indicators) rather than to more major indicators of overall prognosis (e.g. mortality, major clinical events)? Because hard endpoints such as death and myocardial infarction may be few, there is an unfortunate tendency to rely on surrogate endpoints such as coronary artery patency for thrombolytic trials, ejection fraction for heart failure trials, and suppression of arrhythmias for antiarrhythmic trials. As Lipicky and Packer[2] have pointed out, if a physiological variable is to be used as a surrogate, there should not only be a statistical relationship between the proposed endpoint and the clinical outcome, but there must also exist a pathophysiological basis for believing that the surrogate is the primary determinant of the outcome. However, even this is not enough, because, although the variable may be the primary determinant in normal circumstances, this may not obtain in the experimental context. Furthermore, in attempting to limit the necessary size of the trial by using surrogate variables, one may fail to observe some adverse effects that can be appreciated only in large trials.

(c) Was the duration of treatment and length of patient follow-up sufficiently reliable to assess the efficacy and safety of treatment? Trials vary greatly in the duration of follow-up. This may have a profound effect on the assessment of the treatment. Thus in myocardial infarction some trials have been concerned only with 1-week or in-hospital mortality. More commonly, the follow-up is 4–6 weeks, but obviously physicians need to know the effect on prognosis over a much longer period, e.g. at least 1 year. In some cases, a longer follow-up demonstrates that the treatment is more effective than appeared at first sight. In the case of lipid-lowering therapy, no benefit is to be expected for at least 2 years, and one could conclude that any study should have a follow-up of at least 5 years. In terms of safety, much longer follow-up is desirable, as adverse effects may take many years to appear, as has been found with hormone replacement therapy.

(d) Were adequate steps taken to elicit all relevant adverse events and side-effects of treatment? A table should be provided of the main adverse effects encountered, and the report should explain how adverse-event data were collected.

Balanced Discussion and Conclusion

(a) Have the authors given adequate consideration to the limitations of their study in all the above respects? All papers should include a discussion of the limitations of the study being presented. This may reveal aspects of the study that might not be apparent to the reader, and provides insight into the objectivity of the authors.

(1) *The title of the paper.* The title is important as it is this that often attracts attention in the first place. It should not make dramatic claims and it should accurately reflect the content.

(2) *The abstract.* Many readers get no further than the abstract. It is, therefore, essential that the abstract correctly reflects the content of the paper, and is cautious in the claims it makes.

(3) *The methods and material of the study.* The paper should describe in brief the hypothesis

being addressed, the statistical principles upon which it was designed, with power calculations, the inclusion and exclusion criteria, the population being studied, with definitions of the clinical disorders and outcomes being studied, the method of randomization, the handling of data, the way in which blindness was maintained, the role of the committees, and the role of the sponsor.

(4) *Discussion.* In the discussion, authors will normally review their findings and implications of their trial for the kinds of patient included. But, to be of wider interest, they should consider how far their conclusions can be applied to a broader population of related patients. They must bear in mind that those recruited into trials are a selected population, however catholic the inclusion criteria have been. Trials are usually conducted in rather artificial circumstances and with closer observation than is usual, with dedicated physicians and nurses, and compliant subjects. They often have either deliberately, or by circumstances, included a very restricted group of patients, such as predominantly, or only, whites, or men, or Scandinavians. Valid extrapolation to other groups depends upon the statistical strength of the evidence, the biological plausibility of so doing, and the evidence from other sources (both experimental and observational).

(b) Have the authors given a balanced account of evidence from other related studies or have they given undue weight to their own findings? It is essential that the authors consider their results in the light of other publications and give due credit to other research workers in the field. If their estimated treatment effect is (or is not) compatible with previous related studies, then quantitative comparative evidence should be documented together with interpretations as to the reasons for any inconsistencies (including differences in study design and the play of chance).

The goal should be that any trial's main new results are presented clearly, in adherence with previously defined primary hypotheses, study limitations should be discussed openly and the additional knowledge be interpreted in the context of all previous relevant data, so that both clinical investigators planning future research studies and clinicians responsible for future patient care can make rational judgements based on objective evidence.

References

1. Yusuf S, Wittes J, Probstfield J, Tyroler HA. Analysis and interpretation of treatment effects in subgroups of patients in randomized clinical trials. *JAMA* 1991; **266**: 93–8.
2. Lipicky RL, Packer M. Role of surrogate end-points in the evaluation of drugs for heart failure. *J Am Coll Cardiol* 1993; **22**(Suppl A); 179A–84A.

4

Limitations of Clinical Trials

Elliot Rapaport

Introduction

The randomized placebo-controlled clinical trial provides the best scientific approach currently available to establish whether a particular diagnostic, preventive, or therapeutic choice alters a specific outcome. Provided the design is not flawed, such clinical trials offer not only hard evidence as to whether a benefit is seen, but also help establish the quantitative degree of benefit likely to be achieved in one or more predefined primary and secondary endpoints.

Physicians are increasingly dependent on the results of randomized clinical trials in making choices for their patients. Although a physician's past experience in managing a particular condition is important, randomized clinical trials provide unbiased evidence upon which sound medical decisions must be based. When randomized clinical trials have not been extensively undertaken to evaluate important therapies, the clinician can be placed in an awkward position, with uncertainty as to what is best for a particular patient. An illustrative example of this is seen in the recent dramatic controversy over the role of calcium channel blockers in cardiologic practice. After having shown from a meta-analysis that the use of rapid-release nifedipine was potentially harmful to patients with acute coronary syndromes, Furberg et al.[1] have questioned the appropriateness of the chronic use of slow-release forms of this drug and other calcium channel blockers in patients with hypertension. A well-executed case-control study done by these workers suggested that the risk of myocardial infarction was 60% greater in patients taking short-acting calcium channel blockers compared to the risk of those who served as controls.[2] The absence of long-term, large randomized clinical trials looking at mortality and cardiovascular event rates with the calcium channel blockers in hypertension and comparing them to other classes of antihypertensive drugs became startlingly apparent when this controversy arose. Consequently, clinicians are torn between their knowledge that these agents are well tolerated and highly effective in lowering blood pressure and the question of whether lowering blood pressure is an appropriate surrogate for insuring a long-term satisfactory outcome. In the meantime, until the long-term clinical trials, such as INSITE and ALLHAT (Antihypertensive and Lipid Lowering Treatment to Prevent Heart Attack) with their many thousands of patients, report their findings in the years to come, this uncertainty will remain.

The diversity of the patient population suffering from coronary artery disease may mask differing outcomes to interventions in specific subsets of patients. Even good observational data over many years or small clinical trials may fail to identify such variations. In contrast, by insuring baseline comparability and an adequate sample size, the large randomized clinical trial may lead to the identification of certain subsets that appear to behave differently from others. A notable recent example was seen in the BARI (Bypass Angioplasty Revascularization Investigation) trial. This multicenter NHLBI (National Heart, Lung and Blood Institute)-sponsored trial compared bypass surgery with percutaneous transluminal coronary angioplasty (PTCA) in patients with multivessel disease. The primary endpoint was mortality at 5 years. Before conclusion of the trial, a National Institute of Health (NIH) clinical alert was issued in response to the data and safety monitoring board calling attention to a wide difference approaching 16% in absolute mortality after 5 years between PTCA and bypass surgery in the subgroup of patients with diabetes requiring insulin or oral hypoglycemic agents. The 5-year survival among those undergoing coronary artery bypass graft (CABG) surgery was 80.6%, compared to only 65.5% in groups receiving PTCA.[3] When this issue was then examined among the 122 diabetics in another randomized clinical trial, the CABRI study, the mortality rate at 2 years was 15.6% among the PTCA patients but only 3.5% in the CABG group.[3]

Unfortunately, the practicing physician may not have the background or expertise to evaluate critically the data or conclusions of a clinical trial. As a result, the physician is often unduly influenced by excessive enthusiasm or overly optimistic interpretation of the results by the investigators. The results of a clinical trial can be distorted by the investigators' preconceived notions or bias. It can lead to selective use of data presented in the results of the trial. There may also be some distortion in the interpretation of those results. This is particularly likely when a study is negative. Under these circumstances, the investigators may actually choose not to publish the trial. Even if they do publish, they may focus on other issues rather than the original predefined endpoints.

The investigators themselves often become involved in a particular trial because of a specific interest or a prior belief in the value of the proposed intervention. It is one of the major reasons why randomized clinical trials need to be carried out in a double-blind fashion if this is at all technically possible. This issue takes added weight when the difference between two therapeutic alternatives proves to be of small magnitude. For example, in the large GUSTO (Global Utilization of Streptokinase and TPA for Occluded Arteries) I trial, a small but statistically significant absolute mortality reduction of 1% was observed among those with acute myocardial infarction randomized to receive tissue plasminogen activator (t-PA) compared to those receiving streptokinase.[4] In GUSTO, the investigators were not blinded, and it is not difficult to imagine a scenario whereby other treatment decisions on individual patients during the trial, such as, for example, to proceed with CABG surgery or PTCA, may have been influenced, consciously or unconsciously, by knowledge of whether the patient had received t-PA or streptokinase.

Increasingly, authoritative bodies such as national and international professional societies are setting guidelines for the management of particular conditions which are developed by committees composed of experts in the field. In large part, the weight placed on their recommendations is based on the strength of the evidence provided through analysis of clinical trials. Often, the more clear cut the evidence, the stronger the recommendation is made regarding choices of appropriate therapy.

The more clinical-trial protocols restrict concomitant therapy during a trial, the more likely that the results will be less generalizable to the universe of patients having a particular disorder. When beta-blockers were first being evaluated in the postmyocardial infarction patient, there were no other generally accepted concomitant management strategies that were known to influence survival. Consequently, the degree of benefit established from various clinical trials was devoid of any concern that it had been altered by any potential interactions of beta-blockers with other therapy. Today, when one wishes to evaluate a new therapeutic intervention, it is necessary ethically to insure that all patients in both randomized groups receive all other agents that earlier have been demonstrated to be beneficial. The estimate of benefit in a positive trial is then additive to whatever benefits have been contributed through the use of concomitant therapy. It is likely that the risk reduction produced is different from what might have been observed if the intervention under study had been investigated before other agents had been established as beneficial. There is also the possibility that, through interaction, the new agent being evaluated could lessen the beneficial effect established previously for one or more of the concomitantly administered drugs. Unfortunately, this is unlikely to be uncovered in the trial itself.

In many trials, patients are managed far more intensively and seen more often than would be the case for a similar patient under the care of a private physician. Study patients are frequently seen by nurse practitioners and other allied health personnel, to ensure that all data are being collected and to observe the effects of the study drug on the patient. Frequent visits lead to better medication compliance than might otherwise be the case. Often, special ancillary tests are performed that would not normally be routine, and these may lead to the detection of problems from which the patient may benefit because of earlier intervention. The more intensively the patient is managed during the trial, the greater the possibility that the trial results will produce a more favorable outcome than would be the case once the results of the trial are applied to the general population.

The above is one of the major reasons why event rates never seem to meet pretrial expectations. In my experience of sitting on a number of data and safety monitoring boards overseeing clinical trials, control event rates seem to run almost routinely as low as a half of what has been projected prior to the trial. A likely explanation in many cases is the better care that the patient receives in the course of the trial. The better and more attentive the care, the more it seems that the endpoint incidence is decreased.

The underlying strength of the randomized clinical trial is its ability to eliminate bias in the allocation of treatment comparisons and to give a quantitative assessment in terms of a point estimate and associated 95% confidence intervals of any advantage of one therapeutic option over another. However, a randomized clinical trial is not a panacea. There are a number of limitations that arise when trials form the basis of clinical practice.

Inclusion and Exclusion Criteria

Frequently, the clinician will be unaware of the criteria that were used in the recruitment of patients into a trial. Details of the trial protocol are often published years before the conclusion of the trial, and are generally unread. As a result, practitioners often generalize observed favorable results from a clinical trial to all patients with that disorder. Furthermore, issues such as the timing and dose of drug are often overlooked. A classic example was the enthusiasm displayed by cardiologists and internists several years ago when the results of the diltiazem reinfarction trial were published.[5] This trial showed a reduction in the occurrence of reinfarction in patients with acute non-Q-wave myocardial infarctions randomized to diltiazem compared to placebo, and was a major reason for the subsequent widespread use of this calcium channel blocker in non-Q-wave myocardial infarct patients. However, one may speculate on how many clinicians are aware that the trial was only significant statistically, using the usual criterion of $P \leqslant 0.05$, when a one-tailed t-test was used. If a two-tailed t-test is undertaken, the more appropriate statistical test when the intervention is perceived as potentially being worse as well as better than the control, statistical significance is not reached. How many physicians are aware that a significant number of the patients enrolled in this trial presented with ST-segment elevation, not ST-segment depression, on the electrocardiogram at hospital entry, but then qualified for randomization because they failed to develop Q waves? Today such patients are considered immediate candidates for thrombolytic therapy and not a calcium channel blocker. How many physicians are aware that the protocol for this trial required a waiting period of at least 24 and up to 72 hours after hospitalization to insure that a Q wave did not develop and that serum enzymes rose before patients were randomized into the trial? Finally, how many remember that the total trial duration was only 2 weeks?

Generalization of findings from a clinical trial may be inappropriate, and even misleading, unless care is taken to insure that the limitations of any extrapolations are defined. In general, patients randomized into clinical trials are more compliant and have fewer comorbid conditions than the universe of patients with that disease entity. As a result, they constitute a subpopulation that is not always representative of the entire population. Commonly, there are significant exclusions of elderly patients or women in recruitments for trials. In a compilation of 214 trials of specific pharmacotherapies in acute myocardial infarction, over 60% excluded patients over the age of 75 years.[6] Patients with more complex problems or comorbid conditions are often disqualified from incorporation into a trial, or, if not disqualified by the protocol, will frequently be excluded by an individual investigator. On the other hand, if one seeks only patients who are at high risk of the selected endpoint events by adjusting eligibility criteria for trial entrance, one is in danger of sacrificing the ability subsequently to generalize the results for the desired power of the study.

Evidence that clinical trials selectively study subgroups of a larger population with a given disease entity is dramatically portrayed by analysis of myocardial infarction trials. Appropriately, mortality has been a major endpoint in many myocardial infarction trials. When one looks at various randomized clinical trials of thrombolytic agents compared with either a placebo or open controls, one observes among trials as much as a three-fold difference in the 30-day mortality rate. For example, the ASSET (Anglo-Scandinavian Study of Early Thrombolysis) trial had a 9.8% 1-month mortality rate among those receiving t-PA.[7] In contrast, the European Cooperative Study Group data[8] for patients who were also treated with t-PA, 14-day mortality was only 2.82%, while in the trial conducted by White et al.[9] using streptokinase, 30-day mortality was 3.7%. Although some have ascribed the variability in mortality rate among patients receiving different thrombolytic agents as reflecting different management strategies, particularly differences in the thrombolytic agent and anticoagulant regimens used, it is important to appreciate that there has been similar variability in the control populations for these studies. For example, in the GISSI (Gruppo Italiano per lo Studio della Streptochinase nell'Infarto Miocardio) trial[10] control mortality was 13.0%, while in the European Cooperative Study Group trial it was 5.7%. Although, at times, the differences observed in control rates between different trials may reflect changes in overall management with time, they often reflect differences in the baseline characteristics of the population of patients being studied. Even these figures pale, however, when one looks at the worldwide reported mortality as detailed in the comprehensive WHO multinational MONICA (Monitoring Trends and Determinants in Cardiovascular Disease) 10-year study, where 28-day case fatality rates averaged approximately 48% for men (range 37–81%) suffering an acute coronary event.[11] The study demonstrated major differences between populations in nonfatal as well as fatal coronary event rates. The high worldwide mortality, that occurs both in and outside the hospital, of acute myocardial infarct patients who are not seen or hospitalized within the early hours of their infarction is often forgotten when we talk about the benefits that have accrued as a result of the institution of thrombolytic therapy and other types of improved management of the acute infarct patient. Even in mega-trials, study patients represent only a segment of the patients who suffer from the disorder, and clearly comprise a segment in which the prognosis is materially better. To generalize the results of clinical trials taking place within hospitalized populations in industrialized countries with developed medical delivery systems to the overall population of patients with myocardial infarction is unwarranted, and it is clear that much has still to be done in order to improve the life expectancy of patients worldwide who suffer an acute myocardial infarction.

Similarly, even within the hospitalized population of myocardial infarction patients, it is clear that randomized clinical trials have not dealt to any extent with many subsets of patients who present with acute infarction. Today, we know very little about the relative benefits of acute intervention, such as angioplasty or CABG surgery in cardiogenic shock, because it has been difficult clinically to study this subset of patients with infarction. In addition, no major trials specifically looking at the elderly have been undertaken. Although the elderly have been included in some trials, they have been done so only in small numbers, and as a result the conclusions are not all that apparent. An example is the use of thrombolytics in patients over the age of 75 years. Although ISIS-2 suggested a pronounced benefit for thrombolytic therapy in this subset of patients,[12] the meta-analysis carried out by the Fibrinolytic Therapy Trialists showed that the number of lives saved per 1000 patients treated was markedly lower and, in fact, did not prove to be of statistical significance using the usual *P*-value criterion.[13]

Poor study designs and nonrepresentative study cohorts weaken the impact of clinical trials on medical practice. Teaching hospitals and large medical centers tend to participate disproportionately in clinical trials, and it is likely that their patient population differs from those seen in the private outpatient setting or in the small private hospital. This fact is almost never taken into consideration when clinical-trial results are generalized to patient cohorts that may have serious differences in socioeconomic status, degree of comorbid conditions, overall nutritional status, access to medical care, emotional outlook, language barriers, ethnic diversity, and attention to general hygiene measures.

Differences in entry and exclusion criteria also create problems when a systematic overview or meta-analysis of an intervention is undertaken. For example, four major trials looked at the results of oral angiotensin converting enzyme (ACE) inhibitors started within the first 24–36 hours following acute myocardial infarction. In two of these trials, ISIS-4 (International Study of Infarct Survival)[14] and CCS-I (Chinese Cardiac Study),[15] the entry criterion was simply the impression of the admitting physician that the patient was suffering an acute myocardial infarction. In the SMILE (Survival of Myocardial Infarction Long-term Evaluation) trial,[16] however, patients were required to present with ST-segment elevation on the electrocardiogram. In the fourth trial, GISSI-3,[17] the entry into the trial required either 1 mm or more ST-segment elevation, or 1 mm or more of ST-segment depression on the electrocardiogram. Although a systematic overview of these trials suggests that approximately five lives can be saved per 1000 patients treated with oral ACE inhibitors begun on the first day, great uncertainty remains as to which subsets of patients actually benefit, particularly in light of the trials of ACE inhibitors started after several days in which benefit is predominantly among those patients demonstrating significant left ventricular dysfunction following an anterior myocardial infarction.

Randomization is the key to successful clinical trials if unbiased comparison groups are to be generated. However, the quality of randomization can vary greatly from trial to trial. One of the more salient issues that may not be addressed is the question of whether patients who qualified for the trial by the inclusion and exclusion criteria, but refused to enter the trial, introduce a bias in the remaining population that was studied. It is always a matter of concern when tens of thousands of patients are initially screened but only hundreds or a few thousands are included in the eventual randomization. In a recent assessment of the quality of randomization in reported trials,[18] only 32% of published trials in four specialty journals and 48% in four general medical journals reported an adequate method of generating random numbers, and only 9% and 15%, respectively, provided an adequate description of sequence generation and allocation concealment until the point of treatment allocation.

It is important that randomized clinical trials be double-blind whenever this is technically feasible. At times, investigators conclude that the experimental design will become too complex if the protocol requires them to blind the physicians to the form of treatment being administered. Such a conclusion, however, should be subject to rigorous examination and justification before it is accepted. Blinding of the physician caring for an enrolled patient is highly desirable because concomitant therapy and management decisions may be influenced, either subtly or overtly, by a knowledge of which group a patient is in. For example, concern was expressed by some over the absence of physician blinding in GUSTO I. It was suggested that the differences in the rate of early CABG surgery between those receiving t-PA and streptokinase may have been influenced by this knowledge, since the presence of a systemic fibrinolytic state might have discouraged the decision to undertake surgery in some cases.

The patient needs to be blinded merely to avoid the placebo effect. The patient wants to believe that the study drug, for example, is efficacious and, therefore, will tend to bias the endpoint benefits and lead to an underestimate of adverse events. The physician, knowing the group allocation, may be biased in the interpretation of diagnostic tests and may, therefore, tend to underrate an adverse experience or overrate a beneficial one.

Sample Size

Comparison of treatment differences that produce a large effect are unlikely to require a major trial involving tens of thousands of patients. However, most interventions evaluated by clinical trials usually look at an outcome where a potential difference in the primary endpoint of only 10–25% is being examined. The event frequency within the control group influences the sample size required for there to be the same anticipated percentage reduction in event rate in the treated group. For example, the sample size required to detect, with 80% power, a 50% reduction from a control event rate of 10% would require a sample size of approximately 460 patients in each group. On the other hand, an anticipated 50% reduction from a control event rate of 5% would require approximately 960 patients to be enrolled in each group in the trial.[19] For smaller differences between control and intervention, a very large number of patients is required for a randomized clinical trial, which significantly increases the cost and complexity of carrying out the trial. For example, a trial in which one proposes to detect a 10% reduction in mortality rate, with the control group expected to have a 10% mortality, would require over 13 600 patients in each group for 80% power, and over 18 200 patients in each group for 90% power. Failure to use an adequate sample size may lead to a so-called type II error, with an apparent negative result that reflects an underpowered study rather than being a truly negative result.

Some who design randomized clinical trials have labored under the assumption that one should use as large a sample size as possible. The advantage of a huge sample size under these circumstances, apart from insuring that one will have enough endpoint events, is that one need not be concerned about baseline comparability between the experimental and control groups. One assumes that there will be an equal distribution of relevant baseline characteristics under these circumstances. Aside from this, however, one has to be aware of the fact that, regardless of how small the difference may be between two underlying cohorts, provided the difference is not zero, the use of an excessively large sample size virtually guarantees statistical significance of the trial results. For this reason, it is important that investigators define the practically important difference they seek to demonstrate prior to commencing the trial. It is inappropriate simply to set sample sizes so large that they can detect a difference that is of trivial magnitude.

Once one has specified the clinically relevant difference that one seeks to detect, the importance of insuring that a type II error (also known as a beta error) does not occur arises. Such an error occurs when one fails to detect that two cohorts are significantly different when in reality they are. Of paramount importance here is the requirement for the investigators to specify the desired probability of detecting this difference. The specification of such a difference is, obviously, an estimate, but hopefully is based upon earlier trial evidence, a pilot study that has led to a more definitive trial, or the best judgment of an investigator based upon his or her analysis of all relevant previous research carried out in the area. Once one has specified the difference worth detecting, the sample size can be easily determined from tables that define the number of subjects based upon the chosen power of the test; such tables are given in books on statistics and by readily available computer software. The majority of randomized clinical trials generally use a power level of 80% to detect the specified difference with a probability of $P = 0.05$. This translates into a 20% chance that a true difference may be missed, which is generally satisfactory when a new technique is initially being evaluated or a large effect is anticipated. However, when a large mega-trial is contemplated, particularly when it is clearly going to be expensive and time consuming to undertake, a power level of 90% is a more appropriate choice. Furthermore, if one is dealing with a uniformly fatal disorder for which there are few treatment options, a very high power should be chosen. For example, if one is screening drugs for AIDS patients, one would want to use a power level of 90–95%, while at the same time be willing to accept a P value or alpha error of 0.10. In other words, one might be willing to sacrifice statistical significance to obtain evidence that one is not missing a true beneficial effect.

Mega-trials

The mega-trial has evolved to become the gold standard in cardiology for evaluating a therapeutic intervention, particularly where definitive evidence is sought regarding its effect on mortality or serious morbidity. Conceptually, it is appealing to design a randomized clinical trial with a simple protocol algorithm, with minimal need for data collection, and with little or no restrictions on carrying out nontrial treatments. The presumption is that a simple design will encourage investigators in multiple centers to randomize large numbers of patients. This will tend to average out significant variability in non-study-drug management and imprecise data collection. The obvious value of a mega-trial is that it has the power to identify small absolute reductions in important endpoints such as mortality, which potentially can translate into an annual saving of thousands of lives worldwide because of the large number of patients that are at risk. However, studies that have a critical impact on practice, particularly where only small differences have been demonstrated between the trial groups, need confirmation. Similarly, when a secondary, but not the primary, endpoint has a positive outcome or if the outcome is in the opposite direction of the pretrial hypothesis, a confirmatory trial is needed. In the PRAISE (Prospective Randomized Amlodipine Survival Evaluation) trial presented at the Annual

Scientific Sessions of the American Heart Association in November 1995 by Packer, the effects of amlodipine on the combined risk of death or hospitalization for a life-threatening cardiovascular event in patients with severe heart failure was the primary endpoint. At the trial's conclusion, no significant difference was seen. A subgroup analysis, predefined in the protocol, was undertaken of the results observed in patients with dilated congestive cardiomyopathy (DCCM) and those with ischemic cardiomyopathy. This was based on the belief that, because of the known antianginal properties of calcium channel blockers, patients with heart failure due to coronary disease might preferentially benefit from amlodipine. However, at the trial's conclusion, the opposite effect was observed. No reduction was seen in the combined endpoint or in all-cause mortality among patients with coronary artery disease. Unexpectedly, a significant reduction in both the primary and secondary endpoints was seen among the heart failure patients with DCCM randomized to amlodipine. To confirm these observations, a second separate trial, PRAISE II, is now underway, randomizing only patients with DCCM to receive either amlodipine or placebo.

Mega-trials may have other significant problems. In particular, if there are no restrictions on nontrial treatments (i.e. an overly permissive protocol), the ultimate effect of the intervention may be underestimated. That is, a bias towards the null hypothesis is created when concurrent treatments that have similar effects or parallel the pharmacotherapeutic effect of the test intervention are used.

Problems that can arise through such circumstances are not just theoretical, but can have profound implications on the conclusions that are reached. The greater the use of concurrent nontrial interventions that may have effects similar to the trial intervention, the greater the likelihood that the eventual treatment effect under study may be under-estimated. On the other hand, if a standard concurrent treatment is omitted, the therapeutic effect of the study drug can be overestimated. For example, in a trial that looked at the effect of heparin on patency in acute myocardial infarction following thrombolysis, the difference in patency rates was much greater when aspirin was not used in either study group compared to similar trials that included aspirin in both groups.[20,21]

Crossovers

The problem of crossovers from one trial arm to another or of using additional nonprotocol interventions has also been troublesome in several mega-trials and has limited the acceptability of the conclusions drawn from the results. In ISIS-4,[14] in one arm of the study which involved evaluating the influence of the daily use of a long-acting oral mononitrate on 5-week survival, intravenous nitrates were administered to 54% of patients. A total of 60% received nontrial nitrates. Such a large crossover confounds the ultimate conclusions based on an analysis using the intention-to-treat principle that nitrates were not beneficial in reducing 5-week mortality in this trial. Nor is it possible to overcome this problem simply by analyzing those patients in the trial who did not receive nontrial nitrates, since, presumably, the physicians who administered intravenous nitrates to particular patients introduced a bias into the study (i.e. that it was going to be helpful), whereas the opposite bias was introduced with regard to patients who did not receive nitrates (i.e. that such patients were unlikely to benefit from the administration of nitrates). Thus, the more appropriate conclusion from this trial is that stated by Woods:[22] 'the mega-trials have therefore contrasted the general use of nitrates with their liberal use for perceived clinical indications and found no difference in mortality.'

Another example of this type was seen in GUSTO I. In the group of patients randomized to receive streptokinase and subcutaneous heparin, 18% received intravenous heparin on day 1 and 36% had received it by the end of their hospital stay. Clearly, this lessened the ability to determine with confidence whether the group randomized to streptokinase and intravenous heparin behaved significantly differently from those to whom heparin was given subcutaneously.

There are many similar examples of the problems created by crossovers in a number of different clinical trials. This has led to arguments against analyzing the trial data based on the intention-to-treat principle. However, it is clear that intention to treat is a cardinal principle on which one carries out a clinical trial in order to prevent bias, and arguments against its use simply reflect some of the limitations inherent in carrying out a clinical trial rather than a logical reason for changing the way in which trial results are analyzed.

Significance of Findings

One may be readily confused or even misled regarding the quantitative significance of the reported findings from a randomized clinical trial. First, the data may be expressed either in terms of the relative risk of one alternative compared to the other, or as an odds ratio, expressing the odds of the event occurring in one arm compared to the other. Clinicians tend to equate these as being identical, when in reality they are not. The relative risk expresses the ratio of the percentage change from baseline of one arm to the percentage change from the baseline of the other. The odds ratio, however, expresses the odds of the endpoint occurring in the one arm compared to the other.

Table 4.1 presents values from a hypothetical clinical trial in 100 patients. The relative risk with intervention compared to no intervention would be $(10/50) \div (30/50) = 0.333$. The odds ratio, on the other hand, would be $(10/40) \div (30/20) = 0.167$. In this example, the investigators might state that the risk of an event occurring had been reduced by 67% by the intervention. Expressed in terms of the odds ratio, they might say that the event is only 17% as likely to occur as a result of the intervention. Regardless of which means of expressing the data is chosen, the conclusions can still be misleading unless the trialists express their data such that the number of events that are likely to be prevented when a given number of patients are exposed to the intervention is stated explicitly. In the example shown in *Table 4.1*, the frequency of the event with intervention was 20%. With no intervention, the event occurred 60% of the time. Thus, the reduction achieved indicates that for every 100 patients exposed to the intervention, 40 would have been protected from experiencing the event. This provides a perspective not appreciated simply by stating the results in terms of relative risk or odds ratio. The importance of expressing the data in this fashion is best exemplified by looking at a study in which the control mortality is 5%, but

Table 4.1 Results of a hypothetical clinical trial in 100 patients

	Event	No event
Intervention	10	40
No intervention	30	20

Relative risk = $(10/50) \div (30/50) = 0.333$
Odds ratio = $(10/40) \div (30/20) = 0.167$

after intervention becomes 3%. This represents a reduction in mortality of 40%. On the other hand, if the control mortality is 50% and intervention reduces it to 48%, a 4% reduction in mortality has been achieved. However, in both cases, two lives have been saved for every 100 patients treated with the intervention. Thus, expressing the data in terms of a reduction in mortality without expressing it also in absolute terms is likely to distort the significance, particularly when the control mortality is small. The smaller the frequency of an event in the control group, the greater will be the percentage change from the control for an absolute change in event frequency.

The responsibility of insuring that the data are presented in an unbiased and realistic manner resides not only with the trialists but also with the editors of the journals in which these trials are published. It is important that editors publish accompanying editorials from respected authorities in the field that highlight any issues arising from the data. The results of clinical trials, whether one expresses the data as a reduction in relative risk or as an odds ratio, are usually given as a point estimate with 95% confidence intervals. The trial, of course, is considered statistically significant if the 95% confidence intervals do not include the null value. The clinician is unlikely to realize that the conclusions about the effects of the intervention in the case of a positive trial is not necessarily the average relative risk or odds ratio presented in the conclusion by the trialists, but lies somewhere on a bell-shaped curve bounded by the 95% confidence interval. What is not stated, but only inferred, when such results are reported is the fact that were one to repeat the trial in similar fashion 100 times the true estimate would likely duplicate or nearly duplicate the original point estimate in the majority of instances, but would fall outside the two extremes of the confidence interval five times. It is not uncommon for these confidence intervals to be quite large, particularly in smaller trials, or so-called mini-trials. Although the use of meta-analysis will give a more accurate value for the point estimate benefit and will narrow the 95% confidence indices, a significant range may still be present.

Prior Clinical Trials

Conclusions based on clinical-trial data are strictly applicable only during the time during which the trial is being carried out and for a reasonable period thereafter. They may or may not continue to be valid, due to additional observations and changes in practice that may occur subsequently. Yet trial results are often used as the basis for intervention decades later. A classic example is the trials, largely carried out in the 1970s, in which CABG surgery was compared to medical management. The three major trials undertaken during that period were the Veteran's Administration Cooperative Trial (VA),[23] the European Cooperative Surgical Study (ECSS),[24] and the NIH-sponsored Coronary Artery Surgical Study (CASS).[25] Although the results of two of these trials (VA and CASS) individually failed to show an overall reduction in mortality from one approach over the other after 5 years, certain subgroups of patients were identified as having benefited from surgical intervention. These subgroups comprised patients with left main coronary disease and those with multivessel disease and impaired left ventricular function. A recent meta-analysis of these clinical trials and four smaller ones by Yusuf *et al.*[26] gives a further impetus to the suggestion that multivessel coronary disease, even with good left ventricular function, has a more favorable outlook when managed surgically than medically.

It is important to realize, however, that both the surgical and medical management of patients now differs substantially from that carried out at the time when these trials were undertaken. The improvements in myocardial-preservation techniques undertaken at the time of surgery, more complete revascularization procedures, the introduction of the internal mammary artery as a conduit, as well as better overall management of patients pre- and postoperatively, have all significantly improved survival and lessened morbidity with CABG surgery. It is apparent that the current operative mortality for patients with multivessel disease and impaired left ventricular function is markedly less than in the 1970s, when the above described trials were carried out. Despite the fact that the majority of surgical cases today are higher risk cases who are older and frequently have three-vessel disease with decreased left ventricular function, current operative mortality is still lower than that seen among patients studied in those trials, where randomized patients were younger and had less extensive disease and better left ventricular function.

However, medical management has also improved dramatically over that used in the 1970s. One could almost say that the medical-management groups in those trials simply comprised patients who failed to be randomized to the surgical procedure. As was the standard practice at that time, the medically managed patients did not receive many of the major therapeutic interventions with which patients with coronary artery disease are treated today. No significant attention was given to major risk factor intervention, reflecting the philosophy at that time that one was closing the barn door after the horse had bolted and that little benefit would be obtained. Today we know that profound reductions in subsequent mortality and myocardial infarction rates occur with the institution of measures such as the lowering of low density lipoprotein (LDL) cholesterol by means of low cholesterol, low saturated fat diets, and with drugs such as the HMG-CoA reductase inhibitors, cessation of smoking, exercise programs, reducing obesity, and correction of hypertension. In addition, today, aspirin is routinely administered to patients with coronary artery disease, and this in itself lowers mortality. Similarly, patients are now more likely to receive effective antianginal treatment, particularly in the form of beta-blockers and nitrates. In the 1970s and into the 1980s, management of patients with chronic coronary artery disease often consisted mostly of long-acting nitrates, which were usually given without a nitrate-free interval; such a regimen is likely to have produced nitrate tolerance, and thus effectively eliminated the major benefit that can be expected from giving such a drug.

It is interesting to speculate on what the results might be if the same randomized clinical trials as those undertaken in the 1970s were carried out today. Unfortunately, but understandably, such trials are probably no longer possible because of the strong bias that exists today with regard to the relative benefits afforded by surgical revascularization, and the perception that to deny this treatment to a patient (particularly one with multivessel disease and impaired left ventricular function) is unethical. Nevertheless, there are suggestions from recent clinical trials that the potential benefits derived from good medical management of patients with chronic coronary artery disease may be underestimated.

Increasingly, the question is again now being asked as to whether it is necessary to refer symptomatic patients with chronic angina pectoris and one or more demonstrable epicardial stenotic lesions to either angioplasty or bypass surgery rather than to aggressive and complete medical management. This issue still remains to be settled in my judgment, although I admit that the overwhelming practice pattern today is to undertake an interventional procedure to accomplish revascularization. However, studies such as the Scandinavian Simvastatin Survival Study (4S) trial,[27] help to dramatize the fact that conclusions based upon clinical trials carried out decades earlier, even when they are supported through a systematic overview or meta-analysis as showing a benefit in certain populations of patients, are not necessarily valid under the therapeutic options available today.

For example, in the 4S trial, patients who predominantly were suffering from chronic stable angina pectoris, were randomized to good medical management in both arms, but with one group additionally receiving simvastatin and the other placebo. There was a 30% reduction in 5-year mortality among those receiving the HMG-CoA reductase inhibitor. Stated in terms of absolute differences, there were 33 lives saved per 1000 patients treated among those receiving this one antihypercholesterolemic intervention alone. In the meta-analysis done by Yusef et al.[26] of the coronary bypass surgical trials done in the 1970s, the major advantage for surgery was seen after 5 years. Again, translated into absolute differences, 46 lives were saved per 1000 patients randomized to bypass surgery compared to the nonsurgical cohort at the end of 5 years. One can only speculate, but I think it is reasonable to assume that vigorous medical management today, with all the currently available approaches, would result in a markedly improved survival in the medical arm compared to that seen in the 1970s. Although an improved surgical survival would also be expected today, I believe that it is likely that medical management is equally beneficial. In any case, it seems pertinent to reevaluate our assumptions that a bypass surgical trial today would be unethical or unsupportable, particularly in light of our current concern over the cost-effectiveness of various therapeutic strategies.

Some have used changing techniques and results to argue against undertaking clinical trials at an early stage after the introduction of a new therapeutic intervention. For many years this logic was used to defend the failure to carry out randomized clinical trials evaluating PTCA against medical management or bypass surgery. Today, 18 years after PTCA was introduced, there have been only two clinical trials comparing PTCA with medical management: the ACME (Angioplasty Compared to Medicine) trial,[28] which compared PTCA with medical management in patients with chronic stable angina pectoris; and a study that compared management in asymptomatic patients.[29] ACME was a one-vessel coronary artery disease trial involving approximately 200 patients with endpoints of angina frequency and exercise tolerance at 6 months; the other trial involved 88 patients and was also limited to patients with one-vessel disease, which concluded that there was no difference in clinical outcome. Similarly, although, in recent years, trials of PTCA versus bypass surgery, such as RITA (Randomised Intervention Treatment of Angina), EAST (Emory Angioplasty Surgery Trial), GABI (German Angioplasty Bypass Intervention Trial), CAPRI (Coronary Artery Bypass Revascularization Investigation), and BARI, have been completed, only in the last of these was mortality the primary endpoint. A recent meta-analysis of eight trials involving a total of 3371 patients followed for a mean 2.7 years has shown a relative risk of 1.08 (95% CI 0.79–1.50).[30] However, as noted by White,[31] such an analysis is considerably under-powered. For example, to exclude a 20% reduction or a 50% increase in mortality with PTCA would require about 15 800 patients. Therefore, one cannot reach any conclusions about a reduction in mortality associated with one procedure compared to the other. This helps explain why there is still a great variability in actual practice today with regard to choice of which procedure should be undertaken in a given patient with multivessel disease.

I believe it is a mistake to postpone critical analysis of a newly introduced interventional procedure for the reason that early technical approaches change significantly with time and will lead to tests of techniques that are outdated by the time the trial is concluded. Obviously, one has to await the generation of some observational data that point to the potential of an important new therapeutic approach. However, it is also important to insure that important proposed changes in patient management are subjected to a randomized clinical trial before practice bias and customs prevent effective trial participation.

Duration of Benefit

Clinical trials are generally designed with a sample size and trial duration based on the anticipated percentage reduction in the number of events expected to occur with an intervention and an estimate of the total number of events anticipated to occur in the control arm. From these calculations the number of patients that must be recruited, as well as the duration of the trial, are chosen. Failure to enroll an adequate number of subjects may lead to a so-called type II error, i.e. the probability that a real difference could be missed by chance given the chosen sample size. The power of the study defines the probability that a true difference of a given amount will be detected given the proposed sample size. The importance of adequate power is to insure that the failure of a trial to demonstrate a difference truly reflects a negative result and is not a result of an underpowered study in which a difference was missed by chance.

Although a few trials in the field of cardiology may last only for the period of hospitalization or for several weeks, most trials tend to last from 1 to 5 years. Even when a trial has been terminated and a benefit has been demonstrated, the question will arise as to whether one can anticipate that the benefit is likely to continue, increase, decrease, or even disappear in subsequent months or years. Conversely, one cannot exclude the possibility that a trial in which an intervention was not proven effective during the actual course of the trial may demonstrate a benefit years later. A classic example of this was observed following the conclusion of the Coronary Drug Project. In that study, among the various means of secondary prevention tested in the population of postinfarction patients was niacin. Although the ability of niacin to reduce mortality was not demonstrated at the end of 5 years when the trial was concluded, follow-up after 9 years demonstrated that a statistically significant benefit had emerged.[32] This occurred despite the fact that many of those originally randomized to niacin undoubtedly discontinued use of the drug after 5 years. Clearly, such results are likely to occur when interventions are altering a slow, chronic process and thus will not be acutely effective. Nevertheless, they represent a common reason why trialists will often urge continuation of a trial beyond its proposed termination date, i.e. to permit adequate and continuous follow-up of the original randomized populations. However, potential differences may be masked by patients ceasing to take the study medications in the treatment arm and/or crossovers to the study drug by patients originally in the control arm.

The need to follow patients beyond a trial endpoint is particularly important when short-term mortality is the original endpoint. Trials such as GUSTO-1, GISSI-2, ISIS-2, ISIS-3, and ISIS-4 are examples of myocardial infarction trials in which the primary endpoint was survival after 4–6 weeks. Clearly, a mortality benefit over such a short period of time theoretically can be erased in the weeks that follow, and the initial benefit may, therefore, be misleading. This is particularly important where the cost of an intervention that has been shown to be superior may be quite high, and thus, the cost-effectiveness ratio becomes highly dependent on how long one anticipates that the benefit may continue before it may ultimately disappear. Therefore, follow-up for at least 1 year and, preferably, for several years is important. It should be noted that the ISIS and GISSI investigators have done this and confirmed the longer term benefit of the use of a thrombolytic drug.

By their very nature, small randomized clinical trials involve a risk of producing type I and type II errors. However, this fact should not be used as an argument against performing such trials. Small randomized clinical trials are often undertaken early in the course of evaluating a new therapeutic intervention, because it may be difficult to convince many investigators from multiple centers as well as the sponsor that there is sufficient evidence to justify the cost in terms of time and money of a large scale trial. It is sometimes necessary for several small clinical trials together to suggest a beneficial effect before a mega-trial is warranted. Small primary studies are often plagued by inadequate sample size, leading to a type II error where actual differences may be missed. Even when such a trial is positive, with an endpoint that falls below the usually accepted P value of 0.05, the 95% confidence intervals are likely to be very large, leaving uncertainty as to the true magnitude of the benefit.

If a sufficient number of small trials are carried out and show a consistent trend, the performance of a meta-analysis also provides a way of estimating the likelihood of benefit from the intervention being investigated. I personally feel, however, that where decisions that impact on mortality or serious morbidity are involved, such meta-analyses of small trials are insufficient to conclude definitively that the intervention is beneficial. Eventually, a mega-trial is desirable for confirmatory purposes. There are several important examples where the results of such a mega-trial have failed to confirm the conclusions reached from a meta-analysis of earlier smaller trials. For example, based upon the results of a meta-analysis of a number of small trials, cardiologists had for many years assumed that the use of an intravenous nitroglycerin infusion initiated during the early hours following an acute myocardial infarction reduced mortality. The GISSI-3 mega-trial, however, failed to demonstrate a significant mortality benefit from the treatment, although the early frequent crossover in the use of intravenous nitroglycerin during days 0–1 (44%) in the control group[17] may have been a confounding factor.

Type I Error

In addition to considering the possibility of a type II error, when designing a randomized clinical trial one has to recognize the issues surrounding the possibility of a type I error. A type I error arises when investigators declare that the difference demonstrated in a clinical trial is real when, in truth, the difference is zero. It has become standard in clinical trials today to select a P value of 0.05 as the limit beyond which a difference is considered not to have been proven significant. This value seems appropriate if there is a single primary endpoint for the trial. However, when there is more than one primary hypothesis, a lower P value should be chosen. As an analogy, if one rolls a single die, there is a one in six chance that the one spot will come up. If one now asks how likely is it that either the one, two, or three spots will appear in a single throw, there is an even chance.

The P value one selects is actually the type I error. In choosing a P value of 0.05, one is accepting a 5% probability that the true difference is zero. The overall type I error can be expressed mathematically by the probability formula: $1 - (1 - P)^n$, where n is the number of hypotheses to be tested. Normally, when testing a single prespecified endpoint, the type I error $= 1 - (1 - 0.05)^1 = 0.05$. However, if one tests three endpoints, each with a type I error of 0.05, the overall type I error $= 1 - (1 - 0.05)^3 = 0.14$. Thus, what was a 5% likelihood of a zero value becomes a 14% chance. The *Bonferroni correction* permits one to readily determine the equivalent value needed to obtain a significance comparable to a P value of 0.05 when more than one primary hypothesis has been prespecified. The correction is simply the division of the P value by the number of chosen endpoints. In our example, with three separate endpoints, the new P value will be $0.05/3 = 0.017$. One would therefore require that the data for any of the hypotheses demonstrate a P value of $\leqslant 0.017$ before assuming that statistical significance had been shown.

The selection of a P value of 0.05 is entirely arbitrary and, to some extent, represents a compromise. The selection of a P value of 0.05 is another way of expressing the fact that the two extremes of the 95% confidence limits do not cross the null value. However, it does not enable one to make an informed judgment about the range of the actual point estimate of the trial. When the data are expressed as a 95% confidence limit, one can in fact state that there is a 95% probability (and therefore a P value of 0.05) that the actual point estimate of the benefit lies between the two confidence limit extremes. This provides considerably more information to the reader than a simple P value affords.

Most clinicians have developed the concept, in response to the manner in which investigators traditionally report results, that a P value of less than 0.05 means a positive result and that a P value greater than 0.05, for example 0.06, means a negative one. It might be more meaningful when a P value is close to but greater than 0.05, for example 0.06, for the investigator also to present the confidence limit for the point estimate as $(1 - P) \times 100\%$, rather than concluding that the trial was not significant. In this example, the trialists would report that the 94% confidence limit has zero as its lower limit. The reader is then left with the freedom to determine the weight he chooses to give the trial findings.

Equivalence Trials

Another strategy for testing the hypothesis that a new drug is as effective as an established one is to carry out an equivalence trial. Equivalence trials are particularly useful when a new drug is being introduced, and it is felt that the outcome with its use will not be clinically significantly worse than with a currently established drug. The trial may be important because the new drug may cost significantly less or because it has less serious side-effects associated with its use. The trial design requires one to establish a definition of what is a clinically relevant difference. If the difference is small, it is desirable that the power be high (e.g. 90–95%).

A recent example of an equivalence trial is a trial designed to determine if a double bolus injection of a mutant t-PA, r-PA, or reteplase, had a survival rate at least equivalent (defined as within 1% of the fatality rate) to that of streptokinase.[33] The trial was designed to test the one-sided null hypothesis that, if inferior, reteplase is insignificantly so, i.e. the mortality rate with its use would be within 1% of the fatality rate observed with streptokinase. In this double-blind, randomized comparison involving 6010 patients, 35-day outcome was the primary endpoint.

Among the patients receiving reteplase mortality was 8.90%, compared to 9.43% in those given streptokinase. Since the difference in mortality of -0.53% had an upper limit to the 90% confidence interval that crossed the null point (+0.71%), one can conclude that reteplase is as effective as streptokinase. It should be noted that a 90% confidence interval has a narrower distribution around the estimate than does a 95% confidence interval. Therefore, the crossing of the null value with the 90% confidence interval is stronger evidence of equivalence than if a 95% confidence interval had been used. One of the values of this type of clinical trial is that it can appropriately use the one-tailed t-test for statistical significance, and, therefore, one may be able to reduce the sample size required for randomization.

Endpoints

It would seem self-evident that precise definitions of endpoints are extremely important in designing a clinical trial. However, the intuitive interpretation of the endpoint under study frequently may be far removed from the criteria that were actually used in the clinical trial.

return to work was frequently cited as evidence of symptomatic benefit and an improved quality of life. However, many patients who were previously disabled and receiving retirement disability were not concerned with going back to work. Instead, what they wanted was to be able to partake in leisure activities free from angina while continuing to receive their disability benefits. Successful surgery could not be evaluated accurately by measuring the number of patients returning to work. Clearly, if one wishes to evaluate whether an intervention improves the quality of life of a patient, each individual patient needs to be interviewed before the intervention is undertaken and required to define their expectations should the intervention accomplish its purpose. Subsequently, when the intervention is underway or has been completed, the patient needs to be questioned again to see to what extent the intervention has met the original expectations. In this way, one comes much closer to defining whether the intervention improves the patient's quality of life than if one were to utilize a change in a mathematical score from a multipage questionnaire.

The measurement of adverse experiences also presents methodological problems. When sitting on a data and safety monitoring board during a clinical trial, one often sees long lists of potential adverse symptoms comparing the frequency of occurrence between the blinded control and intervention groups. However, such reporting often fails to take into consideration the rate of repetition with which the adverse event is being recorded. Has it occurred once, or is it recurring daily? Furthermore, how severe an effect does it represent? Is it a mild effect that has produced little in the way of discomfort and might not have been monitored at all had the investigator not questioned the patient directly while it was occurring, or is it a severe problem that is incapacitating?

The adverse experience may also be independent of the intervention itself, simply reflecting the underlying disease process or an intercurrent illness. Hopefully, in large mega-trials these effects are effectively cancelled out between the control and intervention groups through randomization. But it is important if attention is to be paid to these events that the trial be designed as a double-blind one.

Meta-analysis

The meta-analysis of trials is not a panacea. There is room for considerable bias when such analyses are undertaken. Of utmost concern is that selection bias be avoided and the criteria upon which trials are included are strictly defined prior to any analysis of the data.

A surprisingly large number of studies incorporated in meta-analyses in the past have included nonrandomized studies. Close to 30% of published meta-analyses have combined results from both randomized and nonrandomized studies. It is obvious that incorporation of nonrandomized studies introduces a potential for unacceptable bias, and those meta-analyses that incorporate such studies need to be identified and the results examined closely.

The issue of homogeneity versus heterogeneity of treatment effect in incorporating studies for pooling is controversial. Statistical methods are available for testing the heterogeneity of different trials being considered for pooling into an overview. Those utilizing such statistical methods as the basis for inclusion in a meta-analysis conclude that it is only valid to pool studies where estimates are close to one another and do not exceed the statistical limits. I side with those who point out that studies differing significantly in magnitude are precisely those studies that need to be included if a meta-analysis is to resolve a controversy regarding a disparity of study results. This approach permits one to pool in an unbiased way all the relevant available information. If one discards studies the results of which deviate significantly or, even in the extreme, are in the opposite direction from the results of other studies based simply upon a test of heterogeneity, one has biased the analysis, with the foregone conclusion that it will demonstrate a difference from the null. Under these circumstances, all that the meta-analysis accomplishes is to define better the point estimate and to narrow the confidence limits of that estimate. However, it would not permit a large mega-trial to reverse the conclusions of earlier small trials giving results in one direction if the mega-trial gives results in the opposite direction. This situation can clearly occur, and was seen in the studies of aspirin use as secondary prevention following recovery from an acute myocardial infarction. In a meta-analysis of five earlier, small, randomized, placebo-controlled studies, an odds ratio for aspirin compared to the control of 0.76 (95% CI 0.65–0.90) was found.[37] In striking contrast, however, the AMIS (Aspirin Myocardial Infarction Study) trial, which randomized more than 2.5 times as many subjects as the largest of the earlier trials, found a 3-year total mortality of 9.6% in the aspirin group and 8.8% among the placebo patients.[38] The odds ratio in the AMIS trial was 1.13, which in itself was not statistically significant. However, when this ratio is added to the earlier pooled odds ratio, the odds ratio for all six studies rises to 0.90 (95% CI 0.80–1.02). Thus, the AMIS trial suggests that the beneficial effect of aspirin under these circumstances is significantly less than had been believed previously, and its value in decreasing mortality in postinfarct patients is in fact of borderline statistical significance. It should be noted that the protocol for AMIS required at least 8 weeks to elapse after the qualifying myocardial infarction for patients to be entered into the study. Thus, the subsequent results of the ISIS-2 mega-trial, which demonstrated a dramatic benefit from the use of aspirin during the acute phase of a myocardial infarction, do not directly contradict the observations from AMIS.

Those who worship at the altar of homogeneity would point out that the odds ratio of 1.13 observed in AMIS was significantly different from the earlier pooled odds ratio of 0.76. Therefore, having failed the test for homogeneity, the AMIS trial should not be incorporated in the pooling of earlier trials. However, there is no obvious basis for excluding AMIS from the pooling of the earlier trials, and in fact quite the opposite may have been true. The AMIS investigators point out that patients in two of the earlier trials were withdrawn owing to side-effects, noncompliance, or other reasons, and were not included in the analysis.[38] This could clearly have biased the results of those studies.

A similar situation arises in relationship to the GUSTO-I trial. GISSI-2 and ISIS-3, involving more than 46 000 patients, failed to demonstrate any significant early mortality difference between the use of t-PA or streptokinase. This contrasts with the GUSTO-I trial, where an approximate 1% absolute mortality reduction was seen with t-PA. Admittedly, GUSTO involved a different method of administering both t-PA and heparin in the t-PA arm than was used in GISSI or ISIS. However, if one pools the 30-day mortality data comparing streptokinase and t-PA from all three trials, the odds ratio for the use of streptokinase compared to t-PA is 1.04 ($P = 0.11$).[39] In other words, the lower mortality advantage for t-PA in GUSTO disappears in the meta-analysis. Thus, the argument for tests of heterogeneity, and when and how they are to be used, becomes an important unresolved question when one looks at the conclusions reached from pooling repetitive clinical trials. In my view, a meta-analysis should generate a total estimate of interventional efficacy by incorporating all appropriate relevant trials. This may include unpublished trials if they conform to the inclusion criteria and have been carried out in a rigorous scientific manner.

An overview of all available randomized clinical trials that have evaluated the same therapeutic intervention in a broadly comparable manner may provide valuable data on the overall benefit to be expected. When only a small number of trials has been performed, rates are frequently undertaken in clinical trials involving the cardiovascular system. Less frequently presented are meta-analyses of adverse reactions. One can find data for some cases where there are well-known, prominent, and serious adverse effects of a particular type of drug, such as intracerebral hemorrhage following the use of thrombolytic agents. However, considering the number of side-effects and adverse experiences that may occur in various drug trials, it is often difficult to weigh up the relative benefits of a particular agent as demonstrated from the primary endpoint without similar accumulated trial experience evaluating its likelihood of producing a significant adverse reaction. There are two possible major outcomes. One is an overemphasis of the occurrence of an adverse effect, which may restrain a physician from using a drug that has been shown otherwise to possess significant benefit. An example is the frequent failure to prescribe a beta-blocker after myocardial infarction owing to concern about producing impotence. Secondly, a drug may actually have a much higher likelihood of producing an adverse reaction than is generally thought to be present by clinicians, as evaluated by their own personal experience. An example of this is the incidence of cough with the chronic use of ACE inhibitors. This effect can be quite distressing to the patient, yet the figures on its incidence generally quoted often appear to be higher than what the practicing physician appears to see. This may reflect the fact that the patient will not necessarily relate an adverse effect to the use of a drug unless specifically questioned about it, such as is customary in a clinical trial. Patients taking an ACE inhibitor who develop a cough may think that the cough is part of the illness and not the result of the medication, particularly if it is being given for congestive heart failure. In a clinical trial, patients are likely to be questioned specifically about the development of a cough, whereas in clinical practice patients given an ACE inhibitor may or may not be asked about this side-effect.

Bayesian Analysis

Recently the desirability of analyzing the results of clinical trials based on a Bayesian analysis has been proposed. The use of Bayesian analysis has become part of the cardiologist's approach to the use of exercise stress tests in the evaluation of patients with suspected coronary artery disease. If one is dealing with a middle-aged male patient who presents with a classic history of exertional angina pectoris, there is already an approximately 90% likelihood that underlying coronary artery disease is present. A positive stress test using the Bruce protocol when the pretest likelihood of coronary artery disease is already 90% results in only a small incremental benefit in concluding that the post-test likelihood of underlying coronary disease may be closer to 95%. In contrast, if one is dealing with a young woman with an atypical chest pain history, the pretest likelihood of coronary artery disease may be closer to 25–30%. Under these circumstances, the sigmoidal shaped Bayesian curve relating the pre- to post-test likelihood would now suggest that a positive stress test would increase the post-test likelihood of coronary disease to perhaps 60–70%; a negative test in the same patient would give such a low post-test probability as to virtually eliminate the diagnosis of underlying ischemic heart disease.

Similarly, one can make a strong case for the use of Bayesian analysis to test a clinical trial hypothesis. Under this concept one begins with a pretrial probability that one arm of the trial is superior to the other. The post-trial calculation of the probability that one treatment is superior is based on both the observed data from the trial and the pretrial probability. If one analyzes the GUSTO trial in terms of the Bayesian approach, one can no longer conclude that there is a distinct advantage to the use of t-PA compared to streptokinase.[45]

Application to Clinical Practice

The overall results of a large randomized clinical trial are not to be taken as a mandate for their automatic application to an individual patient. Rather, they reflect a conclusion that has emerged from group data, and the results must be weighed in their application to any given patient with appropriate clinical judgment based on knowledge of the individual characteristics and circumstances surrounding that patient. Most trials have insufficient power to permit multiple subgroup analysis in order to define better the effect that the intervention might have on that particular group of patients. This creates uncertainty not only in regard to whether the relative risk of change in the endpoint in that group of patients is comparable to the overall trial change in risk, but also in regard to whether the adverse outcomes may also be different. An example of this problem occurred in the ISIS-2 trial on thrombolytic therapy. Patients who presented with ST-segment depression on their initial electrocardiogram failed to demonstrate a benefit in 5-week survival, in contrast to those with either ST-segment elevation or bundle branch block. The ISIS investigators pointed out that the confidence limits for the ST-segment depression subgroup were not statistically significantly different from the confidence limits for the overall group findings. Therefore, they interpreted this failure to demonstrate a benefit as the result of chance. In this interpretation of their data, the fact that the pathophysiology of ST-segment elevation infarction is usually different from that of ST-segment depression infarction was not given sufficient weight, nor was the fact that several earlier trials had also failed to show a benefit in this subgroup. Subsequently, both a meta-analysis of the results in this subgroup of electrocardiographic presentations[13] as well as a mega-trial, TIMI-3 (Thrombolysis in Myocardial Infarction),[46] specifically looking at the use of thrombolytics in non-Q-wave infarction demonstrated that not only is there an absence of benefit, but also there is a likelihood of harm from thrombolysis in these circumstances.

The uncertainty regarding benefit increases when multiple characteristics, each of which may individually affect outcome, are present in the same patient. In GUSTO-1, which compared front-loaded t-PA and intravenous heparin, with streptokinase with either intravenous or subcutaneous heparin, the benefit seen with t-PA was the greatest in patients with an anterior infarct, those treated early, and those aged 55–75 years. Therefore, what should be the decision of the clinician regarding the choice of a thrombolytic if a 77-year-old patient with an inferior myocardial infarct arrives in the emergency department 7 hours after the onset of symptoms? One approach undertaken by the GUSTO investigators is to attempt to model the subgroup results to help define greater or lesser mortality differences with particular combinations of patient characteristics. More knowledgeable clinicians also attempt to integrate and tailor the information to the individual patient, but without assurance necessarily that their choice is wholly defensible in any given situation. Unfortunately, a significant cadre of physicians will simply apply the overall group results to all situations, particularly if the distinctions are blurred by biased physician or pharmaceutical company spokesmen.

Physician behavior is distinctly influenced by market practices. Heavy journal advertisements by the pharmaceutical industry and persistent lobbying by pharmaceutical representatives clearly influence physician choices. Drug companies are frequently the source of physicians' education as it relates to a specific product. It is natural that such companies will present data on their drugs selectively, tending to present those trials that best highlight the advantages of their product and either neglect to mention or minimize the importance of trials that cast the drug in a less favorable light. As a result, the clinician may have a distorted view of what clinical trials have actually demonstrated and, therefore, may prescribe the product inappropriately for their patient. Material presented a promised benefit, and then only at significant financial cost as well as possible symptoms or adverse effects arising from the drugs themselves.

Publication Bias

An examination of the professional journals involving hypothesis testing in cardiology reveals a predominance of reports detailing statistically significant findings. Such findings have been estimated to occur about 85% of the time in various medical journals. It seems unlikely that such a large number of studies reject a prior null hypothesis. It seems far more likely that those studies with negative findings have not been submitted for publication or, less likely, have been rejected by journal editors who want to publish dramatic new findings and not less stimulating articles about negative findings. In an interesting analysis carried out by Dickersin et al.,[48] authors who had published randomized trials were queried about other trials they had undertaken. Fifty-five percent of published trials, as compared with 15% of unpublished trials, had statistically significant results favoring a new intervention. In other words, unpublished trials tend to show little or no effect between an intervention and its control. Such systematic underreporting of negative trials has raised the question of the desirability of requiring registration in a central depository of clinical trials prior to their initiation. This would ensure that such trials, whether positive or negative, would be examined at a later date when meta-analyses are undertaken in a given field.

It is also unfortunate that the zeal for satiating the public's appetite for daily articles detailing the latest research reports continues to grow. Some medical journals vie for public exposure and the results of clinical trials are likely to be aired extensively in the mainstream press or on television the day they appear in the journal. Clinicians often learn of the results in the same manner, i.e. via the mainstream press. This may lead to less attention being paid to the important details surrounding the trial protocol and the limitations detailed in the discussion when the busy practitioner eventually reads the journal publication.

Concluding Thoughts

It is often difficult for the clinician to judge the validity of a reported clinical trial. Many automatically assume that publication in a reputable journal known for its role in publishing important clinical trials, such as *The Lancet* or *The New England Journal of Medicine*, indicates that the trial is probably important and valid. Although this may be true in the majority of circumstances, randomized clinical trials in which significant problems are subsequently identified by knowledgeable readers consistently occur. It is important for the reader to analyze the results with certain principles in mind. The reader has to ask: (1) Is the number of patients eventually randomized such a small fraction of the initially screened cohort, because of extensive inclusion and exclusion criteria, as to result in an unrepresentative cohort of the universe of patients with the clinical disorder being investigated? (2) Were the patients randomized using an appropriate methodology that insured against any potential bias? (3) Was the study double-blind? (4) Were the baseline characteristics of the patients comparable in the various randomized groups? (5) Were all the potential influences of concomitant therapy comparable in the various randomized groups? (6) Were major changes in the protocol undertaken while the trial was in progress and, if so, could they have biased the results? (7) Was the statistical analysis appropriate? (8) Finally, was complete follow-up achieved?

Once the reader has established the validity of the trial, additional questions should be asked regarding the potential applicability of the findings to clinical practice. (1) Were the endpoints chosen in the trial meaningful and important to patient outcome? (2) How large was the treatment effect, not only in terms of changes in relative risk or the odds ratio, but also in terms of absolute differences? (3) Is there a significant cost-effectiveness issue that mitigates against adoption of the favorable treatment? (4) Does the trial present any evidence to suggest that the degree of benefit from the favorable treatment persists significantly over time and, if not, how does this impact on the issue of cost-effectiveness? (5) What is the extent of side-effects or adverse events from the intervention, and are they sufficiently significant to warrant caution or even abandonment of what otherwise appears to be a beneficial treatment strategy? (6) Were all reasonable clinically relevant outcomes considered in choosing the primary and secondary endpoints? (7) Finally, to what extent can the results be generalized?

References

1. Furberg CD, Psaty BM, Meyer JV. Nifedipine. Dose-related increase in mortality in patients with coronary heart disease. *Circulation* 1995; **92**: 1326–31.
2. Psaty BM, Heckbert SR, Koepsell TD, *et al*. The risk of myocardial infarction associated with antihypertensive drug therapies. *JAMA* 1995; **274**: 620–5.
3. Rapaport E. Highlights of the 68th Scientific Sessions of the American Heart Association. *J Myocard Ischemia* 1996; **8**: 9–24, 30–51.
4. The GUSTO Angiographic Investigators. The effects of tissue plasminogen activator, streptokinase, or both on coronary-artery patency, ventricular function, and survival after acute myocardial infarction. *N Engl J Med* 1993; **329**: 1615–22.
5. Gibson RS, Boden WE, Theroux P, *et al*. Diltiazem and reinfarction in patients with non-Q-wave myocardial infarction: results of a double-blind, randomized, multicenter trial. *N Engl J Med* 1986; **315**: 423–9.
6. Gurwitz JH, Col NF, Avorn J. The exclusion of the elderly and women from clinical trials in acute myocardial infarction. *JAMA* 1992; **268**: 1417–22.
7. Wilcox RG, von der Lippe G, Olsson CG, *et al*. Trial of tissue plasminogen activator for mortality reduction in acute myocardial infarction. Anglo-Scandinavian Study of Early Thrombolysis (ASSET). *Lancet* 1988; **ii**: 525–30.
8. Lieu T, Gurley RJ, Lundstrom RJ, Parmley WW. Primary angioplasty and thrombolysis for acute myocardial infarction: an evidence summary. *J Am Coll Cardiol* 1996; **27**: 737–50.
9. White HD, Norris RM, Brown MA, *et al*. Effect of intravenous streptokinase on left ventricular function and early survival after acute myocardial infarction. *N Engl J Med* 1987; **317**: 850–5.
10. Gruppo Italiano per lo Studio della Streptochinasi nell 'Infarto Miocardico (GISSI). Effectiveness of intravenous thrombolytic treatment in acute myocardial infarction. *Lancet* 1986; **i**: 397–402.
11. Tunstall-Pedoe H, Kuulasmaa K, Amouyel P, Arveiler D, Rajakangas A-M, Pajak A. Myocardial infarction and coronary deaths in the World Health Organization MONICA project. Registration procedures, event rates, and case-fatality rates in 38 populations from 21 countries in four continents. *Circulation* 1994; **90**: 583–612.
12. ISIS-2 (Second International Study of Infant Survival) Collaborative Group. Randomised trial of intravenous streptokinase, oral aspirin, both, or neither among 17 187 cases of suspected acute myocardial infarction: ISIS-2. *Lancet* 1988; **ii**: 349–60.
13. Fibrinolytic Therapy Trialists' (FTT) Collaborative Group. Indications for fibrinolytic therapy in suspected acute myocardial infarction: collaborative overview of early mortality and major morbidity results from all randomised trials of more than 1000 patients. *Lancet* 1994; **343**(8893): 311–22.
14. ISIS-4 (Fourth International Study of Infarct Survival) Collaborative Group. ISIS-4: a randomised factorial trial assessing early oral captopril, oral mononitrate and intravenous magnesium sulphate in 58 050 patients with suspected acute myocardial infarction. *Lancet* 1995; **345**: 669–85.
15. Chinese Cardiac Study Collaborative Group. Oral captopril versus placebo among 13 364 patients with suspected acute myocardial infarction: interim report from the Chinese Cardiac Study (CCS-1). *Lancet* 1995; **345**: 686–7.
16. Ambrosioni E, Borghi C, Magnani B, for the Survival of Myocardial Infarction Long-Term Evaluation (SMILE) Study Investigators. The effect of the angiotensin-converting-enzyme inhibitor zofenopril on mortality and morbidity after anterior myocardial infarction. *N Engl J Med* 1995; **332**: 80–5.
17. Gruppo Italiano per lo Studio della Sopravvivenza nell'Infarto Miocardico. GISSI-3: effects of lisinopril and

transdermal glyceryl trinitrate singly and together on 6-week mortality and ventricular function after acute myocardial infarction. *Lancet* 1994; **343**: 1115–22.

18. Schulz KF, Chalmers I, Altman DG, Grimes DA, Dore CJ. The methodologic quality of randomization as assessed from reports of trials in specialist and general medical journals. *Online J Curr Clin Trials* 1995; Doc. No. 197.

19. Califf RM. How should clinicians interpret clinical trials? *Cardiol Clin* 1995; **13**: 459–68.

20. Bleich SD, Nichols TC, Schumacher RR, Cooke DH, Tate DA, Teichman SL. Effect of heparin on coronary arterial patency after thrombolysis with tissue plasminogen activator in acute myocardial infarction. *Am J Cardiol* 1990; **66**: 1412–17.

21. de Bono DP, Simoons ML, Tijssen J, *et al*. Effect of early intravenous heparin on coronary patency, infarct size, and bleeding complications after alteplase thrombolysis: results of a randomised double blind European Cooperative Study Group Trial. *Br Heart J* 1992; **67**: 122–8.

22. Woods KL. Mega-trials and management of acute myocardial infarction. *Lancet* 1995; **346**: 611–14.

23. The Veterans Administration Coronary Artery Bypass Surgery Cooperative Study Group. Eleven-year survival in the Veterans Administration randomized trial of coronary bypass surgery for stable angina. *N Engl J Med* 1984; **311**: 1333–9.

24. Varnauskas E. European Coronary Surgery Study Group. Twelve-year follow-up of survival in the randomized European Coronary Surgery Study. *N Engl J Med* 1988; **319**: 332–7.

25. Coronary Artery Surgery Study (CASS) Principal Investigators and their Associates. CASS: a randomized trial of coronary bypass surgery. Survival data. *Circulation* 1983; **68**: 939–50.

26. Yusuf S, Zucker D, Peduzzi P, *et al*. Effect of coronary artery bypass graft surgery on survival: overview of 10-year results from randomised trials by the Coronary Artery Bypass Graft Surgery Trialists Collaboration. *Lancet* 1994; **344**: 563–70.

27. Scandinavian Simvastatin Survival Study Group. Randomised trial of cholesterol lowering in 4444 patients with coronary heart disease: the Scandinavian Simvastatin Survival Study (4S). *Lancet* 1994; **344**: 1383–9.

28. Parisi AF, Folland ED, Hartigan P, on behalf of the Veterans Affairs ACME investigators. A comparison of angioplasty with medical therapy in the treatment of single-vessel coronary artery disease. *N Engl J Med* 1992; **326**: 10–16.

29. Sievers B, Hamm CW, Herzner A, Kuck KH. Medical therapy versus PTCA: a prospective, randomized trial in patients with asymptomatic coronary single vessel disease. *Circulation* 1993; **88**: I-297.

30. Pocock SJ, Henderson RA, Rickards AF, *et al*. Meta-analysis of randomised trials comparing coronary angioplasty with bypass surgery. *Lancet* 1995; **346**: 1184–9.

31. White HD. Angioplasty versus bypass surgery. Commentary. *Lancet* 1995; **346**: 1174–5.

32. Blakenhorn DH, Nessim SA, Johnson RL, Sanmarco ME, Azen SP, Cashin-Hemphill L. Beneficial effects of combined colestipol–niacin therapy on coronary atherosclerosis and coronary venous bypass grafts. *JAMA* 1987; **257**: 3233–40.

33. International Joint Efficacy Comparison of Thrombolytics. Randomised, double-blind comparison of reteplase double-bolus administration with streptokinase in acute myocardial infarction (INJECT): trial to investigate equivalence. *Lancet* 1995; **346**: 329–36.

34. The CAPS Investigators. The cardiac arrhythmia pilot study. *Am J Cardiol* 1986; **57**: 91–5.

35. Epstein AE, Hallstrom AP, Rogers WJ, *et al*. Mortality following ventricular arrhythmia suppression by encainide, flecainide, and moricizine after myocardial infarction. The original design concept of the Cardiac Arrhythmia Suppression Trial (CAST). *JAMA* 1993; **270**: 2451–5.

36. Furberg B, Furberg C. *All That Glitters is not Gold: What Clinicians Need to Know About Clinical Trials*. Winston-Salem, North Carolina: Dr. Potatta, 1994.

37. Fleiss JL, Gross AJ. Meta-analysis in epidemiology, with special reference to studies of the association between exposure to environmental tobacco smoke and lung cancer: a critique. *J Clin Epidemiol* 1991; **44**(2): 127–39.

38. Aspirin Myocardial Infarction Study (AMIS) Research Group. A randomized, controlled trial of aspirin in persons recovered from myocardial infarction. *JAMA* 1980; **243**: 661–9.

39. Rapaport E. GUSTO: assessment of the preliminary results. *J Myocard Ischemia* 1993; **5**: 21–7.

40. Yusuf S, Collins R, MacMahon S, Peto R. Effect of intravenous nitrates on mortality in acute myocardial infarction: an overview of the randomised trials. *Lancet* 1988; **i**: 1088–92.

41. Jugdutt BI, Warnica JW. Intravenous nitroglycerin therapy to limit myocardial infarct size, expansion, and complications: effect of timing, dosage, and infarct location. *Circulation* 1988; **78**: 906–19.

42. Teo KK, Yusuf S, Collins R, Held PH, Peto R. Effects of intravenous magnesium in suspected acute myocardial infarction: overview of randomised trials. *Br Med J* 1991; **303**: 1499–503.

43. Woods KL, Fletcher S. Long-term outcome after intravenous magnesium sulphate in suspected acute myocardial infarction: the second Leicester Intravenous Magnesium Intervention Trial (LIMIT-2). *Lancet* 1994; **343**: 816–19.

44. Antiplatelet Trialists' Collaboration. Collaborative overview of randomised trials of antiplatelet therapy. I: Prevention of death, myocardial infarction, and stroke by prolonged antiplatelet therapy in various categories of patients. *Br Med J* 1994; **308**: 81–106.

45. Brophy JM, Joseph L. Placing trials in context using Bayesian analysis: GUSTO revisited by Reverend Bayes. *JAMA* 1995; **273**: 871–5.

46. The TIMI IIIB Investigators. Effects of tissue plasminogen activator and a comparison of early invasive and conservative strategies in unstable angina and non-Q-wave myocardial infarction. Results of the TIMI IIIB Trial. *Circulation* 1994; **89**: 1545–56.

47. Grines CL, Browne KF, Marco J, *et al*. A comparison of immediate angioplasty with thrombolytic therapy for acute myocardial infarction. *N Engl J Med* 1993; **328**: 673–9.
48. Dickersin K, Chan S, Chalmers TC, Sacks HS, Smith Jr H. Publication bias and clinical trials. *Controlled Clin Trials* 1987; **8**: 343–53.

5

Ethical Issues in Randomized Clinical Trials

Bertram Pitt

Introduction

Randomized clinical trials are increasingly used as a basis for clinical decision making. In an era of critical pathways, guidelines, and evidence-based medicine, decisions about the use of therapeutic devices, drugs, diagnostic procedures, and length of hospital stay are increasingly made on the basis of randomized clinical trials rather than intuition, experience, and/or expert opinion. This trend and the integration of the results of these trials into clinical practice are particularly common in cardiovascular medicine, as is evident from the several chapters on and recommendations for clinical practice in this volume.

Increased reliance on randomized clinical trials has many benefits in regard to patient care, but also has led to increasing scrutiny of the clinical-trial process, as well as the integrity and ethics of investigators and sponsors.[1-8] The design and conduct of randomized clinical trials and some of their shortcomings have been addressed in several reviews, in individual chapters in this volume, and elsewhere as they apply to particular therapeutic situations. This chapter will focus on ethical issues impacting the investigator and the individual clinician responsible for interpreting and applying the data from randomized clinical trials. It will not attempt to cover all the ethical issues relating to randomized clinical trials, their conduct, and application, but rather will focus on a few selected issues that, in the opinion of the author, need further emphasis. It must also be pointed out that the views in this chapter in regard to ethical issues in randomized clinical trials are those of a clinical investigator and practicing clinician, and not those of a professional ethicist. The opinions in this chapter are not meant to be applied as rules of conduct, but rather as a point of view to stimulate further discussion with the aim of increasing the reliability of data from randomized clinical trials and thereby their application to clinical decision-making.

Investigator Integrity

Recent allegations of data falsification in several large-scale randomized trials have threatened public confidence and affected the willingness of patients to enter and sponsors

Responsibility of the Institutional Review Board

The responsibility of the institutional review board (IRB) should not end with the approval of the protocol and consent to the procedures, but also include at the end of the trial a review of the competence of the investigator in carrying out the trial. There needs to be a greater and more formal dialogue between the local IRB and the data safety monitoring board and/or steering committee of the clinical trial. While auditing of data correctness and completeness may be the responsibility of the FDA, National Institutes of Health, or other funding agencies, the local IRB is often in the best position to judge the competence of individual investigators in their own institution. The local institution must share responsibility for the performance and integrity of their physicians and investigators. Investigators alleged to falsify data should have the opportunity of a formal hearing and, if found guilty, excluded from further participation in clinical research. Similarly, investigators who are found negligent in protocol adherence, patient confidentiality, or data completion should also be formally reviewed by an institutional committee. If failure to adhere to a protocol or complete data forms is found to be willful, these investigators should also be excluded from future clinical trials. There is often a reluctance on the part of institutions to pursue vigorously any allegations of fraud or incompetence in clinical trials, because of a fear of threatening the reputation of their investigators, or losing institutional funding, which in large-scale multicenter trials can be considerable. The institution's reputation is, however, more valuable and its loss far more expensive both in terms of respect and dollars than any single individual or monetary gain from any single project. Repeated violations of the competence or integrity of investigators at a given institution should be cause to place that institution on probation or exclude it from taking part in future multicenter clinical trials until adequate and effective oversight systems have been demonstrated.

There are obvious difficulties with having the IRB assume responsibility for monitoring the integrity and compliance of their colleagues. The time, resources, and will to monitor investigators adequately should not be underestimated; nevertheless, it is unlikely that a national organization such as the NIH or other funding agencies will be in as good a position to detect early warning signs of incompetence or fraud and, therefore, to maintain the integrity of the clinical-trial process. It will be necessary to provide the IRB with additional funding and/or staff support if we are to impose new burdens on their time. Given the increasing temptations and previous failures in our efforts to insure that respected investigators adhere to ethical standards, there is need for vigilance and review, at both a local and a national level. The local IRB and national oversight processes should be independent of each other but, after appropriate review to ensure that their information is correct and due process given, they should be required to share their findings with each other.

Informed Consent

Another issue of ethical concern that has received increasing attention is the matter of informed consent.[18–21] It is now standard practice in most centers to obtain written informed consent from every individual participating in a clinical trial. While the patient may sign an informed consent form it is less certain that they truly understand the nature of the information and the risks associated with participation. In one study it was found that 30% of patients who signed the form had not even read it.[22] There are overt and covert pressures on patients to take part in a clinical trial. These include the fact that the trial may be the only way to obtain access to a new therapy or procedure, access to care that otherwise might not be affordable or available, a desire to please or to help the physician and/or care-givers upon whom they rely, and/or a fear that refusing to enter the trial will jeopardize future care. Regardless of the reason, the patient should have a clear understanding of the potential benefits and risks associated with entering the trial. In the USA, the written informed-consent document is often long and so detailed that the patient loses sight of the overall benefits or risks and relies upon a statement from the nurse or investigator that they will be better off entering the trial. There are certain situations such as acute myocardial infarction where time is of the essence and only a brief outline can be presented to the patient or their family. In most instances, however, there is adequate time and the patient should be given the time to understand the risks and benefits associated with entering the trial. A brief video or audio presentation may be useful to insure that the same information is given to each participant in a balanced manner. Regardless of how the information is presented, the investigator or nurse coordinator should be assured by direct questioning that the patient and/or their responsible family members clearly understand the risks and benefits of entering the trial and any other options available.

The informed-consent form or process should be pretested to ensure that it is truly understood. The consent form may need to be modified on an individual basis according to the level of the subject's education or understanding. Early in the trial it might be useful to pretest a subset of patients to ensure that, under the circumstances of the trial, participants truly understand what they have agreed to in entering the trial. It might also be useful if this process were repeated on a subset of patients at the end of the trial. This information would be useful both to the investigator in planning future trials and to the IRB in approving future studies by the investigator. At the completion of the trial the investigator and IRB should also review the consent form in light of the actual findings in the trial, to determine whether or not the original consent form was accurate in describing the potential risk.

Sniderman[23] has recently suggested that the informed-consent process be modified further by informing the patient during the course of a trial of trends regarding safety or benefit noted by the data safety monitoring board. While I favor a greater role of the local IRB in the governance of clinical trials than currently exists, I do not believe that this suggestion is useful. The data safety monitoring board is charged with monitoring the safety and efficacy of the trial and should have well-defined stopping rules both for safety and efficacy. Premature disclosure of the trends in regard to either safety or efficacy risks a false conclusion being reached that may lead to patient dropout, and in the long run might adversely effect the individual patient in the trial by stopping what might subsequently be proven to be a beneficial strategy, or using what might turn out with further testing to be dangerous. I do, however, agree with his suggestion that the IRB and patients be informed about the results of similar trials completed during the course of an ongoing trial. Sniderman[23] suggests, for example, that after the 4S Trial of simvastatin[16] demonstrated a significant reduction in total mortality in patients with known coronary artery disease and hyperlipidemia, that patients in other trials who had coronary artery disease and hyperlipidemia within the range of the 4S Trial (total plasma cholesterol 5.5–8.0 mmol l^{-1}) be informed. I would, however, be more cautious than Sniderman in the extrapolation of the results beyond the inclusion and exclusion criteria of the reported trial. For example, on the basis of the CARE Trial[24] of patients with moderate hyperlipidemia after infarction it has been suggested that those with a baseline low density lipoprotein (LDL) cholesterol of $\leqslant 125$ mg dl^{-1} do not benefit if treated with an HmG Co-A reductase inhibitor. Regardless of whether this observation stands the test of time, it would be dangerous to conclude from the 4S Trial[16] that all patients with coronary artery disease and hyperlipidemia be treated with HmG CoA reductase inhibitor and to prematurely stop or alter ongoing trials of patients who do not exactly or very closely meet the criteria of the reported trial. One should also be cautious in accepting the results of a single trial, no matter how significant statistically, unless the size of the trial is adequate and the confidence limits are narrow enough to preclude any other conclusions. The overriding principle should be to provide the best currently available information to a potential participant before they enter a trial. Should further information become available during the course of the trial that is relevant and, most importantly, reliable, patients should be informed and have the right to reconsider their participation. Overextrapolation of accumulating data with regard to the safety or efficacy of a given strategy if it results in premature termination of an ongoing trial may, however, not benefit the individual patient or society, and therefore is not ethical. In the long run, an insistence on a rigorous informed-consent process is essential if we are to avoid patient distrust and increased governmental regulation and oversight.

Randomization and Placebo Control

Another threat to the continued ability to carry out clinical trials is a growing uneasiness and skepticism concerning the concept of randomization and placebo-controlled trials.[25–28] It has been argued that randomized clinical trials should not be carried out if the clinician feels that one strategy is superior to another. It has been said that if the choice between two therapeutic options is truly equal, there is no need to randomize.[28] The patient and their physician should choose one strategy or another on the basis of their individual preferences and, after obtaining a sufficient number of patients and events, we need only compare the results in the two arms of the study. Although these arguments deserve discussion they are, in my opinion, not compelling. While randomized placebo-controlled trials may pose ethical difficulties when a new therapy that is perceived to be beneficial is withheld, they should not pose as difficult a problem when the new agent is added to or compared with currently available therapy. More importantly, physician intuition is often proven wrong. The potential efficacy of a new therapeutic approach or procedure is often overexaggerated by our hopes and optimism, as well as by the desire to help our patients. The risks, especially of a new agent, are often unknown or not fully appreciated. Without large-scale placebo-controlled randomized trials it is difficult, if not impossible, to determine the true risks and benefits of a given strategy. For example, flosequinan, an oral vasodilator, was shown to be effective in improving exercise tolerance and patient symptoms of heart failure in several small-scale multicenter randomized placebo-controlled studies.[29–31] It was approved for clinical use by the FDA in March 1993. During the presentation to the FDA Cardiorenal Advisory Committee it was pointed out that the improvement in exercise performance and patient symptomatology with flosequinan was the most consistent of all the known drugs for heart failure, including ACE inhibitors and digoxin. However, in June 1993 flosequinan was withdrawn from the market in the USA because the PROFILE study, a large-scale placebo-controlled randomized study of flosequinan or placebo on top of conventional therapy including angiotensin converting enzyme (ACE) inhibitors, diuretics and digoxin, was prematurely stopped by its data safety monitoring board owing to an excess mortality of $> 40\%$ in those assigned to receive 100 mg flosequinan.[32] Without randomization and a placebo control group progressive cardiac failure and death would have been attributed to the natural history of the underlying cardiac condition.

Many physicians were convinced that type I antiarrhythmic agents were useful in the postinfarction patient with nonsustained ventricular tachycardia or frequent ventricular premature beats. Previous studies had shown that the presence of premature ventricular beats and nonsustained ventricular tachycardia after infarction were significantly associated with an increased risk of sudden cardiac death, especially in patients with concurrent systolic left ventricular dysfunction.[33,34] Intuition on the part of many physicians suggested that randomization to placebo would place their patients at increased risk compared to those receiving a type I antiarrhythmic agent such as encainide or flecainide. History has, of course, shown otherwise.[35,36] Only a well-designed large-scale placebo-controlled randomized study could have shown the true risk of this therapeutic strategy. Sudden cardiac death in a postinfarction patient with left ventricular dysfunction and nonsustained ventricular arrhythmias receiving a type I antiarrhythmic agent would likely have been attributed to the risk of the disease process, rather than to the drug itself. Numerous other examples exist where decisions based on intuition, prior knowledge, current understanding, the experience of the clinician, as well as the results from small randomized trials have failed.

Randomized placebo-controlled clinical trials may benefit society but potentially sacrifice the subjects' individual good. Societal good is an important reason for carrying out a clinical trial. If, however, the results of a clinical trial have little or no impact on clinical practice, then societal good has not been served. The investigator may argue that his or her role is to provide 'scientific truth' and that the dissemination and application of the results are the concern of others. Clinical practice may change slowly or not at all despite the results of a large-scale randomized trial. There is often a lag time of up to several years between the end of a major trial and the adaptation of its results to clinical practice.[37] For example, despite the overwhelming evidence of a benefit of ACE inhibitors in chronic heart failure[39–43] it is estimated that less than 50% of patients in the USA with chronic heart failure are currently receiving an ACE inhibitor.[44] This has been attributed to an inadequate educational effort and the lag time between reporting the trial results and their implementation in clinical practice.

Lag time or lack of education may, however, not be the only cause for the failure of physicians to adopt the results of large-scale randomized studies. Perceptions of risk/benefit and cost/benefit may prevent application of the results of statistically significant interventions in clinical practice. For example, over 15 000 patients have been randomized to intravenous beta-adrenergic blocking agents during the acute phase of myocardial infarction[45] and many thousands more to oral beta-blocking agents during the convalescent phase of myocardial infarction.[46] Data accumulated over the last several years have shown that, despite the clinically and statistically significant effects of beta-adrenergic blocking agents in myocardial infarction, less than one-quarter of patients with myocardial infarction are currently treated acutely and chronically with a beta-adrenergic receptor blocking agent.[47,48] When used they are often given to relatively low-risk patients in whom the absolute benefit is small. The failure to use either intravenous or oral beta-adrenergic receptor blockers in a larger number of patients after infarction has several likely explanations. In the case of intravenous beta-adrenergic receptor blocking agents, despite the data from large-scale randomized trials, clinicians may fear that administration of an intravenous beta-blocker within the early hours of acute infarction is potentially hazardous. These risks, and/or the perception of these risks, are great enough to outweigh the statistically significant reduction in mortality.[45] In the case of oral-adrenergic blocking agents during the convalescent and late phase of acute myocardial infarction, the clinician may also perceive that the side-effects (including fatigue, depression, nightmares, cool extremities, and impotence) associated with oral beta-adrenergic blocking agents are frequent and severe enough to outweigh the benefits of reducing mortality and recurrent myocardial infarction. In some trials with the statistical power to detect relatively small differences between strategies, such as GUSTO,[49] in which a mortality difference of 7.2% was detected between intravenous streptokinase and tissue plasminogen activator in over 50 000 patients, we need to ask if the cost/benefit will be justified and whether, with these differences, clinicians, healthcare organizations, and/or society will be willing to bear the cost. The finding of a statistical difference, no matter how small in absolute terms, places pressure on the clinician and healthcare system to provide that therapy. In the era of the mega-trial we need to consider carefully the importance of clinical relevance and cost-effectiveness separately from statistical significance. Perceptions as to the risks, side-effects, and costs of a given drug or strategy are, for the most part, known prior to the institution of a major trial. It can be argued that a randomized clinical trial asking a valid scientific question that fails to alter clinical practice, in a positive or negative sense, either because of inadequate dissemination of results, or a low benefit/risk or benefit/cost ratio, is unethical. In these cases societal good has not been altered, despite exposing the patient to potential, and often actual, risk.

Before beginning a large-scale randomized trial there should be a survey of current clinical practice with regard to the issues being tested in order to determine the impact of the postulated results of the trial. We need to develop and apply methodology to predict the impact of the trial results on clinical practice. For example, if we postulate a 10–15% reduction in mortality for a given intervention in acute myocardial infarction and power the trial to detect this difference, will clinicians, knowing the side-effect profile, potential risks, and cost of the drug, use it? If not, at what level of benefit or cost would they use it? Given the knowledge concerning the risks of a given therapeutic strategy or the cost of an agent, clinicians may or may not feel that they would alter their practice based on a statistically significant change or difference in mortality of 10–15%, whereas they might for a 30–50% benefit. While the failure of clinicians to state that they would alter their practice on the basis of projected trial results should not prevent a trial from taking place, it should raise some concern to the investigators and the IRB as to the relevance of the trial and the power calculations. When deciding upon the acceptable level of risk they will allow for a given trial, the IRB should consider the potential quantitative benefits and costs, as well as the potential impact on current practice and society. In situations where the results of a randomized trial are unlikely to result in a major change in clinical practice or where the results from a societal point of view do not appear to be justified because of cost, the IRB should require assurance that the risks to patients are minimal. While we cannot hope to predict the future use of trial results, failure to attempt to apply current techniques, such as decision analysis, that are being developed for use in outcomes research and develop new technology to predict the impact of results may result in an unethical exposure to risk for research subjects.

Basic science may result in unanticipated societal benefit. Clinical investigation is, however, not basic science and should not be carried out to determine 'scientific truth' without regard to patient risk. There is a need to justify the risk to the patient by the postulated impact of the results on society, and to be assured that the patient truly understands the risks.

These considerations are not necessarily new or original but need emphasis since, to my knowledge, they have not been widely adopted or adhered to. Increasing reliance on meta-analysis for clinical decision-making makes it even more compelling that care be taken to insure that even relatively small clinical trials take into account these recommendations. A number of small trials, or even a mega-trial, may provide answers that are biased, quantitatively misleading, or quantitatively wrong unless care is taken to insure that the principles outlined above are followed. In the last analysis, however, no rules or regulations will solve all the problems that have recently surfaced regarding clinical trials. The training and integrity of the individual physician and investigator remains the most important factor in any clinical trial.

References

1. Kassirer JP. The frustrations of scientific misconduct. *N Engl J Med* 1993; **328**: 1634–6.
2. Dingell JD. Shattuck Lecture – Misconduct in medical research. *N Engl J Med* 1993; **328**: 1610–15.
3. Special New Reports. Problems in clinical trials go far beyond misconduct. *Science* 1994; **264**: 1538–41.
4. Friedman PJ. Research integrity. *Academic Med* 1993; **68**: S1.
5. Angell M, Kassirer JP. Setting the record straight in the breast-cancer trials. *N Engl J Med* 1994; **330**: 1448–9.
6. News and Comment. NIH tightens clinical trials monitoring. *Science* 1994; **264**: 499.
7. News and Comment. How not to publicize a misconduct finding. *Science* 1994; **263**: 1679.
8. Marwick C. Ethicist faults human research subject population. *JAMA* 1994; **16**: 1228–9.
9. Thompson DF. Understanding financial conflicts of interest. *N Engl J Med* 1993; **329**: 573–6.
10. Kassirer JP, Angell M. Financial conflicts of interest in biomedical research. *N Engl J Med* 1993; **329**: 570–1.
11. Healy B, Campeau L, Gray R, *et al.* Special report. Conflict of interest for a multicenter clinical trial of treatment after coronary artery bypass graft surgery. *N Engl J Med* 1989; **320**: 949–51.
12. Freestone DS, Mitchell H. Inappropriate publication of trial results and potential for allegations of illegal share dealing. *Br Med J* 1993; **306**: 1112–14.
13. Levin C, Dubler NN, Levine RJ. Building a new consensus: ethical principles and policies for clinical research on HIV/AIDS. *IRB* 1991; **13**: 194–210.
14. Sutherland HJ, Meslin EM, Till JE. What's missing from current clinical trial guidelines? A framework for integrating science, ethics, and the community context. *J Clin Ethics* 1994; **5**: 297–302.
15. Pinching AJ. Publication of clinical trial results: a clinician's view. *J R Soc Med* 1995; **88**: 12–16.
16. Scandinavian Simvastatin Survival Study Group. Baseline serum cholesterol and treatment effect in the Simvastatin Survival Study (4S). *Lancet* 1995; **345**: 1274–5.
17. National Research Act. *Public Law 93–348.*
18. Ingelfinger FJ. Informed (but uneducated) consent. *N Engl J Med* 1972; **287**: 465–6.
19. Lynoe N, Sandlund M, Dahqvist G, Jacobson L. Informed consent: study of quality of information given to participants in a clinical trial. *Br Med J* 1991; **303**: 610–13.
20. Gallo C, Perrone F, DePlacido S, Giusti C. Informed versus randomised consent to clinical trials. *Lancet* 1995; **346**: 1060–4.
21. Sulmasy DP, Lehmann LS, Levine DM, Faden RR. Patient's perceptions of the quality informed consent for common medical procedures. *J Clin Ethics* 1994; **5**: 189–94.
22. Caplan AL. Consent to randomised treatment. *Lancet* 1982; **ii**: 164.
23. Sniderman AD. The governance of clinical trials. *Lancet* 1996; **347**: 1387–8.
24. Pfeffer M, Braunwald E, *et al.*, for the Cholesterol and Cardiac Events (CARE) Investigators. Presented at the 45th Annual Scientific Session of the American College of Cardiology, March 24–27, 1996.
25. Taubes G. Use of placebo controls in clinical trials disputed. *Science* 1995; **257**: 25–6.
26. Lilford RJ, Jackson J. Equipoise and the ethics of randomization. *J R Soc Med* 1995; **88**: 552–9.
27. Rothman KJ, Michels KB. The continuing unethical use of placebo controls. *N Engl J Med* 1993; **331**: 394–8.
28. Freedman B. Equipoise and the ethics of clinical research. *N Engl J Med* 1987; **317**: 141–5.
29. Packer M, Narahara KA, Elkayam V, *et al.* Double-blind, placebo controlled study of the efficacy of flosequinan in patients with chronic heart failure. *J Am Coll Cardiol* 1993; **22**: 65.
30. Pitt B, for the Reflect II Study Group. A randomized, multicenter, double-blind, placebo-controlled study of the efficacy of flosequinan in patients with chronic heart failure. *Circulation* 1991; **84**: II-311.
31. Massie BM, Berk MR, Brozena SC, *et al.*, for the FACET Investigators. Can further benefit be achieved by adding flosequinan to patients with congestive heart failure who remain asymptomatic on diuretic, digoxin, and an angiotensin-converting enzyme inhibitor? Results of the flosequinan-ACE inhibitor trial (FACET).
32. Packer M. Personal communication.
33. Ruberman W, Weinblatt E, Goldberg JD, Frank CW, Shapiro S. Ventricular premature beats and mortality after myocardial infarction. *N Engl J Med* 1977; **297**: 750–7.
34. Bigger Jr JT, Fleiss JL, Kleiger R, Miller JP, Rolnitzky LM. The relationship among ventricular arrhythmias, left ventricular dysfunction, and mortality in the 2 years after myocardial infarction. *Circulation* 1984; **69**: 250–8.
35. Echt DS, Liebson PR, Mitchell LB, *et al.* Mortality and morbidity in patients receiving encainide, flecainide, or placebo: the Cardiac Arrhythmia Suppression Trial. *N Engl J Med* 1991; **324**: 781–8.
36. The Cardiac Arrhythmia Suppression Trial II Investigators. Effect of the antiarrhythmic agent moricizine on survival after myocardial infarction. *N Engl J Med* 1992; **327**: 227–33.

37. Antman EM, Lau J, Kupeinick B, Mosteller F, Chalmers TC. A comparison of results of meta-analyses of randomized control trials and recommendations of clinical experts. Treatments for myocardial infarction. *JAMA* 1992; **268**: 240–8.
38. Dzau VJ, Gibbons GH, Cooke JP, Omiogui N. Vascular biology and medicine in the 1990s: scope, concepts, potentials, and perspectives. *Circulation* 1993; **87**: 705–19.
39. The SOLVD Investigators. Effect of enalapril on survival in patients with reduced left ventricular ejection fractions and congestive heart failure. *N Engl J Med* 1991; **325**: 293–302.
40. Pfeffer MA, Braunwald E, Moye LA, *et al.*, on behalf of the SAVE Investigators. Effect of captopril on mortality and morbidity in patients with left ventricular dysfunction after myocardial infarction. Results of the Survival and Ventricular Enlargement Trial. *N Engl J Med* 1992; **327**: 669–77.
41. Cohn JN, Johnson G, Ziesche S *et al.* A comparison of enalapril with hydralazine-isosorbide dinitrate in the treatment of chronic congestive heart failure. *N Engl J Med* 1991; **324**: 303–10.
42. The Acute Infarction Ramipril Efficacy (AIRE) Study Investigators. Effect of ramipril on mortality and morbidity of survivors of acute myocardial infarction with clinical evidence of heart failure. *Lancet* 1993; **342**: 812–28.
43. Gruppo Italiano per lo Studio delia Sopravvivena nell'infarcto Miocardico. GISSI-3: effects of lisinopril and transdermal glyceryl trinitrate singly and together on 6-week mortality and ventricular function after acute myocardial infarction. *Lancet* 1994; **343**: 1115–22.
44. Flaherty J. Personal communication.
45. ISIS-1 Collaborative Group. Randomized trial of intravenous atenolol among 16,027 cases of suspected acute myocardial infarction: ISIS-1. *Lancet* 1986; **ii**: 57–66.
46. Yusuf S, Peto R, Lewis J, Collins R, Sleight P. Beta-blockade during and after myocardial infarction. An overview of the randomized trials. *Prog Cardiovasc Dis* 1985; **27**: 335–71.
47. Latini R, Avanzini F, Zuanetti G, *et al.*, on behalf of the GISSI Investigators. Changing patterns of pharmacological treatment after myocardial infarction. The GISSI experience. *J Am Coll Cardiol* 1994; 1A–484A, 210A.
48. Lamas GA, Pfeffer MA, Hamm P, *et al.*, for the SAVE Investigators. Do the results of randomized clinical trials of cardiovascular drugs influence medical practice? *N Engl J Med* 1992; **327**: 241–7.
49. The GUSTO Investigators. An international randomized trial comparing four thrombolytic strategies for acute myocardial infarction. *N Engl J Med* 1993; **329**: 673–82.

SECTION II

Clinical Topics

6

Lipid-lowering Agents

Jacques E. Rossouw

Introduction

The evidence that elevated serum cholesterol is related to coronary heart disease (CHD) incidence is extensive, and includes animal data, genetic conditions, pathologic studies, detailed knowledge of biologic mechanisms, epidemiologic evidence, and angiographic studies. However, the most direct and convincing evidence that lowering cholesterol reduces CHD risk comes from clinical trials. The clinical trials of cholesterol lowering are conventionally categorized as primary prevention if performed in ostensibly healthy individuals and secondary prevention if performed in individuals with pre-existing clinical CHD. These distinctions are somewhat artificial in that many of the 'healthy' middle-aged and older healthy primary trial participants (and particularly those who developed clinical symptoms during the trial) had underlying coronary atherosclerosis at baseline, and conceptually the inferences drawn from the primary and secondary trials are rather similar. These kinds of trial evidence can best be regarded as being complementary to each other. Nevertheless, there is some merit in examining them separately, in that the CHD event rates are much higher in secondary prevention trials. The higher absolute risk of CHD in patients with existing coronary disease leads naturally to a more intensive therapeutic approach to elevated cholesterol in such patients, so there is some clinical relevance in evaluating secondary prevention trials separately.[1]

Methods

The trials included in this chapter have been selected because they influenced (whether positively or negatively) the acceptance of cholesterol lowering as a preventive treatment for CHD. Only randomized placebo-controlled trials with single interventions were considered. For uniformity, the differences between placebo and active treatments are expressed throughout as a percentage of

$$\text{Value on placebo} - \text{Value on active treatment}$$

Value on this method of calculation will, on occasion, yield results that differ slightly from the original report. Unless otherwise specified, statistical significance implies a two-sided P value of <0.05.

Primary Prevention Trials

The World Health Organization Cooperative Trial on Primary Prevention of Ischaemic Heart Disease Using Clofibrate to Lower Serum Cholesterol (WHO)[2-5]

The WHO trial was a monumental undertaking at the time it was launched in 1965, and even today it remains the largest published clinical trial of lipid lowering to prevent CHD. Three centers (Prague, Budapest, and Edinburgh) randomized 10 627 men aged 30–59 years in the upper third of the serum cholesterol distribution to receive clofibrate 1.6 g daily or placebo, and treated them for an average of 5.3 years. They also followed a third untreated group of 5118 controls in the lower third of the cholesterol distribution for outcomes, but these men will not be considered further, since they are not comparable to either the active treatment or the placebo treatment group.

The trial had a number of good design features. It had a large number of subjects and it was double-blind and randomized. Mortality outcome ascertainment was essentially complete. However, there were also deficiencies in the design and in the reporting of the results, which have complicated interpretation. The drug clofibrate did not lower serum cholesterol by the expected 15% (the actual fall relative to placebo was 8%), and this reduced the ability of the trial to test the cholesterol hypothesis. It is now recognized that the fibrate class of drugs is more effective at lowering triglycerides than at lowering serum cholesterol.

Secondly, and potentially more importantly, the design allowed for the withdrawal of participants for a variety of reasons, and these participants were excluded from the analyses of the in-trial treatment effect in the initial report[2] and in two subsequent follow-up reports.[3,4] These reports were essentially equivalent to on-treatment analyses rather than on intention-to-treat analyses. About 10% of study participants were withdrawn from treatment when they developed a variety of medical conditions, including nonfatal myocardial infarction (MI), hypertension, and diabetes, and another 24% withdrew from treatment for nonmedical reasons. Omission of clinical outcome data for the in-trial period for this large number of withdrawn participants has complicated the interpretation of the trial results. Participants who withdraw may have a higher rate of clinical events, and if there is differential withdrawal (either in overall number or cause for withdrawal) across treatment groups then the disease incidence may be biased in the groups being compared. For example, more participants in the fibrate group than in the placebo group withdrew because of the development of diabetes mellitus, and fewer withdrew because of nonfatal MI and hypertension.

However, the recent publication of in-trial intention-to-treat mortality data[5] have alleviated concerns that such biases had a major influence on the interpretation of the trial results for mortality, even though results for nonfatal events remain open to question. The potential for obtaining erroneous results is illustrated by the fact that the intention-to-treat analysis reported on a total of 417 deaths 'before closure', compared to only 210 'in-trial' deaths in the original publication.

Because of the design flaw referred to above, only on-treatment data are available for nonfatal MI and for combined nonfatal MI and CHD death. Clofibrate appeared to reduce the primary outcome of combined nonfatal MI and CHD death by a significant 20% (167 in the clofibrate and 208 in the placebo group, $P < 0.05$). All of the reduction was accounted for by nonfatal MI, which decreased by 25% (131 versus 174, $P < 0.05$). However, the original report also notes that there was an apparent excess of non-CHD mortality (especially from cancer and from conditions related to the liver, biliary, and intestinal systems), and an excess of all-cause mortality in the clofibrate group compared to the placebo group. The cholecystectomy rate was also higher in the clofibrate group. The authors speculated that the excess mortality in the clofibrate group may have been due to chance, to drug toxicity, or to the excretion of biliary sterols.

Two subsequent reports of mortality follow-up at a mean duration of 9.6 years[3] and 13.2 years[4] indicated that, combining the 'in-trial' and 'out-of-trial' data, there was a progressive decrease in the excess non-CHD mortality and total mortality, so that in the final mortality report these were no longer significant. This was because most of the excess mortality occurred in the 'in-trial' period, so that the longer the follow-up continued, the more the excess was diluted. The data are compatible with a toxic effect of clofibrate or of cholesterol lowering which does not persist after the end of treatment.

The clarification of the mortality data published in 1992 presented true intention-to-treat in-trial and post-trial data for the first time. During the in-trial period ('before closure' in the terminology used by the authors), there were 91 CHD deaths in the clofibrate group and 77 in the placebo group, a nonsignificant increase of 18%. There were 145 versus 104 non-CHD deaths, an excess of 39% in the clofibrate group, and a 30% excess of all-cause mortality (236 versus 181). The increases in non-CHD and all-cause mortality in the clofibrate group were less than those previously reported, but nevertheless remained significant. Among the non-CHD causes of excess death the major contributors were cancer (75 versus 55) and 'other medical' causes, including diseases of the liver, biliary system, and intestines (22 versus 6). As before, there was no significant excess mortality in the post-trial follow-up period.

Over the years since the WHO trial results were reported in 1978, they have played a significant role in raising the level of skepticism about the value of cholesterol lowering. The finding that CHD mortality was not lowered (in fact it increased somewhat), and that non-CHD mortality was increased, overshadowed the finding that nonfatal CHD was significantly decreased. Because of the ambiguous findings in the WHO trial, it was clear that further studies with improved designs and using different agents were needed.

Lipid Research Clinics Coronary Primary Prevention Trial (LRC-CPPT)[6,7]

The LRC-CPPT can be regarded as the first of the new generation of well-designed trials of primary prevention by cholesterol lowering. Procedures developed during the LRC program set the standard for subsequent cholesterol-lowering prevention studies. The LRC adhered to just about all the tenets of what a well-designed trial should be. It was double-blind and placebo controlled, outcomes were rigorously and completely ascertained, and the primary analysis was on an intention-to-treat basis. As part of a comprehensive quality-assurance program, a number of LRC-standardized lipid laboratories were set up. The trial did have some deficiencies in that it was somewhat underpowered because of unrealistic assumptions about adherence to study medication and the degree of lipid lowering that would be obtained. The statistical test for the primary outcome was a one-sided test ($P < 0.05$), rather than the more appropriate two-sided test. Like the WHO trial, its external validity was limited by the fact that only middle-aged men with high blood cholesterol were included; on the other hand, it did offer a test of a pure cholesterol-lowering agent rather than one which primarily lowered triglycerides.

This 12-center study randomized 3806 men aged 35–59 years who were free of CHD but at high risk because they had serum cholesterol levels $> 6.89 \text{ mmol l}^{-1}$ (the 95th percentile) and low-density lipoprotein (LDL) cholesterol levels $> 4.94 \text{ mmol l}^{-1}$. Men with triglycerides $> 3.3 \text{ mmol l}^{-1}$ were excluded, as were those with secondary hypercholesterolemia, or whose elevated LDL cholesterol levels responded to a prerandomization diet. The study

Side-effects were mainly limited to the gastrointestinal system. The number of gallstone operations was not significantly increased on gemfibrozil (18 versus 12), but the number of abdominal operations was (81 versus 53; $P < 0.02$).

The HSS results were published in 1987 and encouraged the use of gemfibrozil in patients with dyslipidemic syndromes, including those with elevated triglycerides and low HDL cholesterol levels. Riding on the coattails of the study, a number of other newer fibrates have also gained acceptance. One of the attractions of the fibrates was the apparent low incidence of unpleasant symptoms such as those associated with the resins and niacin. However, the HHS did not provide reassurance that fibrates were indeed safe. As in the WHO clofibrate trial, there was an excess of noncardiac deaths, although in this instance it was not significant. Also, the study did not resolve another issue raised by the WHO results, i.e. that fatal MI was not reduced. The subsequent results of a secondary prevention component of the HSS (in men screened out because they had prevalent CHD) have suggested that, if anything, gemfibrozil may increase rather than decrease the risk of fatal CHD.[11]

West of Scotland Coronary Prevention Study (WOSCOPS)[12]

WOSCOPS was the definitive trial of primary prevention in middle-aged men (35–64 years) with moderate high blood cholesterol. It established beyond reasonable doubt that cholesterol lowering with effective and safe drugs will reduce CHD incidence without incurring a penalty of increased noncardiac deaths or unacceptable side-effects. It is likely that the results will have a considerable effect on medical practice by increasing the prescription of lipid-lowering agents in men without CHD but with high serum cholesterol levels. The findings will likely be extrapolated to women, given the positive results for women in the secondary prevention Scandinavian Simvastatin Survival Study (4S).[13]

WOSCOPS was a randomized double-blind placebo-controlled trial of 6595 men followed for an average of 4.9 years. To be eligible, men had to be free of a history of MI and have no electrocardiographic evidence of previous MI; however, men with stable angina or other evidence of vascular disease were eligible (there were 1066 such men, forming 16% of the trial cohort). The Scottish men were a high-risk cohort; apart from the fact that 16% had some evidence of vascular disease, their mean body mass index was 26 kg m^{-2}, 3% reported diabetes, 15% reported being hypertensive, and 44% were current smokers. They had to have LDL cholesterol levels above 4.0 mmol l^{-1} on two occasions (with at least one level at or above 4.5 mmol l^{-1}) and at least one level at or below 6.0 mmol l^{-1}. The lipid eligibility criteria selected a group of men with moderate type IIA hyperlipoproteinemia (mean serum cholesterol 7.07 mmol l^{-1}, LDL cholesterol 4.99 mmol l^{-1}, HDL cholesterol 1.14 mmol l^{-1}, and triglycerides 1.80 mmol l^{-1}).

The study drug was a fixed dose of pravastatin 40 mg daily (a hydroxymethylglutaryl coenzyme A reductase inhibitor) or placebo. In participants who continued to receive pravastatin, the drug reduced serum cholesterol levels by 20%, LDL cholesterol by 26%, and triglycerides by 12%, and increased HDL cholesterol by 5%. By the end of the fourth year, 25% of both the pravastatin and the placebo group had stopped taking the study medications.

The primary outcome in WOSCOPS was combined definite nonfatal MI and death from CHD. There were 174/3302 (5.3%) events in the pravastatin men and 248/3293 (7.5%) events in the placebo group, a significant reduction of 30%. Cox proportional hazards model analyses yielded a relative risk estimate of 0.69 (95% confidence interval 0.57–0.83; $P < 0.001$). If definite and suspected coronary events were combined, there were 215

(6.5%) events in the pravastatin group and 295 (9.0%) events in the placebo group, a significant reduction of 27%. Deaths from definite and suspected CHD were significantly reduced, by 33% (41 versus 61). There were no increases in deaths from noncardiac causes; there was a total of 65 deaths from noncardiac causes in the pravastatin group versus 74 in the placebo group. There was no trend in cause-specific noncardiac deaths: strokes occurred in 9 versus 12, suicide and trauma in 5 versus 6, cancer in 44 versus 49, and all other causes were 7 in each arm. Even though the study was not designed to estimate the effect on all-cause mortality, because of the decrease in deaths from cardiac causes and the lack of effect on noncardiac deaths, deaths from all causes tended to decrease (106 or 3.2% versus 135 or 4.1%, an almost significant reduction of 22%; $P = 0.051$).

Nonfatal definite and suspected coronary events decreased by a significant 26% (182 versus 246), and coronary revascularization procedures decreased by a significant 36% (51 versus 80). There was little apparent effect on fatal plus nonfatal stroke (46 versus 51) or on incident cancer (116 versus 106).

Subgroup analyses indicated that the benefit for the primary outcome of definite nonfatal MI and CHD death was not dependent on initial serum cholesterol, LDL cholesterol, HDL cholesterol, or triglyceride level. Benefit was seen in men above or below age 55 years, in smokers and nonsmokers, in men without multiple risk factors, and in men without evidence of prior vascular disease.

Pravastatin appeared to be safe. As noted above there was no trend for an increase of noncardiac deaths or of incident cancers. Equal numbers of men reported myalgia (20 versus 19) and, although there was some increase in the number with asymptomatic elevations of creatine kinase (4 versus 1), alanine aminotransferase (26 versus 20), and aspartate aminotransferase (16 versus 12), these were not significant.

The finding that pravastatin reduced coronary disease incidence in men with and without evidence of prior vascular disease is important to the interpretation of WOSCOPS as a primary prevention trial. As can be expected, men with prior vascular disease had a considerably higher rate of coronary disease during the trial, and if benefit had been shown in this subgroup only the criticism could have been leveled that no efficacy of primary prevention had been shown. As it turned out, the risk reduction was approximately equal in men with and without prior vascular disease, and there was a sufficient number of events in men without vascular disease (125 pravastatin versus 183 placebo) for the reduction to be significant (by Cox proportional hazards model the relative risk was 0.67, 95% CI 0.54–0.85; $P < 0.001$).

Secondary Prevention Trials

The Newcastle and Edinburgh Trials of Clofibrate in the Treatment of Ischemic Heart Disease[14,15]

Both these secondary prevention trials were unusual in that they included patients with angina, and a small proportion of women. Participants were unselected with regard to lipid levels, except that in Newcastle those with serum cholesterol levels exceeding 400 mg dl^{-1} or with xanthomata were excluded. Participants were aged less than 65 years in Newcastle[14] and 40–69 years in Edinburgh.[15] Both trials were double-blind placebo-controlled studies of rather small size: there were 244 participants on clofibrate and 253 on placebo in the Newcastle trial, and 350 on clofibrate and 367 on placebo in the Edinburgh trial. The dose of clofibrate was 1.5–2.0 g per day, and the duration was 5 years in Newcastle and 6 years in Edinburgh.

The total cholesterol levels in Newcastle fell by 10% compared to controls, and in Edinburgh by 15%. In Newcastle there were significantly fewer nonfatal MI plus CHD deaths in the clofibrate compared to the placebo group (52 versus 81, a 33% decrease; $P < 0.01$). The reduction in CHD deaths (but not that in nonfatal MI) was significant. In Edinburgh the 21% reduction in combined nonfatal MI and CHD death was not significant (54 versus 72). In both studies the subgroups who had angina at entry had significantly fewer sudden deaths on treatment than the controls, and there were more such patients in Newcastle than in Edinburgh, possibly accounting for the more favorable results in regard to all CHD events in the Newcastle trial.

The reports of these early studies created some interest at the time of their publication, because both concluded that the beneficial effects in regard to MI were relatively independent of the initial level of cholesterol and of the response to treatment. If true, this would suggest a nonlipid mode of action for clofibrate. However, these studies were far too small to allow for meaningful conclusions to be drawn from such subgroup analyses, so that they could not adequately test this hypothesis. In the subsequently reported and much larger WHO clofibrate primary prevention trial, benefit was more marked in those with highest levels of serum cholesterol at baseline and in those who had the greatest fall on treatment.

The Coronary Drug Project (CDP)[16,17]

The CDP belongs to the same era as the WHO primary prevention trial, and commenced recruitment in 1966. The major results were reported in 1975.[16] As in the WHO trial, the trial design had many good features in that it was large (but not large enough for the primary outcome of all-cause mortality), randomized, double-blind, and placebo-controlled. In retrospect, it can be said that the main problem that the CDP suffered from is that, at the time, there were no really good choices of lipid-lowering drugs available. Of the drugs tested in the CDP (estrogen, dextrothyroxine, clofibrate, and niacin), only clofibrate and niacin were ever used in practice to any degree, and even these have been superseded by newer drugs. The CDP can also be faulted for initially reporting mortality results based on death certificates received from the investigators, rather than awaiting the more reliable determination of cause-specific mortality from its mortality classification committee. The subsequent report of the long-term mortality follow-up published in 1986 also had revised data on cause-specific in-trial mortality.[17] A small number of additional deaths were reported, but the important difference was that the causes of death were frequently reassigned. The main consequence was that, whereas there was a significant excess of non-CHD mortality for the clofibrate treatment group in the original report, this was no longer the case. Conversely, a previously missed excess of stroke in the clofibrate group was now apparent. The deaths discussed here are from the second report.[17]

Men aged 30–64 years ($N = 8341$) with at least one electrocardiographically documented previous MI were recruited in 53 centers.[16] They were unselected with regard to serum cholesterol level. Originally, they were randomized into five treatment groups and a placebo group; the allocation schedule was designed to ensure approximately five patients in the placebo group for every two in any other group. The statistical significance level was adjusted upwards to compensate for the fact that five drug–placebo comparisons were to be undertaken. The two estrogen groups and the dextrothyroxine group were discontinued early in the trial because of an unacceptably high incidence of toxic effects. The clofibrate and niacin active-treatment groups completed the planned 6.2 years of treatment and follow-up. The primary outcome of the study was total mortality.

Clofibrate was given at a total daily dose of 1.8 g to 1103 men. Compared to the 2789 men in the placebo group, clofibrate reduced total cholesterol by 6% and triglycerides by 22%. Combined definite nonfatal MI and CHD deaths decreased by 7% (309 or 28% in the clofibrate group versus 839 or 30% in the placebo group; not significant). Neither nonfatal MI (144 or 13.1% versus 386 or 13.8%) or CHD death (240 or 21.7% versus 632 or 22.6%) were decreased significantly. All-cause mortality was unchanged (288 on clofibrate and 723 on placebo, 26% in each case). Non-CHD deaths occurred in 42 (3.8%) of the clofibrate group compared with 86 (3.1%) in the placebo group. Among the non-CHD deaths there was a marginally significant excess of cerebrovascular deaths (14 or 1.3% versus 14 or 0.5%, $P < 0.05$). Overall, this large and well-conducted study failed to provide evidence in favor of using clofibrate in unselected patients with CHD, perhaps because of the modest decrease in serum cholesterol obtained.

Niacin was given to 1119 patients in a total daily dose of 3 g. The niacin-treated subjects experienced net decreases (compared to the 2789 men on placebo) of 10% in total cholesterol and 26% in triglycerides. At the end of 6 years the combined nonfatal MI and CHD death had decreased by 15% (287 or 25.6% on niacin versus 839 or 30.1% on placebo; $P < 0.05$). The decrease in nonfatal MI was significant (114 or 10.2% versus 386 or 13.8%), while that in fatal MI (238 or 21.3% versus 632 or 22.7%) was not. Other cardiovascular endpoints also tended to decrease, significantly so for stroke and new angina, except that there was a significant excess of cardiac arrhythmias. During the trial non-CHD deaths occurred in 39 (3.5%) of the niacin group versus 86 (3.1%) of the placebo group. All-cause mortality was similar during the 6-year in-trial period (277 or 24.7% versus 723 or 25.9%), but during a post-trial follow-up of a further 9 years the 11% decrease in mortality became statistically significant.[17]

Thus, the results of the CDP niacin group suggested somewhat more benefit for niacin than for clofibrate, and less indication of potential toxic effects. However, the results were not so striking that they had any great influence on the practice of preventive cardiology; in fact they were more frequently used to make the case that, while nonfatal MI may be reduced by cholesterol lowering, fatal CHD is not. The results for estrogen did bring an end to hopes that this might be an acceptable treatment for men, and may have held up trials of estrogen for the prevention of CHD in women. After the CDP, dextrothyroxine disappeared as a viable treatment for high blood cholesterol.

The Stockholm Ischemic Heart Disease Secondary Prevention Study[18]

This trial was a small, randomized comparison of a combination of clofibrate (2 g daily) plus niacin (3 g daily) with no treatment in consecutive survivors of MI below 70 years of age. There were 279 participants in the active-treatment group and 279 in the control group. One-fifth of subjects were women, but these were not analyzed separately. The treatment period was 5 years.

The net decrease in total cholesterol was 13% in the actively treated group, while serum triglycerides declined by 19%. Nonfatal MI plus CHD death decreased by 28% (72 in the treated group versus 100 in the control group; $P < 0.05$). The reduction in CHD death was significant, while that in nonfatal MI was not. Unique among the early trials, in-trial all-cause mortality was also significantly lower in the treated group (61 versus 82; $P < 0.05$). Subgroup analyses seemed to indicate that individuals who had elevated triglycerides, and those who showed the greatest decline in triglycerides, had the greatest reductions in MI. No such relationships were noted for total cholesterol. The findings might suggest that the role of triglycerides in the etiology of MI needs to be reassessed, and the results of the

Helsinki primary prevention trial offer some support that lowering triglycerides may be beneficial. While provocative, the subgroup analyses are not sufficient to make the case, owing to the small numbers in each of the subgroups. Subgroup analyses that are not prespecified in the protocol are always suspect, since a number will be significant by chance alone.

The Program on the Surgical Control of the Hyperlipidemias (POSCH)[19-21]

This was a randomized single-blind clinical outcome trial (the primary endpoint was total mortality) with some unique characteristics.[19] The intervention was partial ileal bypass, which is the surgical equivalent of administering a bile acid binding resin with near-complete compliance. The duration of intervention was long, almost 10 years. Finally, POSCH also recorded the angiographic appearance of the coronary vessels at intervals, and therefore provides an opportunity to compare directly angiographic and clinical responses to treatments. POSCH documented that angiographic change was highly predictive of subsequent clinical CHD events.[20]

The trial was fairly large, although not large enough for the primary outcome of all-cause mortality. There were 421 patients (90% men) aged 30–64 years in the surgery group and 417 in the control group. Baseline serum cholesterol levels were 6.49 mmol l^{-1}, LDL cholesterol was 4.62 mmol l^{-1}, HDL cholesterol 1.05 mmol l^{-1}, and triglycerides 2.30 mmol l^{-1}. The mean net reduction in serum cholesterol was 23%, and that in LDL cholesterol was 38%. HDL cholesterol and triglycerides increased by 4% and 20%, respectively. Although the 28% reduction in CHD deaths (33 versus 47) was not significant, the 35% reduction in combined nonfatal MI plus CHD death was highly significant (82 or 19.5% in the surgery group versus 125 or 30% in controls; $P < 0.001$). The incidences of coronary revascularization, unstable angina, and peripheral vascular disease were also significantly reduced. Non-CHD mortality was not affected by the intervention (16 versus 15). All-cause mortality was decreased (49 versus 62), but this was not significant. Because the active treatment is permanent, further follow-up of the trial cohort is of particular interest, and the result for total mortality has become marginally significant.[21]

Published in 1990, POSCH offered the most convincing evidence up to that time that lowering serum cholesterol in patients with CHD would decrease their reinfarction rate. The POSCH results contributed largely to the favorable results for secondary prevention observed in analyses of pooled data. The actual treatment modality used in POSCH (partial ileal bypass) has never found wide application. In 1975, when POSCH was launched, there were no really effective lipid-lowering drugs available, but since then the hydroxymethylglutaryl coenzyme A reductase inhibitors alone or in combination with bile acid binding resins have superseded surgical approaches for the treatment of the vast majority of patients with high blood cholesterol.

Scandinavian Simvastatin Survival Study (4S)[13]

Published in 1994, the 4S study is the definitive secondary prevention trial of cholesterol lowering to prevent coronary disease. Like POSCH, the primary outcome was total mortality, but unlike POSCH, the 4S trial could prove that cholesterol lowering would in fact reduce total mortality. The two studies showed similar percentage changes in serum cholesterol, MI, and mortality, but because of a larger sample size (and correspondingly larger numbers of clinical events) the results in the 4S trial were more precise, and therefore statistically significant.

To qualify for inclusion, patients had to have had a documented MI more than 6 months previously or a history of stable angina pectoris with documentation of coronary atherosclerosis. They also had to have serum cholesterol levels of 5.5–8.0 mmol l^{-1} after 8 weeks on a lipid-lowering diet. Patients with hypertriglyceridemia were excluded, and therefore the study population comprised men and women aged 35–69 years (mean age: men 58 years; women 61 years) with CHD and moderate type IIA hyperlipidemia (average serum cholesterol 6.75 mmol l^{-1}, LDL cholesterol 4.87 mmol l^{-1}, HDL cholesterol 1.19 mmol l^{-1}, and triglycerides 1.51 mmol l^{-1}). Patients with cardiac failure or with arrhythmias were excluded because they were at high risk of dying before the effects of lipid lowering could begin to be manifest. The patients frequently had other risk factors: 26% reported hypertension, 6% reported diabetes, and 26% were smokers. With regard to concomitant therapy: 37% were on aspirin, 57% were on beta-blockers, 31% were on calcium antagonists, and 32% were on nitrates.

This was a multicenter, double-blind, randomized, placebo-controlled trial of the hydroxymethylglutaryl coenzyme A reductase inhibitor simvastatin. The initial dose of simvastatin was 20 mg daily, but in accordance with the protocol this dose was doubled to 40 mg daily in 37% of patients who did not achieve the target serum cholesterol of <5.2 mmol l^{-1} in the first 6 months. Only two patients had to have their simvastatin dose lowered to 10 mg daily because their cholesterol levels fell below the floor level of 3 mmol l^{-1}. Thirteen percent of patients in the placebo group and 10% in the simvastatin group stopped taking the tablets during the study period. The study was designed to detect a 30% reduction in total mortality. The design called for 4000 patients to be followed for at least 3 years, and about 440 deaths had occurred. The 94 centers eventually randomized 4444 patients and follow-up was extended to a median 5.4 years, by which time 438 deaths had occurred. The extended follow-up was needed because event rates were somewhat lower than originally predicted. The ascertainment of vital status (alive or dead at the end of the study) was complete.

The results of the study were very close to those predicted during the planning phase. Compared to placebo, in the simvastatin group serum total and LDL levels dropped by 26% and 36% respectively, HDL cholesterol rose by 7%, and triglycerides dropped by 17%. Total mortality decreased by 29% (182/2221 or 8.2% in the simvastatin group compared to 256/2223 or 11.5% in the placebo group). Cox proportional hazards model estimates yielded a relative risk of 0.70 (95% CI 0.58–0.85, $P = 0.0003$). The reduction in mortality was accounted for entirely by a 41% reduction in coronary deaths (111 or 5% in the simvastatin group, 189 or 8.5% in the placebo group). The relative risk estimate for coronary death was 0.58 (95% CI 0.46–0.73). There were no significant differences in noncoronary deaths (71 simvastatin versus 69 placebo), including no differences in cerebrovascular deaths (14 versus 12), violent deaths (6 versus 7), or cancer (33 versus 35).

The results were also encouraging for the secondary endpoint of any major coronary event (coronary death, nonfatal definite or probable MI, silent MI, and resuscitated cardiac arrest). There were 431 (19%) major coronary events in the simvastatin group and 622 (28%) in the placebo group, a significant reduction of 31%. Nonfatal definite or probable MI was reduced (279 or 12.6% simvastatin versus 418 or 18.8% placebo, a significant reduction of 33%), as was silent MI (88 versus 110, a significant reduction of 20%), and coronary surgery or angioplasty (252 versus 383, a significant reduction of 34%). Non-MI acute CHD events (e.g. unstable angina) were not significantly reduced (295 versus 331), but fatal plus nonfatal cerebrovascular events were (70 versus 98, a significant 29% reduction).

Subgroup analyses indicated that benefit for any major coronary event extended to women (59/407 or 14.5% on simvastatin versus 91/420 or 21.7% on placebo, a significant 33% reduction) and to older patients. Patients aged 60 years and older had a significant 26% reduction in major coronary events (243/1156 or 21% on simvastatin versus 319/1126 or 28.3% on placebo), even though the magnitude was smaller than the 36% reduction in patients younger than 60 (188/1065 or 17.6% versus 303/1097 or 27.6%). Older patients also had a significant 26% reduction in deaths (127 versus 167), this again being somewhat smaller than the 36% reduction for younger patients (55 versus 89). There was no observed reduction in deaths for women (27 versus 25), but there were too few deaths in women to draw any firm conclusions. Another important subgroup observation was that major coronary events decreased equally in patients on aspirin or on beta-blockers, as well as in those not receiving these medications. This suggests that the benefit of lipid lowering may be additive to the benefit from these agents.

Simvastatin appeared to be very safe. Only 6% of patients in either the simvastatin or placebo groups discontinued the study drug because of adverse events. As noted above, there were no excess cancer deaths. The incidence of nonfatal cancers was also similar (57 on simvastatin versus 61 on placebo). There was only one case of reversible rhabdomyolysis on simvastatin. Increases in creatine kinase were rare (6 versus 1), and increases in aspartate aminotransferase (20 versus 23) or alanine aminotransferase (49 versus 33) were unusual and did not necessitate discontinuation of the study drug.

The most important contribution of the 4S trial is the demonstration that lipid lowering reduces total mortality in patients with CHD. Secondary prevention with a highly effective cholesterol-lowering agent reduced the burden of recurrent coronary disease. Because most of the deaths in patients with existing coronary disease are due to recurrent coronary disease (77% of deaths in the 4S placebo group), and because there was no increase in noncoronary deaths, the overall mortality was also reduced. The only other secondary prevention trial that has shown a significant reduction in total mortality during the in-trial period was the small Stockholm trial of clofibrate and niacin, where the finding could well have been a chance occurrence. The niacin arm of the CDP showed a significant reduction in mortality during the follow-up period, but not during the in-trial period.

The 4S trial validates the recommendations of the European Atherosclerosis Society (EAS)[22] and the National Cholesterol Education Program (NCEP)[23] that high blood cholesterol in patients with existing coronary disease should be treated aggressively. Those recommendations were based on the high risk for recurrent disease, on the projected benefit from meta-analyses combining results of previous secondary prevention trials, and on the favorable effects of aggressive lipid lowering on the angiographic appearance of coronary arteries. Now that benefit has been confirmed, and it has been demonstrated that this class of agents is safe, lipid lowering should take its rightful place on a par with and in addition to low-dose aspirin and beta-blockers as a standard treatment of coronary disease.

One area the 4S trial did not address is whether the benefit will be present also in patients with less severe degrees of high blood cholesterol. The entry criteria for the 4S trial excluded patients who had serum cholesterol levels below 5.5 mmol l^{-1}. However, many patients with coronary disease have levels lower than 5.5 mmol l^{-1}. Will they benefit to the same extent as those with higher levels? The angiographic studies have provided conflicting results; the Harvard Atherosclerosis Reversibility Project (HARP)[24] suggested that they will not benefit, while the larger Regression Growth Evaluation Statin Study (REGRESS)[25] suggested that they will. The Cholesterol and Recurrent Events (CARE)[26] trial of CHD patients without elevated cholesterol levels was due to report results on clinical CHD outcomes in 1996. Analyses within the 4S cohort indicate that benefit is obtained irrespective of the quintile of the cholesterol level in the range 5.5–8.0 mmol l^{-1} at baseline, and it seems reasonable to extrapolate benefit to both higher and lower levels.[27] The 4S results also provide reassurance that lowering cholesterol in older persons and in women with CHD is beneficial.

Discussion and Conclusions

The idea that lowering serum cholesterol will reduce CHD is an old one. Until recently it has also been a controversial one. It has taken almost 30 years and almost 40 clinical trials to settle the controversy. We now know that lowering serum cholesterol is beneficial. We know that CHD, both fatal and nonfatal, is reduced. We know that total mortality is reduced, and we know that cholesterol lowering is safe. Why has it taken so long? In part it was because the early trials were too small or were confounded by the use of drugs that were either ineffective (clofibrate), or toxic (estrogens, dextrothyroxine), or both (clofibrate). Other drugs used in the earlier trials may have been effective if only patients could have been persuaded to take them (niacin, bile acid binding resins). Because of the general apparent lack of success in these earlier trials and the toxic effects of some of the drugs, the hypothesis became a favored target of skeptics.

The skepticism began to give way in the 1990s. Secondary prevention was the first to turn the corner and gain wide acceptance. The POSCH results, the pooled analyses of the secondary prevention trials, and angiographic trials were persuasive. Guidelines to physicians were modified to emphasize the benefits of cholesterol lowering in those with existing CHD.[22,23] Such patients have a very high rate of reinfarction (3–5% per year), and more than half of the MI events in secondary prevention trials were fatal, compared to about one-quarter of the MI events in primary prevention trials. Because CHD accounts for more than three-quarters of all deaths in patients with existing CHD, there was also a trend towards a reduction for all-cause mortality. Finally, in 1994 it was shown that the reduction in all-cause mortality was significant when an effective drug (simvastatin) was used in a sufficiently large trial (4S).

Primary prevention had to wait until 1995 before the benefit could be said to be incontrovertible. WOSCOPS, again using a highly effective drug (pravastatin) in a sufficiently large study cohort, demonstrated that not only nonfatal MI, but also CHD death, and very likely all-cause mortality, would be reduced by lipid lowering. Prior to that, the primary prevention trials were particularly confounded by the ineffective and/or toxic drugs available. While all the large primary prevention trials (WHO, LRC-CPPT, and HSS) could point to some benefit for CHD, there was no indication of any benefit for all-cause mortality. The effect on CHD mortality was small, and in all these earlier trials there was some excess of non-CHD mortality (significant in the case of WHO); given that non-CHD mortality accounted for more than half the deaths, there was no decrease in, or even an increase in, all-cause mortality. A selective meta-analysis of the primary prevention trials indicated that the excess non-CHD mortality in primary prevention trials was significant and mainly due to deaths from accidents and violence.[28] It was suggested that lowering cholesterol was somehow toxic.

The lack of benefit for all-cause mortality and the suggestion that lowering cholesterol was dangerous led to a questioning of primary prevention. For a long time the debate ignored two factors: first, that there was a logical inconsistency in postulating an increased non-CHD mortality in primary prevention but not in secondary prevention (since rates of non-CHD mortality are approximately the same in both situations); and, secondly, that any increase in non-CHD mortality may not be due to cholesterol lowering itself, but rather to the drugs used to obtain the cholesterol lowering. A meta-analysis that examined these specific issues predicted that cholesterol lowering itself would not increase non-CHD mortality in either primary or secondary prevention, but that certain drugs would (estrogen, dextrothyroxine, and fibrates).[29] Conversely, if a drug that was effective and safe were used, it could be anticipated that CHD mortality would decrease, non-CHD mortality be unaffected, and all-cause mortality would decrease. The hydroxymethylglutaryl coenzyme A inhibitors appear to fit this profile, as shown by the WOSCOPS and 4S results. Use of a class of drugs that apparently does not have severe intrinsic toxic effects allowed for a demonstration that cholesterol lowering itself is beneficial, reducing CHD mortality and all-cause mortality without any indication of adverse trends in non-CHD mortality. One caveat is that, while the recent trials had adequate statistical power to address CHD mortality (and all-cause mortality in the case of 4S), they did not have sufficient power to address non-CHD mortality specifically. It is unlikely that any single trial can be done that will address non-CHD mortality, because the sample size would need to be very large indeed. In order to overcome the sample-size constraints of individual trials, a prospective meta-analysis of all current and planned lipid-lowering trials has been initiated.[30]

If cholesterol lowering with modern drugs is effective for reducing CHD and all-cause mortality, questions of cost-effectiveness still remain to be answered. These drugs are expensive, and potentially have to be used for life in order to reduce CHD. While it is not the purpose of this chapter to address cost-effectiveness, it is somewhat interesting to look at the relative utility of cholesterol lowering in primary and secondary prevention, using data from WOSCOPS and 4S (*Table 6.1*). From an examination of the absolute reductions in events, the number of patients who would have to be treated for approximately 5 years to prevent one event can be calculated. The numbers look very favorable for secondary prevention: only 12 patients would need to be treated to prevent one major CHD event (nonfatal MI or CHD death). In addition, one revascularization procedure would be avoided for every 17 patients treated. When compared to other standard therapies (e.g. drug treatment of hypertension) the numbers for primary prevention of patients at high

Table 6.1 Absolute risk reduction attributable to treatment and the number of patients that must be treated to prevent one event

	No. of events per 100 patients over approx. 5 years			No. treated to prevent one event (100/number prevented)
	Placebo	Active	Prevented	
Primary prevention (WOSCOPS)				
Death from any cause	4.10	3.21	0.89	112
CHD death	1.85	1.24	0.61	164
Nonfatal MI	7.47	5.51	1.96	51
Nonfatal MI or CHD death	8.96	6.51	2.54	41
CABG or PTCA	2.43	1.54	0.89	112
Secondary prevention (4S)				
Death from any cause	11.52	8.19	3.33	30
CHD death	8.50	5.00	3.50	29
Nonfatal MI	18.80	12.56	6.24	16
Nonfatal MI or CHD death	27.98	19.41	8.57	12
CABG or PTCA	17.23	11.35	5.88	17

CABG, coronary artery bypass graft; PTCA, percutaneous transluminal coronary angioplasty.

risk also look quite favorable: for every 41 patients treated one major CHD event would be avoided, and in addition treating 112 patients would avoid one revascularization procedure.

Now that the questions of the efficacy and safety of lipid-lowering therapy have been resolved, the question of cost-effectiveness will become paramount. From these calculations, the preliminary indications are that cholesterol lowering is likely to be very cost-effective in secondary prevention, and moderately cost-effective in high-risk primary prevention.

References

1. Rossouw JE, Lewis B, Rifkind BM. The value of lowering cholesterol after myocardial infarction. *N Engl J Med* 1990; **323**: 1112–19.
2. Committee of Principal Investigators. A cooperative trial in the primary prevention of ischaemic heart disease using clofibrate. *Br Heart J* 1978; **401**: 1–118.
3. Committee of Principal Investigators. WHO cooperative trial on primary prevention of ischaemic heart disease with clofibrate to lower serum cholesterol: mortality follow-up. *Lancet* 1980; **ii**: 379–85.
4. Committee of Principal Investigators. WHO cooperative trial on primary prevention of ischaemic heart disease with clofibrate to lower serum cholesterol: final mortality follow-up. *Lancet* 1984; **ii**: 600–4.
5. Heady JA, Morris JN, Oliver MF. WHO clofibrate/cholesterol trial: clarifications. *Lancet* 1992; **340**: 1405–6.
6. Lipid Research Clinics Program. The Lipid Research Clinics Coronary Primary Prevention Trial results. I. Reduction in incidence of coronary heart disease. *JAMA* 1984; **251**: 351–64.
7. Lipid Research Clinics Program. The Lipid Research Clinics Coronary Primary Prevention Trial results. II. The relationship of reduction in incidence of coronary heart disease to cholesterol lowering. *JAMA* 1984; **251**: 365–74.
8. Frick MH, Elo O, Haapa K, *et al*. Helsinki Heart Study: primary-prevention trial with gemfibrozil in middle-aged men with dyslipidemia. Safety of treatment, changes in risk factors, and incidence of coronary heart disease. *N Engl J Med* 1987; **317**: 1237–45.
9. Manninen V, Elo O, Frick MH, *et al*. Lipid alterations and decline in the incidence of coronary heart disease in the Helsinki Heart Study. *JAMA* 1988; **260**: 641–51.
10. Manninen V, Tenkanen L, Koskinen P, *et al*. Joint effects of serum triglyceride and LDL cholesterol and HDL cholesterol concentrations on coronary heart disease risk in the Helsinki Heart Study. *Circulation* 1992; **85**: 37–45.
11. Frick MH, Heinonen OP, Huttunen JK, Koskinen P, Manttari M, Manninen V. Efficacy of gemfibrozil in dyslipidaemic subjects with suspected heart disease: an ancillary study of the Helsinki Heart Study frame population. *Ann Intern Med* 1993; **25**: 41–4.
12. Shepherd J, Cobbe SM, Ford I, *et al*., for the West of Scotland Coronary Prevention Study Group. Prevention of coronary heart disease with pravastatin in men with hypercholesterolemia. *N Engl J Med* 1995; **333**: 1301–7.
13. Scandinavian Simvastatin Survival Study Group. Randomized trial of cholesterol lowering in 4444 patients with coronary heart disease: the Scandinavian Simvastatin Survival Study (4S). *N Engl J Med* 1994; **344**: 1383–9.
14. Group of Physicians of the Newcastle upon Tyne Region. Trial of clofibrate in the treatment of ischaemic heart disease. *Br Med J* 1971; **4**: 767–75.
15. Research Committee of the Scottish Society of physicians. Ischaemic heart disease: a secondary prevention trial using clofibrate. *Br Med J* 1971; **4**: 775–84.
16. Carlson LA, Rosenhammer G. Reduction in mortality in the Stockholm Ischaemic Heart Disease Secondary Prevention Study by combined treatment with clofibrate and nicotinic acid. *Acta Med Scand* 1988; **223**: 405–18.
17. Coronary Drug Project Research Group. Clofibrate and niacin in coronary heart disease. *JAMA* 1975; **231**: 360–81.
18. Canner PL, Berge KH, Wenger NK, *et al*. Fifteen year mortality in Coronary Drug Project patients: long-term benefit with niacin. *J Am Coll Cardiol* 1986; **8**: 1245–55.
19. Buchwald H, Varco RL, Matts JF, *et al*. Effect of partial ileal bypass surgery on mortality and morbidity from coronary artery disease in patients with hypercholesterolemia. *N Engl J Med* 1990; **323**: 946–55.
20. Buchwald H, Matts JP, Fitch LL, *et al*., for the Program on the Surgical Control of the Hyperlipidemias (POSCH) Group. Changes in sequential coronary arteriograms and subsequent coronary event. *JAMA* 1992; **268**: 1429–33.
21. Matts JP, Buchwald H, Fitch LL *et al*. Subgroup analyses of the major clinical endpoints in the Program on the Surgical Control of the Hyperlipidemias (POSCH): overall mortality, atherosclerotic coronary heart disease (ACHD) mortality, and ACHD mortality or myocardial infarction. *J Clin Epidemiol* 1995; **48**: 389–405.
22. European Atherosclerosis Society. Prevention of coronary heart disease: scientific background and new clinical guidelines. *Nutr Metab Cardiovasc Dis* 1992; **2**: 113–56.
23. Expert Panel. Summary of the Second Report of the National Cholesterol Education Program (NCEP) Expert Panel on Detection, Evaluation, and Treatment of High Blood Cholesterol in Adults (Adult Treatment Panel II). *JAMA* 1993; **269**: 3015–23.
24. Sacks FM, Pasternak RC, Gibson CM, Rosner B, Stone PH, for the Harvard Athererosclerosis Reversibility Project

(HARP). Effect on coronary atherosclerosis of decrease in plasma cholesterol concentrations in normocholesterolemic patients. *Lancet* 1994; **344**: 1182–6.

25. Jukema JW, Bruscke AVG, van Boven AJ, *et al.*, on behalf of the REGRESS study group. Effects of lipid lowering by pravastatin on progression and regression of coronary artery disease in symptomatic men with normal to moderately elevated serum cholesterol levels. The Regression Growth Evaluation Statin Study (REGRESS). *Circulation* 1995; **91**: 2528–40.

26. Sacks FM, Pfeffer MA, Moyle L, *et al.* Rationale and design of a secondary prevention trial of lowering normal plasma cholesterol levels after acute myocardial infarction: the Cholesterol and Recurrent Events Trial (CARE). *Am J Cardiol* 1991; **68**: 1436–46.

27. Scandinavian Simvastatin Survival Group. Baseline serum cholesterol and treatment effect in the Scandinavian Simvastatin Survival Study (4S). *Lancet* 1995; **345**: 1274–5.

28. Muldoon MF, Manuck SB, Matthews KA. Lowering cholesterol concentrations and mortality. A quantitative review of primary prevention trials. *Br Med J* 1990; **301**: 309–14.

29. Gould AL, Rossouw JE, Santanello NC, Heyse JF, Furberg CD. Cholesterol reduction yields clinical benefit. A new look at old data. *Circulation* 1995; **91**: 2274–82.

30. Cholesterol Treatment Trialists' (CTT) Collaboration. Protocol for a prospective collaborative overview of all current and planned randomized trials of cholesterol treatment regimens. *Am J Cardiol* 1995; **75**: 1130–4.

7

Dietary Fat Intake

Michael F. Oliver

Introduction

Most national and international recommendations[1–3] for the prevention of coronary heart disease (CHD), whether for primary prevention or for patients who have already developed clinical manifestations of CHD, have made dietary restriction of total and saturated fats the first advice and often the *sine qua non* in relation to all other forms of management. Yet trial evidence provides little support for such a policy.

Of course, it can be argued that it is virtually impossible to design and conduct an adequate dietary trial. The alteration of one dietary ingredient invariably leads to a change in another or other changes in lifestyle, and it is often impossible to assume that the effects of a prescribed dietary change on any endpoint are solely related to that which is under test. In addition, compliance over many years by large population samples to dietary advice is poor. 'Blinding' of a diet can seldom be achieved, and this leads to a confounding factor in the control population, usually recruited from the same geographic area, which may be so serious that the conduct of the study is irrevocably flawed. While these problems may be overcome by the random use of food supplements, such as antioxidant vitamins, good dietary trials not involving supplements are few. Thus the national recommendation and policies regarding the optimum diet for preventing CHD are based more on the numerous epidemiological surveys, which have amply confirmed the seminal observation of Keys in the Seven Countries Study[4] that there is a positive correlation between the intake of dietary fat and CHD; although a recent cohort study has demonstrated that this is not independent of fiber intake.[5]

It is now tacitly assumed that a reduction of total fat, especially saturated fat, in the diet will lead to less CHD. But no large long-term trial of the effect of reducing total and saturated fat on the primary prevention of CHD has ever been conducted. In reality, only those trials with some other concurrent intervention, such as a reduction of cigarette smoking, or those in which the quality of dietary fat was altered, have made any impact on the incidence of CHD. Such trials that have been conducted on reducing total and saturated fats alone, or with restriction of dietary cholesterol, either in primary or secondary prevention, have not led to lower CHD. In short, the many projected estimates, using simulated models of the effects of dietary restriction, of what (or will, in the minds of some) be achieved by reducing CHD risk through dietary measures have not been confirmed by formal long-term clinical trials.

Background and Questions

The data incriminating raised concentrations of plasma low-density lipoproteins (LDL) as an important pathogenic factor in the development of atherosclerosis, and hence CHD, are overwhelming. They are derived from: extensive evidence that induction of atherosclerosis occurs in experimental animals as a result of raising plasma LDL; the powerful relationship in man between raised LDL in familial hypercholesterolemia, both homozygote and heterozygote varieties, with coronary atherosclerosis and premature CHD; the moderately strong epidemiological relationship between raised LDL in communities with a high incidence of CHD in contrast to those with a low incidence; and the fact that in individuals raised LDL increases the relative risk of CHD.

None of these facts are any longer arguable, but the relations of different dietary fats to the mechanisms through which plasma LDL concentrations lead to atheroma are far from clear.[6] As we shall see, a biologically significant reduction of plasma LDL is difficult to achieve through dietary means, and lower plasma LDL concentrations *alone* will not necessarily lead to less atheroma. We need to understand the precise mechanisms through which oxidized LDL is taken up by monocyte-macrophages,[6,7] how LDL/macrophages interact with endothelial functions and the role of cytokines in these interactions, how and why LDL oxidation occurs and to what extent unstable long-chain polyunsaturated fatty acids (which are liable to undergo peroxidation) may be involved, and whether local antioxident forces are relevant.

Furthermore, we do not understand how high concentrations of high-density lipoproteins (HDLs) protect against CHD and the factors influencing 'reverse cholesterol transport',[8,9] or the mechanisms through which cholesterol leaves the arterial wall. We know even less about dietary factors that favor removal of deposited lipid.

Trials of Reducing Dietary Saturated Fat and Altering CHD Risk in High-risk People

There have been six trials designed to prevent the development of CHD by various dietary regimens in high-risk but otherwise healthy people. They have comprised a reduction of total and saturated fat intake in conjunction with additional advice regarding cigarette smoking, management of blood pressure, and increasing exercise[10–15] (*Table 7.1*). Most of these trials showed no significant reduction in either all-cause or CHD mortality. There are, however, two exceptions.

The first exception is the 6-year Helsinki Mental Hospital Study,[10] a trial of complex design conducted in mental institutions, in which exact control of the ingested diet was possible because of the institutional environment, and the dietary regimens given to the test and control populations remained separate as they were inmates in different institutions. A crossover design was used, such that the mental hospital which initially gave the test diet for the first 6 years then gave the control diet for the next 6 years. However, unfortunately, the inmates of these hospitals changed over the 12 years of study, with at least 33% being different. However, a polyunsaturated/saturated fatty acid (P/S) ratio of about 1.5 was achieved and, as a measure of compliance, adipose linoleic acid increased by more than three times (to 33%) in the treated group compared with the control group. The greatest benefit was the reduction of major coronary events ($P < 0.001$), rather than coronary deaths.

The other exception is a Norwegian study[11] which requires special comment not only because it was the only trial which showed a significant reduction in CHD events ($P <$

Table 7.1 Six primary prevention trials of low fat, low cholesterol diets and risk-factor changes

Trial	No. (diet/control)	Age range (years)	Follow-up (years)	Serum cholesterol Baseline (mmol l^{-1})	Serum cholesterol Difference[a] (%)	Odds ratio Death	Odds ratio CHD
Helsinki Mental Hospital[b10]	300/309	34–64	4	6.8	16	?	0.61*
Hjermann et al.[c11]	604/628	40–49	6–7	7.5–9.8	13	0.69	0.55*
MRFIT[12]	6428/6438	35–57	6–8	6.5	2	1.02	0.99
WHO factories[13]	24 615/25 169	40–59	5–6	5.8	4	1.11	1.05
Frantz et al.[14]	4922/4853	All	5	5.3	14	1.03	1.02
Strandberg et al.[15]	612/610	40–55	5 (+10)	7.0	6	1.45	2.42**

*$P = 0.028$; **$P = 0.01$.
[a]Difference between mean serum cholesterol in the diet and control groups at the end of the trial.
[b]An institutional trial with polyunsaturated/saturated fatty acid ratios of 1.4–1.55.
[c]Also a trial of reducing cigarette smoking: $P = 0.028$.

0.05) and a favorable trend in CHD mortality (*Table 7.1*), but also because it was not solely a dietary trial. It was established in hypercholesterolemic men and included more high-risk men than did any of the other studies. The intervention group was instructed to decrease or stop smoking and, by the end of 4 years, the tobacco consumption in this group had decreased by 45% more than in the control group. There were significant decreases in total cholesterol and weight, and an increase in HDL cholesterol in the intervention group. A subsample of the intervention group showed that the P/S ratio at the end of the trial was 1.01 compared with 0.39 for the control group. Calculations were made in an attempt to determine how much of the beneficial effect might be due to decreasing smoking and how much to a reduction of serum cholesterol, and it was concluded that the former was responsible for about 25% of the difference in CHD and the latter about 60%. However, it was not possible to separate the effects of these two interventions. This was really a trial of the *combined* effects of reducing smoking and of a high P/S ratio diet.

When considering the trials listed in *Table 7.1*, attention should be drawn to the fact that the two positive results were associated with the greatest reduction in serum cholesterol. The other trials summarized in *Table 7.1* were disconcertingly negative, and one study[15] showed a significant *adverse* effect on all-cause and CHD mortality. In this trial the subjects were 1222 business executives with one or more risk factors. Men in the intervention group were seen regularly and underwent intensive dietary and hygiene measures (low saturated fat and low cholesterol), physical activity, cigarette smoking reduction, and were treated by drugs for hypercholesterolemia or hypertension. After 5 years, the predicted risk of CHD had fallen by almost half in the intervention group (there was a 6% fall in serum cholesterol), but there were more nonfatal myocardial infarctions ($P < 0.01$) and an adverse trend for cardiac deaths. All subjects were followed for 10 years after the end of the 5-year intervention period; all-cause mortality, cardiac deaths, and deaths associated with violence were all significantly increased. While various attempts have been made to rationalize the results of this study, no plausible explanation has been forthcoming; we should not ignore these results.

Brief mention is needed, because of its size and the apparent effectiveness of the dietary

A stringent lipid-lowering diet was used in another angiographic regression trial.[37] The diet comprised 27% energy, 8–10% saturated fats, 8% polyunsaturated fats, dietary cholesterol in the region of 200 mg, and an increase in plant-derived fiber. In the 26 patients allocated to this regimen there was a significant reduction in total and LDL cholesterol and triglycerides. After 3 years, there was an improvement in coronary artery diameter and fewer clinical events than in the 24 patients given the usual care. While these encouraging findings are consistent with those more recently derived from cholesterol-lowering drug trials,[38] the regimens used were rigorous and not easily translatable to the more general health advice usually given.

Responsiveness to and Compliance with Dietary Recommendations

It is relevant to emphasize how little appears to have been achieved in terms of altering serum cholesterol and lipoproteins by the type of dietary advice given in these trials (and also in some of those listed in *Table 7.1*). In the community as a whole, the situation is worse. The Step 1 diet, recommended by the US National Cholesterol Education Program Expert Panel,[2] leads to a reduction in serum cholesterol concentration of 0–4%.[39] This diet recommends less than 30% of calories from fat, a P/S ratio of 1.0, and less than 300 mg cholesterol daily. However, over 4–10 years, even when population and individual dietary advice were combined, changes in serum cholesterol ranged from a fall of 2% to a rise of 1%. Intensive healthcare advice, aimed at improving lifestyle and including dietary advice along the lines of the Step 1 diet, for those with initial cholesterol concentrations >250 mg dl^{-1} has been unsuccessful in achieving a significant reduction in serum cholesterol.[40] Dietary advice is equally ineffective when given by a dietician, nurse, or by leaflet, and results in a reduction of LDL cholesterol of less than 5%[41] (*Table 7.4*). The more intensive Step 2 diet[2] aims for a P/S ratio of 1.4 or more and a cholesterol intake of less than 200 mg daily; it does better by reducing serum cholesterol by 13% over 5 years in high-risk men and by 6.5–15% over 2–5 years in hospital outpatients,[40] but the Step 2 diet also lowers HDL cholesterol by about 6%.[42]

The poor compliance with these diets should be a matter of concern, particularly since the more desirable the diet in terms of lowering atherogenic lipoproteins the worse the compliance. It appears to be unrealistic, outside the conditions of a rigorous trial (e.g. atherosclerosis regression studies) to expect to achieve changes in LDL concentrations that are likely to be of long-term benefit to the general population. However, an interesting

Table 7.4   Pooled mean concentrations at the start and end of a 6-month trial of intensive lipid-lowering dietary advice in general practice[14]

	Serum lipid (mmol l^{-1})		
	Start of study	After 6 months	Change (%)
Total cholesterol	7.13 (0.64)	7.00 (0.71)***	−2
LDL cholesterol	5.17 (0.64)	5.02 (0.67)***	−3
HDL cholesterol	1.21 (0.27)	1.24 (0.29)*	+2.5
Triglycerides[a]	1.53	1.52	−0.6

*$P < 0.05$; ***$P < 0.001$.
[a]Geometric mean (ranges are given in the paper[41]).

natural experiment has been reported recently.[43] In 1987, the government of the island of Mauritius changed the composition of the commonly used cooking oil from being mostly palm oil to wholly soya bean oil. There was a 14–15% decrease in total cholesterol in a cohort studied 5 years later. Thus, a single public health intervention with obligatory compliance can have a lasting effect.

Recently published seminal drug trials in the primary[44] and secondary[45] prevention of CHD make it clear that the reduction in incidence is proportional to the degree of reduction in LDL. The success of the statins in this regard is because reductions in LDL of 25% or more were achieved consistently over 5–6 years.[46]

Summary of Diet Trials

Randomized controlled clinical trials of the effects of diet on the incidence of CHD have been disappointing,[47] (*Table 7.5, Figure 7.1*), probably because the extent of the reduction in LDL cholesterol has been too small. Holme[47] concludes his meta-analysis by suggesting that total cholesterol must be reduced by more than 10%. When rigorous control of dietary fat intake, leading to decreases in LDL cholesterol of 25% or more, is achieved angio-

Table 7.5   Randomized controlled clinical trials of diet and CHD

Primary prevention
- Six trials of low saturated fat + low cholesterol and risk factor changes
  No benefit, except when combined with halving of smoking

Secondary prevention
- One trial of low saturated fat + low cholesterol
  No benefit
- Six trials of low fat + increased polyunsaturated fats
  Significant reduction of recurrence of myocardial infarction and CHD mortality. Favorable trend for all-cause mortality
- One trial of fish supplementation
  Significant and rapid reduction of CHD mortality. Adverse trend for reinfarction

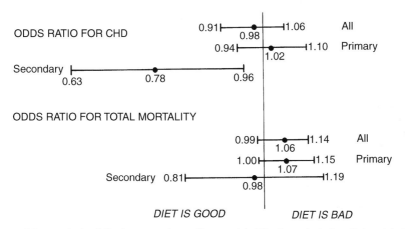

Figure 7.1   Meta-analysis of diet/coronary heart disease trials. The figure includes all the trials listed in *Tables 7.1–7.3*, except the Lyon Diet Heart Trial.[22] (From Ref. 47 with permission.)

graphic improvement in the diameter of diseased coronary arteries has been demonstrated. Trials which led to a marked increase in P/S ratio in conjunction with a reduction in other risk factors also showed less CHD. Trials in patients with CHD on diets rich in n-3 fatty acids show a decrease in CHD incidence without altering plasma lipoprotein concentrations.

There is persuasive nontrial evidence from clinical studies[48] that oleic acid supplementation has the most beneficial effect on atherogenic lipoproteins, and this is supported by studies of the eating habits of Mediterranean farmers, such as in Crete where the incidence of CHD is particularly low.[49] However, there has never been a formal randomized trial of the effects of monounsaturated fatty acid supplementation.

Conclusions

Controlled clinical trials of the *primary prevention* of CHD using diets low in saturated fat and cholesterol, also accompanied by changes in other risk factors, have been unsuccessful in reducing the incidence of CHD. However, trials in which the polyunsaturated fat content was increased leading to a P/S ratio in the region of 1.5, or where cigarette smoking was almost halved concurrently, led to a reduction in CHD incidence.

There has only ever been one very small clinical trial of the *secondary prevention* of CHD using diets low in saturated fats and cholesterol. It had no significant impact on the CHD recurrence rate. In contrast, five out of seven secondary prevention trials in which diets low in saturated fats were supplemented with polyunsaturated fats reduced CHD deaths and, to a lesser extent, all-cause mortality.

No formal trial of the effects of monounsaturated fats has been made. One trial of the effects of a diet with increased oleic acid and α-linolenic acid suggested a reduction in CHD incidence.

Diets supplemented with n-3 fatty acids appeared to reduce CHD mortality, and this benefit was independent of changes in plasma lipoproteins, but further confirmatory trials are needed.

Dietary advice along the lines of Step 1 recommendations does not reduce atherogenic lipoproteins sufficiently in free-living communities. The continued recommendation of such diets as a means of reducing CHD should be reconsidered. The compliance to Step 2 diets is poor and, in general, the more rigorous the diet the lower the compliance.

The evidence from formal controlled long-term clinical trials indicates that more emphasis should be given in national and international dietary recommendations to supplementation with monounsaturated fats and also with polyunsaturated fats, including n-3 fatty acids, rather than to diets low in total and saturated fats. The aim is to reduce LDL cholesterol to levels equivalent to those achieved by drugs, namely 20–25%.

It is high time that this anomalous situation was addressed. Governments, health departments, and many health educationalists are rigid in the belief that reducing dietary saturated fat is beneficial and all that is necessary. The agricultural industry has been persuaded to adjust to the received wisdom. Vast sums of money are being spent on nutritional programs, dietician advice, and nurse counselling in pursuing diets that may be ineffectual.

References

1. Department of Health and Social Security (DHSS). *Diet and Cardiovascular Disease (COMA Report) 1984*. Report on Health and Social Subjects, No. 28. HMSO: London.
2. National Cholesterol Education Program Expert Panel on Detection, Evaluation and Treatment of High Blood Cholesterol in Adults. First report. *Arch Intern Med* 1988; **148**: 36–9. Second report, *Circulation* 1994; **89**: 1329–445.
3. Pyörälä K, De Backer G, Poole-Wilson P, Wood D. Prevention of coronary heart disease in clinical practice. Recommendations of the Task Force of the European Society of Cardiology, European Atherosclerosis Society and European Society of Hypertension. *Eur Heart J* 1994; **15**: 1300–31.
4. Keys A. *Seven Countries. A Multivariate Analysis of Diet and Coronary Heart Disease*. Cambridge: Harvard University Press, 1980.
5. Ascherio A, Rimm EB, Giovannucci EL, *et al*. Dietary fat and risk of coronary heart disease in men: cohort follow up study in the United States. *Br Med J* 1996; **313**: 84–90.
6. Reaven P. The role of dietary fat in LDL oxidation and atherosclerosis. *Nutr Metab Cardiovasc Dis* 1996; **6**: 57–64.
7. Steinberg D, Parthasarathy S, Carew TE, *et al*. Beyond cholesterol: modifications of low-density lipoprotein that increase its atherogenicity. *N Engl J Med* 1989; **320**: 915–24.
8. Miller NE. *High Density Lipoproteins and Atherosclerosis*. Amsterdam: Elsevier, 1989; Vol. II.
9. Durrington PN. How HDL protects against atheroma. *Lancet* 1993; **342**: 1315–16.
10. Turpeinen O, Karvonen MJ, Pekkarinen M, *et al*. Dietary prevention of coronary heart disease: the Finnish Mental Hospital Study. *Int J Epidemiol* 1979; **8**: 99–118.
11. Hjermann I, Velve Byre K, Holme I, Leren P. Effect of diet and smoking on the incidence of coronary heart disease. *Lancet* 1981; **ii**: 1303–10.
12. Neaton JD, Blackburn H, Jacobs D, *et al*. Serum cholesterol level and mortality: findings for men screened in the Multiple Risk Factor Intervention Trial. *Arch Intern Med* 1992; **152**: 1490–1500.
13. World Health Organisation European Collaborative Group. European collaborative trial of multifactorial prevention of coronary heart disease. *Lancet* 1986; **i**: 869–72.
14. Frantz ID, Dawson EA, Ashman PL, *et al*. Test of effect of lipid lowering by diet on cardiovascular risk. The Minnesota Coronary Survey. *Arteriosclerosis* 1989; **9**: 129–35.
15. Strandberg TE, Salomaa VV, Naukkarinen VA, *et al*. Long-term mortality after 5 year multifactorial primary prevention of cardiovascular diseases in middle-aged men. *JAMA* 1991; **266**: 1225–9.
16. Research Committee to the Medical Research Council. Low fat diet in myocardial infarction. A controlled trial. *Lancet* 1965; **ii**: 501–4.
17. Dayton S, Pearce ML, Hashimoto S, *et al*. A controlled clinical trial of a diet high in unsaturated fat preventing complications in atherosclerosis. *Circulation* 1969; **39/40** (Suppl II): 63.
18. Research Committee to the Medical Research Council. Controlled trial of soya-bean oil in myocardial infarction. *Lancet* 1968; **ii**: 693–700.
19. Leren P. The Oslo Heart Study: eleven year report. *Circulation* 1970; **XLII**: 935–42.
20. Woodhill JM, Palmer AJ, Leelarthaepin C, *et al*. Low fat, low cholesterol diet in secondary prevention of coronary heart disease. *Adv Exp Med Biol* 1978; **109**: 317–30.
21. Burr ML, Fehily AM, Gilbert JF, *et al*. Effects of changes in fat, fish, and fibre intakes on death and myocardial reinfarction: diet and reinfarction trial (DART). *Lancet* 1989; **ii**: 757–61.
22. de Lorgeril M, Renaud S, Mamelle N, *et al*. Mediterranean α-linolenic-acid-rich diet in secondary prevention of coronary heart disease. *Lancet* 1994; **343**: 1454–9.
23. Singh RB, Rastogi SS, Verma R, *et al*. Randomised controlled trial of cardioprotective diet in patients with recent myocardial infarction: results of one year follow up. *Br Med J* 1992; **304**: 1015.
24. Burr ML, Sweetnam PM, Fehily AM. Diet and reinfarction. *Eur Heart J* 1994; **15**: 1152–3.
25. Dart AM, Riemersma RA, Oliver MF. Effects of MaxEPA on serum lipids in hypercholesterolaemic subjects. *Atherosclerosis* 1989; **80**: 119–24.
26. Kromhout D, Bosschieter EB, Coulander C de L. The inverse relation between fish consumption and 20-year mortality from coronary heart disease. *N Engl J Med* 1985; **312**: 1205–9.
27. Shekelle RB, Missell L, Paul O, *et al*. Fish consumption and mortality from coronary heart disease. *N Engl J Med* 1985; **313**: 820.
28. Vollset SE, Heuch I, Bjelke E. Fish consumption and mortality from coronary heart disease. *N Engl J Med* 1985; **313**: 820–1.
29. Curb JD, Reed DM. Fish consumption and mortality from coronary heart disease. *N Engl J Med* 1985; **313**: 821.
30. Kromhout D, Katan MB, Haveke L, *et al*. The effect of 26 years of habitual fish consumption on serum lipid and lipoprotein levels (the Zutphen Study). *Nutr Metab Cardiovasc Dis* 1996; **6**: 65–71.
31. Aschierio A, Rimm EB, Stampfer MJ, *et al*. Dietary intake of marine n-3 fatty icids, fish intake, and the risk of coronary disease among men. *N Engl J Med* 1995; **332**: 977–82.
32. Guallar E, Hennekens CH, Sacks FM, Willett WC, Stampfer MJ. A prospective study of fish oil levels and incidence of myocardial infarction in US male physicians. *J Am Coll Cardiol* 1995; **25**: 387–94.
33. Goodnight SH, Cairns JA, Fisher M, Fitzgerald GA. Assessment of the therapeutic use of n-3 fatty acids in vascular disease and thrombosis. *Chest* 1992; **102**: 374S–84S.
34. Weber PC. Atherosclerosis risk factor modification by n-3 fatty acids. *Atherosclerosis Rev* 1990; **21**: 91–102.

35. McLennan PL, Abeywardena MY, Charnock JS. Influence of dietary lipids on arrhythmias and infarction after coronary artery ligation in rats. *Can J Physiol Pharmacol* 1985; **63**: 1411–17.
36. Ornish D, Brown SE, Schwerwitz LW, *et al*. Can lifestyle changes reverse coronary heart disease? *Lancet* 1990; **336**: 129–33.
37. Watts GF, Lewis B, Brunt JNH, *et al*. Effects on coronary artery disease of lipid-lowering diet, or diet plus cholestyramine, in the St Thomas' Atherosclerosis Regression Study (STARS). *Lancet* 1992; **339**: 563–9.
38. Vos JW. Retardation and arrest of progression or regression of coronary artery disease: a review. *Prog Cardiovasc Dis* 1993; **35**: 435–54.
39. Ramsay LE, Yeo WW, Jackson PR. Dietary reduction of serum cholesterol concentration: time to think again. *Br Med J* 1991; **303**: 953–7.
40. Lindholm LH, Ekbom T, Dash C, *et al*. The impact of health care advice given in primary care on cardiovascular risk. *Br Med J* 1995; **310**: 1105–9.
41. Neil HAW, Roe L, Godlee JW, *et al*. Randomised trial of lipid lowering dietary advice in general practice: the effects on serum lipids, lipoproteins, and antioxidants. *Br Med J* 1995; **310**: 569–73.
42. Hunninghake DB, Stein A, Dujovne CA, *et al*. The efficacy of intensive dietary therapy alone or combined with lovastatin in outpatients with hypercholesterolemia. *N Engl J Med* 1993; **328**: 1213–19.
43. Uusitalo U, Feskens EJM, Tuomilehto J, *et al*. Fall in total cholesterol concentration over five years in association with changes in fatty acid composition of cooking oil in Mauritius: cross sectional survey. *Br Med J* 1996; **313**: 1044–6.
44. Shepherd J, Cobbe SM, Ford I, *et al*. Prevention of coronary heart disease with pravastatin in men with hypercholesterolemia. *N Engl J Med* 1995; **333**: 1301–7.
45. Scandinavian Simvastatin Survival Study Group. Randomised trial of cholesterol lowering in 4444 patients with coronary heart disease: the Scandinavian Simvastatin Survival Study (4S). *Lancet* 1994; **344**: 1383–9.
46. Oliver MF. Statins prevent coronary heart disease. *Lancet* 1995; **346**: 1378–9.
47. Holme I. Relation of coronary heart disease incidence and total mortality to plasma cholesterol reduction in randomized trials: use of meta-analysis. *Br Heart J* 1993; **69**: S42–S50.
48. Mattison FH, Grundy SM. Comparison of effects of dietary saturated, monounsaturated, and polyunsaturated fatty acids on plasma lipids and lipoproteins in man. *J Lipid Res* 1985; **26**: 194–202.
49. Stamler J. Assessing diets to improve world health: nutritional research on disease causation in populations. *Am J Clin Nutr* 1994; **59**: 46S–56S.

8

Hypertension

J. Ian S. Robertson

Introduction

The purpose of antihypertensive treatment is clear: to prevent or correct the cardiovascular complications associated with raised arterial pressure. These complications comprise the following.[1]

Most baleful is the malignant phase, in which the blood pressure has risen so high, especially if the increase has been very rapid, that fibrinoid arterial and arteriolar necrosis is occurring. Clinically, malignant hypertension can be recognized by the presence of bilateral retinal hemorrhages and exudates and, in the later stages, papilledema also. If untreated, the patient in the malignant phase will inevitably die within months of progressive renal failure, although the course may be terminated more abruptly by cardiac failure or cerebral hemorrhage. An even more dire consequence of very marked hypertension, and almost always superimposed on the malignant phase, is hypertensive encephalopathy, in which cerebral edema leads to confusion, clouding of consciousness, coma, and epileptiform fits. Severe hypertension can also be accompanied by overt cardiac congestive and/or left ventricular failure. This is to be distinguished from the more subtle impairment of cardiac function which can follow hypertension-associated coronary artery disease.

Hypertension predisposes to both brain hemorrhage and infarction. With raised arterial pressure, even short of the malignant phase, the decline of renal function with age is more rapid. An especially prevalent complication of hypertension, of increased importance since recent attention has been drawn to modest blood pressure elevation, is coronary artery disease and its sequelae. Aortic dissection, although a declared endpoint in some treatment trials, is uncertain as a complication of hypertension.

The distribution of blood pressure values, both systolic and diastolic, in populations, is continuous and roughly bell-shaped, being skewed at the upper end of the distribution. The accompanying cardiovascular risk follows the blood-pressure distribution, and also is consequently continuous; there is no threshold above which risk starts and below which it is absent. Most of the early epidemiological and intervention studies focused on diastolic pressure. It is now recognized that systolic hypertension also carries cardiovascular risk, although the comparative importance of systolic and diastolic blood pressure remains controversial.[2–5] Systolic pressure is said to be the more closely related to stroke in persons aged over 60 years.[6] Throughout this chapter, diastolic blood pressures are given as taken at the Vth Korotkoff phase (the point of disappearance of sounds), unless stated otherwise.

Several of the complications of hypertension appear to be a direct consequence of the raised arterial pressure *per se*; these include the malignant phase, encephalopathy, overt heart failure, brain hemorrhage, and possibly aortic dissection. Trials of antihypertensive treatment have, as will be shown, demonstrated most clear efficacy against these conditions. Other manifestations are related less directly to hypertension, via arterial atheroma (atherosclerosis). It has been proposed that hypertension promotes the advance of atheroma by causing increased arterial blood flow turbulence and shear, and both histological and biochemical lesions of arterial endothelium. Atheromatous consequences of hypertension include coronary artery disease and brain infarction. These sequelae are, as will be seen, less susceptible, but not wholly unresponsive, to prevention by antihypertensive therapy.

The benefits of blood-pressure lowering in limiting the adverse consequences of hypertension have so far been shown only with antihypertensive drugs. Surgical procedures such as dorsolumbar sympathectomy and adrenalectomy are now of historical interest only. While a range of nonpharmacological approaches, including weight reduction, physical exercise, restriction of the intake of sodium salts and of alcohol, and a variety of psychological techniques, including relaxation procedures, biofeedback, yoga, and trancendental meditation, have been advocated with varying success as antihypertensive measures, neither their ability to limit morbidity, nor indeed the safety of some, have yet been evaluated. One study[7] has even raised the possibility that dietary salt restriction can increase the risk of myocardial infarction in drug-treated hypertensive men. Moreover, it has been argued that emphasis on nonpharmacological measures may deprive some patients of necessary drug treatment.[8] Nevertheless, several guidelines to the treatment of hypertension advise a number of these nonpharmacological methods, both as a prelude and accompaniment to antihypertensive drug therapy.[9]

In the trials to be considered herein, hypertension is taken to be 'primary' ('essential') in nature, i.e. without evident cause. Throughout, the trial organizers have taken pains to exclude subjects in whom hypertension has an identified, and hence potentially correctable, cause ('secondary' hypertension). Also excluded almost invariably from trials are patients with malignant hypertension, uremia, carcinoma, drug or alcohol addiction, or mental disorder.

Early Uncontrolled Studies

The introduction of effective antihypertensive drugs was soon followed by the observation that their use could correct both the malignant phase, provided that serious renal failure had not supervened, and overt hypertensive heart failure.[10–13] Indeed, the course of these conditions when left untreated was so consistently and rapidly adverse that controlled trials were considered to be unnecessary and ethically dubious. In the malignant phase, prognosis was seen to be closely related to the effectiveness of the control of blood pressure.[14] Clinical experience through subsequent years has repeatedly sustained these assumptions.[1]

Leishman[12] reported on the progress of 211 untreated severely hypertensive patients followed for 13 years and compared with 73 similarly hypertensive patients treated by dorsolumbar sympathectomy plus 118 given ganglion-blocking drugs. In the absence of the malignant phase, mortality among the treated patients was only one-third that of those left untreated. The reduction in mortality was mainly due to prevention of cerebral hemorrhage and renal failure.[12,13]

Controlled Trials of Drug Treatment in Hypertension

Demonstration of the ability of antihypertensive drug treatment to prevent complications in hypertension which had not progressed to the malignant phase or to cardiac failure required the prosecution of controlled trials. It is with an evaluation of these that the present chapter will mainly be concerned. The principal characteristics of the studies to be considered are summarized in *Tables 8.1* and *8.2*. Additional aspects are described in the text dealing with each trial. The various trials have been arranged in six groups as follows: marked hypertension, poststroke hypertension, mild-to-moderate hypertension in young or middle-aged persons, hypertension in the elderly, trials comparing different systems of healthcare (including multiple-risk-factor interventions), and trials comparing different drug regimens. Whilst this arrangement has some convenience, there is inevitably occasional overlap between groups.

Trials in Marked Hypertension

Hamilton *et al.* 1964

This pioneering British trial[15] recruited patients who showed diastolic blood pressures (IVth phase) of at least 110 mmHg over a period of outpatient observation of 3 months. All were free from overt cardiovascular disease at entry and were symptomless. Subjects were then assigned alternately to the control group, which entailed simply outpatient review, or to antihypertensive drug therapy.

At the conclusion of the trial, three cases were excluded, one being over the defined entry age limit of 60, and two because of possible secondary hypertension. The initial declared endpoint was stroke, but the final analysis included also myocardial infarction and incipient cardiac failure. Results for men and women were analyzed separately.

There were no complications amongst the 10 treated men, as compared with eight endpoints, including four strokes, with one death, among the 12 male controls ($P < 0.025$).

Amongst the women, 8 of the 19 controls suffered complications, including three strokes, compared with 5 of the 20 treated patients, including three strokes (difference not significant). Therapy had, however, been notably less effective in lowering blood pressure in those women developing complications.

This trial is vulnerable to the obvious criticism that the allocation of patients to control and therapeutic groups was alternate rather than random. However, the conduct of the study was described in detail and much care was evidently taken to minimize bias. All patients were apparently followed closely, although compliance with therapy could not always be fully substantiated, and may have been responsible for the inadequate blood pressure control in some women. The predefined primary outcome, stroke, was clearly reported, albeit the eventual statistical analysis included additional endpoints. The trial ran its full course, antedating monitoring committees. Although the numbers were small the severity of the hypertension and the 2–6 years' duration of the study largely offset that limitation. The patients included were probably representative of those attending outpatient departments for the treatment of hypertension in the early 1960s.

This trial is not usually included in meta-analyses of antihypertensive treatment, because allocation was alternate rather than random. Nevertheless, it was the first prospective controlled study to be performed in this field, and showed that drug therapy could, at least in men, prevent complications in hypertension.

Table 8.1 Main characteristics of the principal trials considered in the text. (Adapted and expanded from Gueyffier et al.[27] with permission)

Trial	No. of patients Treated	Control	Follow-up (years)	Men (%)	Age (years) Min.	Max.	Ave.	Type of trial[a]	Inclusion criteria SBP (mmHg)	DBP (mmHg)	No. of baseline measures	Mean baseline BP (mmHg)	Δ BP between groups (mmHg)	Study drug[b] Basic	Supplementary	Lost to follow-up[c] (%)	Withdrawal due to increasing BP Treated	Control	Reason
Marked hypertension																			
Hamilton[15]	30	31	4.0	32	?	60	47	Open		>109 (phase IV)	3	229/132	?	G	M, T	0	1	8	?
VA (Part 1)[17]	68	63	1.5	100	?	?	51	DB vs PL		115–129	2	186/121	40//30	T, H, R	–	8		?	
Wolff[16]	45	42	2.0	47	?	?	49	DB vs PL		100–130	>3	177/109		R	T, G	<6		?	
Barraclough[19]	58	58	1.5	43	45	69	55	SB vs PL		100–120	2	/109	//13	T, M, D	–	?		9	>130 × 1
Poststroke hypertension																			
Carter[20]	50	49	3.6	57	?	80	?	Open	>160	>110	>2			T, M	Be, G, D	2	?	?	?
US Stroke[21]	233	219	2.3	59	?	75	?	DB vs PL	140–220	90–115	6	167/100	25//12.3	T, R	–	0?		6	>220/125 × 2
Mild-to-moderate hypertension in young or middle-aged people																			
VA (Part 2)[22]	186	194	3.3	100	24	75	51	DB vs PL		90–114	2	164/104	31//19	T, H, R	–	15	0	20	>/124
Smith[25]	193	196	7.0	80	21	55	44	DB vs PL		90–114	>2	148/99	16//10	T, R	–	7	0	24	>130 (×3 or symptoms)
Perry[28]	508	504	1.4	81	21	50	38	DB vs PL		85–105	3	/93	//6.6	T	R, U	?	0	12	>130 × 1 or 120 × 2 or 110 × 4
Australian[30]	1721	1706	4.0	63	30	69	50	SB vs PL	<200	95–109	4	157/100	//5.6	T	B, Cl, H, M	3	4	198	>200/110 × 4
Oslo[29]	406	379	5.5	100	40	49	45	Open	150–179	90–109	6	155/97	17/10	T	B, M, U	0	?	65	>180/110 × 3
MRC-1[32]	8700	8654	4.9	52	35	64	52	SB vs PL	<200	90–109	6	161/98	11.5//5.5	B, T	G, M	0	76	1011	>210/115 × 2 then 200/110
TOMHS[39]	668	234	4.4	62	45	69	55	DB vs PL		85–99	3	140/91	6.8//3.7	A, ACE, B, C, T	U	0.4	121	60	?

Hypertension in old people

Trial																		
Kuramoto[40]	44	55	4.0	55	60	>90	76	SB vs PL	160–199	90–109	11	169/86	T	R, M, H	13	0	8	>200/100
Sprackling[41]	61	61	7.5	74	60	>90	80	Open		>100 (phase IV)	1	200/107 12//4	M	–	2		?	?
Australian (elderly)[31]	293	289	4.0	55	60	69	64	SB vs PL	<200	95–109	4	//6.7	T	B, Cl, H, M	2		?	?
EWPHE[35]	416	424	4.7	30	60	?	72	DB vs PL	160–239	90–119	3	182/101 19//8	T	M	0	2	19	Plus 40/20 or >250/130 × 3
Coope[46]	419	465	4.4	31	60	79	69	Open	>170 or	105–120	3	196/99 16//10	B	C, M, T, U	0	?	9	>280/120
SHEP (pilot)[48]	443	108	2.8	47	60	?	72	DB vs PL	160	<90	4	172/75 15//3	T	B, H, R	0	?	?	?
SHEP[49]	2365	2371	4.5	43	60	≥80	72	DB vs PL	160–219	<90	7	170/77 12//14	T	B, R	<1	?	356	>220/90 × n or 240/115 × 1
STOP[50]	812	815	2.1	37	70	84	76	DB vs PL	180–230	>90 or 105–120	3	187/104 19.5//8.1	B, T	–	0	10	75	? ≥230/120 × 2
MRC-2[6]	2183	2213	5.8	42	65	74	70	SB vs PL	160–209	<115	13	185/91 15//7	B, T	C, U	0	13	175	>210/115 × 2
STONE[56]	891	741	3.0	47	60	79	66	SB vs PL	160–200	96–124	3	169/98 9.3//5.6	C	ACE, T	2	0	74	Realloc. >109 diastolic × 1
Multiple risk factor interventions plus special care																		
HDFP (stratum I)[57]	3903	3922	5.0	55	30d	69d	51d	Open	<161	90–104	3	152/96 //5	T, S	G, H, M, R, U	1d	?	3164d	?
HDFP (stratum II)[57]	1048	1004	5.0	51	(see stratum If)			Open	<161	105–114	3	169.5/109 //7	T, S	G, H, M, R, U	(see Stratum 1)	(see Stratum 1)	?	?
HDFP (stratum III)[57]	534	529	5.0	61	(see stratum If)			Open	<161	>114	3	190/122 //6	T, S	G, H, M, R, U	(see Stratum 1)	(see Stratum 1)	?	?
MRFIT (high BP subgroup)[73]	4019	3993	7.0	100	35	57		Open		90–114 (or on antihypertensive drug)	3	?/96 (for whole SI vs UC) //4	T	G, H, R, U	0.4	?	2595	?

BP, Blood pressure; SBP, systolic blood pressure; DBP, diastolic blood pressure.

DB, Double blind; SB, single blind; PL, placebo; ?, information not available.

[b] A, alpha-blocker; ACE, ACE inhibitor; B, beta-blocker; Be, bethanidine; C, calcium antagonist; Cl, clonidine; D, debrisoquine; G, ganglion blocker; H, hydralazine; M, methyldopa; R, rauwolfia; S, spironolactone; T, thiazide (including chlorthalidone), with or without potassium-conserving agent; U, other unspecified drug.

[c] The number given concerns mortality.

[d] HDFP overall.

Table 8.2 Number of observed outcomes in the trials shown in *Table 8.1*. (Adapted from Gueyffier et al.[27] with permission)

Trial	No. patients Treated	No. patients Control	No. deaths Treated	No. deaths Control	No. CV deaths Treated	No. CV deaths Control	No. strokes Treated	No. strokes Control	No. major coronary events Treated	No. major coronary events Control	No. congestive heart failure Treated	No. congestive heart failure Control
Marked hypertension												
Hamilton[15]	30	31	2	2	1	2	3	7	1	3	0	2
VA (Part 1)[17]	73	70	0	4	0	4	1	4	0	3	0	4
Wolff[16]	45	42	4	2	4	1	2	1	2	0	0	8
Barraclough[19]	58	58	1	2	0	1	0	0	1	2	0	1
Poststroke hypertension												
Carter[20]	50	49	13	22	10	16	10	21	2	2	3	4
US Stroke[21]	233	219	26	24	15	19	37	42	6	6	0	6
Mild-to-moderate hypertension in young or middle-aged people												
VA (Part 2)[22]	186	194	10	21	8	19	5	20	11	13	0	11
Smith[25]	193	196	2	4	2	4	1	6	15	18	0	2
Perry[28]	508	504	2	0	2	0	0	0	8	5	0	0
Australian[30]	1721	1706	25	35	8	18	13	22	33	33	3	3
Oslo[29]	406	379	10	9	7	6	0	5	14	10	0	1
MRC-1[32]	8700	8654	248	253	134	139	60	109	222	234	?	?
TOMHS[39]	668	234	{9}		{4}		{4}		26 (3.89%)	12 (5.13%)	{2}	
Hypertension in old people												
Kuramoto[40]	44	55	7	7	3	3	3	4	1	2	0	2
Sprackling[41]	61	61	50	47	?	?	?	?	?	?	?	?
Australian (elderly)[31]	293	289	7	9	2	5	7	9	7	9	?	?
EWPHE[35a]	416	424	135	149	67	93	–	–	–	–	–	–
Coope[46]	419	465	60	69	35	50	20	39	35	38	22	36
SHEP (pilot)[48]	443	108	32	7	14	5	11	4	15	4	6	2
SHEP[49]	2365	2371	213	242	90	112	103	159	104	141	56	109
STOP[50]	812	815	36	63	17	41	29	53	29	40	19	39
MRC-2[26]	2183	2213	301	315	161	180	101	134	128	159	2	?
STONE[56]	891	741	15	26	11	14	16	36	3	4	2	6
Multiple risk factor interventions plus special care												
HDFP (stratum I)[57]	3903	3922	232	292	122	165	59	88	307	355	?	?
HDFP (stratum II)[57]	1048	1004	70	78	45	41	25	36	84	103	?	?
HDFP (stratum III)[57]	534	529	48	51	28	34	18	35	40	55	?	?
MRFIT (high BP subgroup)[73]	4019	3993	169	174	88	91	32	38	276	254	?	?

[a] Intention-to-treat data only.

Wolff and Lindeman 1966

In this American trial,[16] outpatients, most of whom were black, were assigned in a random and double-blind fashion to active antihypertensive drug therapy or to matching placebo. Eight patients with a history of heart failure who were considered to need digitalis plus thiazide were allowed to continue with these agents, even though allocated to placebo. Predeclared endpoints were heart failure, retinal evidence of malignant hypertension, encephalopathy, stroke, myocardial infarction, angina, peripheral arterial disease, advancing uremia, severe headache, or symptomatic diabetes mellitus. Clinical assessment was made by independent observers blinded to therapy.

The two groups were broadly similar at the outset, although those assigned to placebo initially had more prevalent overt coronary artery disease, while those allocated to treatment had more frequent cerebrovascular disease or headache. During the trial 10 patients in the treated group and one in the placebo group defaulted; six of these were later traced and assessed, but were not included in the final analysis. Blood pressure was significantly lower in those on active therapy.

There were six endpoints, including three deaths, in the treatment group, compared with 19, including one death and eight patients with congestive heart failure, in the placebo group. These figures also include two patients with diabetes and four with severe headache in the placebo group. The authors did not present a formal statistical analysis of the trial outcome. Interestingly, although patients on placebo were allowed, if necessary, to continue digitalis plus diuretic, there were eight patients with congestive heart failure as an endpoint in the placebo group against none among those on antihypertensive drugs.

This was the first randomized double-blind prospective trial of antihypertensive drug treatment. Patients and those evaluating outcome, but not therapists, were ostensibly unaware of treatment prescribed. Comparability of the groups was clearly stated, while defaulting patients, and those showing endpoint complications, were described in detail. Safety was evidently a prominent consideration, although there was no independent monitoring committee. The statistical approach would nowadays be regarded as naive, although the number of endpoints was sufficient to indicate benefit from active therapy. The patients who were entered seemed representative, and therapy was appropriate for the date of the trial. Presentation was clear and relevant.

Veterans Administration Trial 1967

The US Veterans Administration (VA) Trial was conducted in men only.[17,18] Entry diastolic pressure was required to be in the range 90–129 mmHg. Patients were initially admitted to hospital for 1 week, during which blood pressure was recorded five times daily, and were then returned to the outpatient clinic for 3 weeks, during which blood pressure was again checked. Those still eligible were entered into a prerandomization single-blind evaluation lasting 2–4 months, when compliance with placebo therapy was assessed by tablet count and by the urinary excretion of riboflavin incorporated in the tablets. Unreliable subjects, totalling nearly half of those initially entered, were excluded.

The trial proper involved double-blind randomization to placebo or active therapy. At the end of the first year of the study, evidence emerged that patients taking placebo, and with entry diastolic pressures between 115 and 129 mmHg, showed excessive mortality, and consequently the study was terminated in those subjects. The trial was continued as planned in the remaining patients, who had baseline diastolic pressures between 90 and 114 mmHg, for an everage period of 2 more years. The two resulting subgroups were then

The prior declaration of trial size, duration, and major endpoints was followed. While unreliable patients were excluded, those entered were relevant to clinical practice. Treatment was appropriate for the date of the trial.

Summary of Trials in Poststroke Hypertension

The negative findings concerning stroke recurrence in the US multicenter trial[21] contrast with the earlier but smaller study by Carter.[20] The two studies are, however, disparate in several aspects. In particular, Carter's trial was open, under the continuous personal supervision of one physician, and entered patients with more severe hypertension, while still in hospital shortly following a stroke. In the US trial, patients were entered up to a year after their stroke, and these survivors appear to have been at lesser risk, since the recurrence rate was higher in the English study. The prevention of congestive heart failure with therapy in the US trial is noteworthy.

Trials in Mild-to-Moderate Hypertension in Young or Middle-aged Persons

VA Part 2: Patients with Entry Diastolic Pressures of 90–114 mmHg 1970, 1972

The design of the US Veterans Administration study has been outlined above.[17,18] As stated, during its course the trial was split into two parts. Described here is the subgroup containing patients with less severe hypertension, in whom the trial was pursued as originally planned.[22,23]

A total of 380 male patients had entry diastolic pressures averaging 90–114 mmHg; of these, 186 received active drugs and 194 placebo. As in the group with more severe hypertension in the VA trial, at entry overt cardiovascular disease was already very prevalent. The control and treatment groups were well matched at the outset. Trial observation ranged from 1 to 5.5 years. Active therapy was accompanied by a substantial and significant fall in blood pressure from starting values, by mean values of 27 mmHg systolic and 17 mmHg diastolic pressure at 4 months, while there were slight rises in blood pressure in the control subjects. Fifty-six patients (29 on active drug and 27 on placebo) dropped out during the trial for various reasons, and were not followed.

Case records of patients reported as developing assessable morbid events were reviewed by two independent physicians. Of the cardiovascular complications attributable to hypertension, 22 occurred among the treated patients versus 56 among the controls. The number of deaths was 8 and 19, respectively.

Although the trial authors calculated that the difference in morbidity between the groups at 5 years would be significant, others have been less convinced.[24–27] In this part of the VA study, patients with prerandomization diastolic pressures in the range 90–104 mmHg derived little benefit from therapy unless they had cardiovascular lesions at entry or were over 50 years of age;[23] treatment was more effective in those with higher entry diastolic pressure.

Taken as a whole, although for many years it provided much of the case for treating hypertension with drugs, the VA trial has been severely criticised and some now regard it as of historical interest only.[26] Concerns have included the splitting of the study into two parts after its commencement, the loss of many patients to follow-up, that those studied were unrepresentative, and that the results were seemingly inspected continually and the trial discontinued arbitrarily when an apparently significant result was obtained.[24] The second part of the VA study has been of particular concern,[24–27] and has been omitted from a recent meta-analysis.[27] In 1983, Hampton[24] wrote: 'the US Veterans study broke almost every rule of trial design and analysis, and if it were offered to a medical journal today it would probably not be accepted for publication'.

The US Public Health Service Hospitals Cooperative Trial 1977

The US Public Health Service Hospitals Cooperative Trial in mild hypertension[25] was prospective, randomized, placebo-controlled, and double-blind, being conducted in six centers. Potential trial subjects qualifying on initial screening proceeded to 3 months of single-blind placebo and were excluded if their diastolic pressure fell below 90 mmHg on two of the three clinic visits made in that time. Patients entering the trial proper were randomized to placebo or to active drug therapy. Blood pressure was measured bimonthly, and compliance assessed by pill count. More detailed clinical evaluation was performed 6-monthly. Specified primary statistical endpoints were death from any cardiovascular cause, nonfatal stroke, or nonfatal myocardial infarction.

Of over 1600 subjects initially referred, 422 were randomized, of which 33 were erroneous inclusions, leaving 389 for follow-up and analysis. The two groups were well matched in all relevant characteristics. There were 132 dropouts, of whom 75 were lost to regular follow-up and 26 were untraced. There was no differential dropout between the control and treated groups.

The average reduction in blood pressure, comparing the treated with control groups, was 16 mmHg systolic and 10 mmHg diastolic. Even in the control group, blood pressures were not very high, averaging about 145/95 mmHg at 7 years. Major morbid events during this trial were few, and were equally distributed between the actively treated and placebo groups (8 versus 9). Less severe features of coronary artery disease were also equally distributed.

This apparently carefully conducted trial in mild hypertension in an initially largely healthy population was too small to reveal any effects of antihypertensive therapy.

Perry *et al.* 1978

Perry *et al.*[28] reported in detail on a prospective, double-blind, randomized multicenter trial in mild hypertension, sponsored jointly by the US Veterans Administration and the National Heart, Lung and Blood Institute. This was a feasibility study for a larger trial which seems not to have materialized. Even so, the data are of interest.

Potential candidates underwent three outpatient screening tests at monthly intervals. Compliance was confirmed by checking the urinary excretion of riboflavin administered in placebo tablets, and relevant physical examination and investigations were performed. Subjects with evident cardiovascular, renal, or other serious disease, and those thought likely to comply poorly, were excluded. Of 4188 subjects who attended the first screening, 1012 entered the trial proper.

Participants were randomly assigned double-blindly to placebo or to active treatment. A data monitoring and safety committee operated independently of the physicians managing the patients. Predefined major morbid events were death, stroke, myocardial infarction, angina pectoris, and congestive heart failure.

The placebo and treatment groups were initially well matched. Ninety-eight patients on bendrofluazide group, 42% of the propranolol group, and 47% of the placebo group; the corresponding figures for women were 33%, 40% and 40%, respectively. The cumulative percentage of patients lost to follow-up at 5.5 years was 19%. The records of all those who defaulted were checked at the National Health Service central registry to ensure notification of any death.

An aspect which diminished the planned statistical power of the trial was that the average blood pressure fell immediately after entry in all groups, including those on placebo. The fall was steepest in the first 2 weeks and continued more gradually for about 3 months. Thereafter, average pressure changed little. Subsequent annual measurements showed that between one-third and one-half of all those taking placebo had a diastolic blood pressure below 90 mmHg. Thus the trial examined hypertension of lower severity than that assumed in the design. A converse problem, which also confounded later analysis, was that a cumulative 611 men and 400 women were withdrawn from placebo and placed on active therapy because their blood pressure exceeded the defined trial range.

Thirty-four percent of men and 24% of women initially allocated to bendrofluazide took supplementary antihypertensive drugs. The corresponding figures for those randomized to propranolol were 25% and 19%, respectively. In 5% of patients the two primary drugs were given together.

The main results were analyzed by 'intention to treat'.

Active treatment was accompanied by a substantial reduction in stroke ($n = 60$ versus 109 in the placebo group; $P < 0.01$). Cardiovascular events of all kinds were also significantly fewer in the actively treated group ($n = 286$ versus 352; $P < 0.05$). However, although coronary events predominated amongst cardiovascular events, considerably exceeding stroke incidence, coronary events taken in isolation were not significantly fewer with active treatment ($n = 222$ versus 234).

Deaths from all causes were similarly frequent in the actively treated ($n = 248$) and placebo ($n = 253$) groups. However, the pattern was different in men, who appeared to gain protection from active treatment ($n = 157$ versus 181 on placebo) compared with women, who fared better on placebo ($n = 91$ versus 72). The difference between the sexes in this respect was significant ($P = 0.05$).

The further stated aim of the first MRC trial, a comparison of the two primary drugs, was unavoidably confounded by withdrawals, supplementary therapy, and the combining of bendrofluazide with propranolol. Supplementary drugs were more often needed with bendrofluazide, although that group then achieved better blood-pressure control. While both primary drugs caused a reduction in stroke rate (per 1000 patient-years: 0.8 with bendrofluazide, 1.9 with propranolol, and 2.6 with placebo), the effect of bendrofluazide was significantly better than that with propranolol ($P = 0.002$). This superiority of bendrofluazide versus propranolol remained when the comparison was restricted to patients showing similar control of blood pressure.[34] The stroke rate was lower in both smokers and nonsmokers taking bendrofluazide, but only in nonsmokers on propranolol.

The coronary-event rate as defined was not influenced by treatment in women, in male smokers or nonsmokers on bendrofluazide, or in male smokers on propranolol. However, the rate was lowered substantially in male nonsmokers on propranolol, from 7.5 to 5.0 per 1000 patient-years of observation.

Sudden-death rates in men (in which sex most of these events occurred) were (per 1000 patient-years) 2.6 for bendrofluazide, 1.1 for propranolol, and 1.8 for placebo. Neither comparison against placebo was significant, but the rate was significantly lower when comparing propranolol with bendrofluazide ($P = 0.01$).

A retrospective analysis of the main report conducted independently by Green,[36] originally a member of the trial steering committee, in which both overt and latent coronary events were examined (the latter assessed using Minnesota coding), showed age-adjusted rates per 1000 patient-years of 27.4 on bendrofluazide, 20.4 on propranolol, and 23.9 on placebo. The rate on propranolol was significantly lower than that on either bendrofluazide ($P < 0.001$) or placebo ($P < 0.05$).

The rate of all defined cardiovascular events taken together was not reduced by bendrofluazide whatever the smoking habit, or in smokers taking propranolol, but was lower in nonsmokers on propranolol. The difference in this respect between the drugs was significant ($P = 0.01$).

This, the first MRC trial, is the largest so far conducted in hypertension. As mentioned, it was restricted to British general practices dealing predominantly with higher social classes, thus limiting its relevance. The chosen daily dose of the thiazide, bendrofluazide 10 mg, would now be regarded as excessive, and may have been responsible for some of the adverse cardiac comparisons with propranolol, as well as for several prevalent side-effects.[37,38] Moreover, there was notable contamination of the original treatment allocations during the trial. As mentioned earlier, the projected statistical power was weakened by unpredicted falls in pressure in many patients on placebo, as well as by the initiation of active therapy in another 1011 in the placebo group. In these circumstances it was probably unwise of the Working Party to conclude their original report[32] by stating that 'if 850 mildly hypertensive patients are given active antihypertensive drugs for one year about one stroke will be prevented'. Such treatment would almost certainly be more beneficial than that.[27]

This important trial illustrates the advantages and limitations both of very large, but hence necessarily crude, studies, and especially of the intention-to-treat method of statistical analysis when extensive contamination of the initial treatment allocations has occurred.

Treatment of Mild Hypertension Study 1993

The US Treatment of Mild Hypertension Study (TOMHS)[39] was not strictly controlled, as all trial entrants were given advice on nonpharmacological means designed to lower blood pressure. Against this background, there was then random double-blind allocation to one of several active antihypertensive drugs, or to placebo.

Men and women aged 45–69 years, either untreated, or with prior antihypertensive therapy withdrawn, could be entered. Previously untreated subjects were eligible if their diastolic blood pressure was in the range 90–99 mmHg at each of two initial visits, and averaged 90–99 mmHg over three screening visits. Those in whom previous drugs were withdrawn could enter the study if their diastolic pressure averaged 85–99 mmHg over three consecutive visits at least 8 weeks after stopping such treatment.

All trial entrants received intensive advice aimed at reducing weight by means of a fat-modified diet, lowering their consumption of alcohol and sodium chloride, and increasing their leisure-time physical activity. They were then randomly assigned to placebo ($n = 234$), chlorthalidone ($n = 136$), acebutolol ($n = 132$), doxazosin ($n = 134$), amlodipine ($n = 131$), or to the angiotensin converting enzyme (ACE) inhibitor enalapril ($n = 135$). If the diastolic pressure was 95 mmHg or more on three successive clinic visits, or 105 mmHg or more at a single visit, the drug dose was doubled. If elevated blood pressure persisted, chlorthalidone, in two increasing doses, was added, the original placebo group being included in this procedure, unless the patient was already on chlorthalidone, when enalapril was added instead. If the pressure remained uncontrolled in the above terms, open medication was begun.

Participants were seen at least 3-monthly for 4 years. Some were followed for up to 63 months. The trial was monitored, and clinical events evaluated, by independent scruti-neers. Analysis was by intention to treat.

All groups showed similar responses to the nonpharmacological measures. Weight loss averaged 2.6 kg after 4 years, overnight average urinary sodium excretion fell from 54 mmol l^{-1} per 8 hours at entry to 48 mmol l^{-1} per 8 hours (those on doxazosin had less of a reduction in sodium excretion than the others), reported alcohol consumption was less, and reported exercise was more. Total cholesterol, low-density lipoprotein (LDL) choles-terol, and triglyceride in plasma decreased in all groups, while high-density lipoprotein (HDL) cholesterol increased. The decreases in total and LDL cholesterol in the doxazosin group were more than with placebo ($P < 0.01$). An increase in plasma total cholesterol in the chlorthalidone group at 1 year was no longer evident at 4 years. There was a significant decrease in serum potassium concentration in the chlorthalidone group throughout.

At 4 years, 59% of those assigned to placebo and 72% of those on active drug continued on their allocated medication alone, while 33% of the initial placebo group were taking also an active antihypertensive drug outwith the trial protocol.

Blood pressure decreased from initial values in all groups, but to a significantly greater extent in those allocated to an active drug. At 4 years the averages were 126.7/79.4 mmHg in the combined active drug groups, against 132.6/81.9 mmHg in the placebo group ($P < 0.001$).

The groups assigned to individual active drugs were too small for worthwhile between-group analyses concerning cardiovascular morbidity to be possible. Thus the statistical evaluation was confined to a comparison of these drug-treated groups combined against the group randomized to placebo. The only significant finding to emerge was that, when both the major and minor declared cardiovascular events (the latter including transient cerebral ischemic attack, angina, and peripheral arterial occlusive disease) were combined, they were seen to be significantly fewer on active drug ($n = 74$, 11.08%) versus placebo ($n = 38$, 16.24%) ($P = 0.03$, 95% CI 0.44–0.97).

Any conclusions drawn from this trial must be very limited. No control group was included, so there is no certainty that the nonpharmacological methods alone lowered blood pressure. Neither here nor elsewhere has evidence been provided that such nonpharmacological approaches diminish morbidity in hypertension. The groups allo-cated to different active drugs were too small for any worthwhile comparisons to be made. Moreover, the placebo group was contaminated during the trial by the addition of active drug in one-third of patients. Nevertheless, these very modest data do reinforce the case for antihypertensive drug therapy limiting cardiovascular complications.

Summary of Trials in Mild-to-Moderate Hypertension

This group of trials is dominated in size by the first MRC study. Overall, the clearest, albeit numerically modest, benefit was in preventing stroke, even though coronary events outnumbered strokes in the subjects studied.[27] Therapeutic advantages were most obvious in men.

Trials in Hypertension in the Elderly

Kuramoto *et al.* 1981

A prospective single-blind, controlled trial was performed in elderly hypertensive men and women recruited from old peoples' homes in Tokyo, Japan.[40] One-hundred potential trial entrants had any current antihypertensive treatment stopped and were observed for approximately 1 year; during this run-in phase, six subjects dropped out because their blood pressure exceeded 200/110 mmHg and three for other reasons. The remaining 91 patients, with blood pressures of 160/90–200/110 mmHg, were then allocated to matched groups, 47 to receive placebo and 44 to receive active therapy comprising initially thiazide diuretic, to which latter were added stepwise as needed reserpine, methyldopa, and hydralazine. The trial was planned to continue for 4 years, in which time patients were reviewed at least monthly. Stated trial endpoints were blood pressure exceeding 200/110 mmHg, cerebrovascular or cardiac complications, other diseases needing hospital admission, or death.

The two groups were matched rather than randomly allocated, and thus were initially comparable, with an overall age range of 60–90 years (mean 76 years), and containing 50 men and 41 women. In the actively treated group, average blood pressure fell from an initial 171/87 mmHg to 151/80 mmHg in the fourth year. In the placebo group comparative figures were 166/86 and 150/78 mmHg, but the low latter readings were derived from only seven subjects remaining on placebo at the end of the study.

Cerebral plus cardiac morbid events totalled four (10.5%) in those actively treated, versus nine (22.0%) in those on placebo, an insignificant difference. However, when dropouts due to the need for treatment of severe hypertension were added, the figures changed to four (10.5%) versus 17 (41.5%) ($P < 0.01$). Deaths from all causes numbered seven in each group.

This trial was too small to show any treatment effect, unless the questionable endpoint of severe hypertension was allowed. Moreover, the allocation to treatment and control groups by matching rather than randomization has usually (but not always) led to the omission of this study from meta-analyses. The patients were apparently typical residents in homes for the aged in Japan. The drugs used were appropriate for the date, except that in nine patients reserpine and methyldopa were seemingly given together, a combination not now advised.[1]

Sprackling *et al.* 1981

Sprackling *et al.*[41] conducted a simple prospective study of mortality plus some aspects of morbidity in elderly hypertensive subjects who were randomly allocated to treated and observed groups; also recorded was the survival of comparable normotensive elderly persons not entered into the trial. Subjects were resident in geriatric hospitals or nursing homes in or near Nottingham, England, and were recruited on the basis of a single IVth phase diastolic blood pressure of 100 mmHg or more. Pre-entry examination was confined to seeking a history or signs of heart failure or stroke. No conditions incompatible with antihypertensive treatment were found. No routine investigations were done. Of 549 candidates screened, 123 qualified for the study and were allocated at random to either simple observation or to methyldopa, which was titrated so as to bring the standing diastolic pressure towards the target of 90 mmHg. Other antihypertensive drugs were not to be prescribed without withdrawing patients from the trial. Of the initial 123 subjects, one, with a diastolic pressure over 145 mmHg, was withdrawn at once and started on therapy. Two others, one from each group, were lost to follow-up, leaving 60 in each group for comparison.

The two groups were well matched in relevant criteria at entry. Analysis was by intention to treat; survival data were available for all subjects apart from the three mentioned above.

There were no significant differences in mortality between the treated and untreated hypertensive patients at any time up to 90 months from entry. Mortality in this elderly population was high, with only 10.3% of those treated and 9.9% of those untreated still alive at 90 months. Interestingly, survival was not significantly better at 90 months (12.4%) in the normotensive subjects of the population from which the trial patients had been recruited. Nonfatal cardiovascular morbidity (stroke, myocardial infarction, or heart failure) was no different in the treated and untreated hypertensives, with four and six such events, respectively, being recorded.

This trial was conducted in a group of elderly subjects apparently eminently representative of those defined. Statistical methods were declared at the start, and follow-up was thorough.

Clearly, the study was too small to demonstrate any benefit from therapy. Equally clearly, the negative results colored the views of those conducting the trial.

Australian Trial in Elderly Subjects 1981

The Australian Therapeutic Trial in Mild Hypertension has already been described.[30] Included were 582 subjects over the age of 60 years at entry, one-third of whom were aged 69–74 years at the end of the study. The results on these elderly patients were additionally reported on separately.[31]

Comparing active therapy with placebo by intention to treat, there was no significant reduction in trial endpoints ($n = 37$ versus 48) or in all-cause mortality ($n = 7$ versus 9). The on-treatment analysis did, however, reveal with therapy a significant reduction in trial endpoints ($n = 27$ versus 42; $P < 0.025$), but not in deaths ($n = 3$ versus 5).

This was the first report of a beneficial effect of antihypertensive drug therapy in a substantial group of subjects aged over 60 years, albeit a separate analysis in these elderly subjects was not apparently declared in the original trial design.

The European Working Party Trial on Hypertension in the Elderly 1985

The multicenter European Working Party trial (EWPHE)[35] was devoted specifically and exclusively to hypertension in subjects over 60 years of age. Prospective patients of both sexes were placed on placebo for a single-blind run-in period and entered the trial proper if the sitting blood pressure was in the range 160/90–239/119 mmHg. Those with a previous history of stroke or cardiac failure, with severe retinopathy, evident secondary hypertension, or other serious disease were excluded. Entrants were randomly assigned double-blindly to active therapy or to matching placebo. Trial endpoints and complications were preset and were reviewed throughout by an independent monitoring committee. Notably, a rise in blood pressure above the defined entry limits was a declared endpoint. The study ran from 1972 to 1984, being stopped on the recommendation of the monitoring committee when certain predefined endpoints had been reached. The results were analyzed by both intention-to-treat and on-treatment methods, the former evaluation being restricted to mortality.

At entry the two groups were similar in gender ratio, blood pressure, cardiovascular complications, and other relevant characteristics. A total of 256 patients defaulted or left the trial prematurely for various reasons, and in one center 29 patients stopped double-blind treatment after completing an agreed 5 years. A total of 291 patients remained in the study to its termination.

The overall intention-to-treat analysis revealed with therapy a nonsignificant fall in total mortality rate (-9%). There was a significant reduction in cardiovascular mortality rate (-27%; $P = 0.037$) made up of an insignificant fall in cerebrovascular mortality (-32%; $P = 0.16$) plus a significant fall in cardiac mortality (-38%; $P = 0.036$).

The on-treatment (per protocol) analysis also examined nonfatal endpoints. Total mortality rate was not significantly reduced by active treatment (-26%; $P = 0.077$). Cardiac deaths overall were reduced by treatment (-47%; $P = 0.048$), as were deaths from myocardial infarction (-60%; $P = 0.043$), but the decrease in cerebrovascular mortality was not significant (-43%; $P = 0.15$). Nonterminating cerebrovascular events were substantially fewer with active treatment (-52%; $P = 0.026$). Subset analysis showed benefit in both women and men.[42] Renal impairment was unusual, most often being associated with therapy; greater falls in blood pressure appeared to cause greater rises in serum creatinine.[43]

In a later detailed evaluation of the EWPHE data[44] concerning blood lipids, a high serum cholesterol at entry was found to be accompanied by longer survival. There was a lower noncardiovascular mortality with a high serum cholesterol, and an absence, in this elderly population, of a positive correlation between serum cholesterol and cardiovascular mortality.

The EWPHE trial clearly illustrated the benefits to be obtained from treating hypertension in elderly subjects, as had been earlier indicated in the analysis on the elderly subgroup of the Australian trial.[31] Moreover, EWPHE was the first controlled trial to show that antihypertensive therapy could lower the incidence of fatal myocardial infarction, in which regard the use of a potassium-conserving diuretic, triamterene, could be relevant.[45] The patients entered appear to have been representative of European elderly populations, and the treatment appropriate to practice that was current when the trial started. For a multicenter study this was small, indicating problems of recruitment, and thus needed to be prolonged. Partly perhaps for these reasons, the results were more impressive analyzed by the on-treatment rather than the intention-to-treat basis.

Coope and Warrender 1986

Coope and Warrender[46,47] reported on a British multicenter open trial of antihypertensive treatment in elderly men and women in primary care. Screening was performed in 10 718 men and women aged 60–79 years, comprising 78% of that total age range in 13 general practice lists. Those with a systolic pressure over 169 mmHg and/or diastolic pressure over 104 mmHg were asked to attend again on two further occasions. If the blood pressure remained at these levels, subjects were eligible for trial entry.

Those with blood pressures over 280 mmHg systolic or 120 mmHg diastolic or already on antihypertensive therapy (together $n = 1165$) were excluded, as were those with serious disease ($n = 1871$). A further 302 subjects declined to participate. A total of 884 patients (273 men and 611 women) entered the trial and were randomly assigned either to no treatment with the STOP-Hypertension study[50] in which patients with isolated systolic hypertension were excluded. The treatment employed in SHEP has contemporary relevance, notably the attention paid to sustaining serum potassium concentration during chlorthalidone administration. No information was provided concerning any precautions being taken at blood sampling to ensure an accurate estimation of serum potassium concentration;[45] presumably, therefore, these aspects were generally neglected. With the consequent attendant caveats, active therapy did not lower serum potassium unduly (4.1 ± 0.5 SD mmol l^{-1} on treatment versus 4.4 ± 0.4 mmol l^{-1} in the placebo group at 1 year).

Concern has been expressed that those entering the trial may have been unrepresentative of the American population as a whole.[51] Only 4736 of some 450 000 individuals screened were eventually studied.

Staessen *et al.*[52] have further drawn attention to a seeming anomaly in the SHEP results, in that there was a surprising progressive reduction in the treatment benefit regarding stroke with higher entry systolic pressure, the converse of what would be expected. This has, however, been discounted by members of the SHEP Research Group.[52]

STOP-Hypertension 1991

The Swedish Trial in Old Patients with Hypertension (STOP-Hypertension)[50] was multi-center, randomized, double-blind, and placebo controlled. Men and women having a systolic pressure above 180 mmHg with a diastolic pressure of at least 90 mmHg, or a diastolic pressure above 105 mmHg, irrespective of the systolic pressure, on each of three separate occasions during a 1-month placebo run-in period were entered. Any previous antihypertensive treatment was required to be discontinued at least 1 month before the run-in phase. Those with systolic pressures over 230 mmHg or diastolic pressures above 120 or below 90 mmHg were excluded. Altogether, 1627 patients were recruited and were randomly allocated to placebo or to active therapy.

Primary endpoints were defined at the outset, and were reviewed, while the conduct of the trial was monitored, by an independent committee. Statistical analysis was by intention to treat.

The two comparison groups were well matched in relevant characteristics at the outset.

The trial was stopped earlier than planned on the advice of the monitoring committee because clear results had emerged. All surviving patients were then recalled and examined; no patient was lost to follow-up.

The principal declared analysis, performed on grouped primary endpoints (fatal and nonfatal myocardial infarctions plus fatal and nonfatal strokes plus other cardiovascular deaths) were highly significantly reduced with active treatment (n = 58 versus 94; P = 0.0031). Stroke morbidity plus mortality was also reduced (n = 29 versus 53; P = 0.0081), as was all-cause mortality (n = 36 versus 63; P = 0.0079). No significant advantage was seen with active therapy concerning fatal or nonfatal myocardial infarction. The authors did not consider sudden deaths as myocardial infarction deaths, and did not regard it as proper to alter this view retrospectively. There were 4 sudden deaths on active treatment against 12 on placebo; these have, despite the view of the trial authors, been counted as 'major coronary events' in *Tables 8.1* and *8.2*. In this population treatment benefits were as distinct, or more distinct, in women compared with men.

This well-conducted and clearly reported trial seems to have been conducted on a representative Swedish elderly population, being performed in 116 of a total of 846 health centers. The drugs employed are those in current use; the use of a potassium-conserving diuretic, amiloride, together with a thiazide diuretic, is noteworthy.[45]

The Second Medical Research Council Trial 1992

The Second MRC trial[6] had the declared objective to examine whether treatment initially with a diuretic or beta-blocker in hypertensive subjects aged 65–74 years at entry could diminish the risk of stroke, coronary heart disease, or death. As in the first MRC trial,[32] the second was conducted in British general practices dealing predominantly with patients in the upper socioeconomic strata. Invitations to attend screening were sent to 184 653 people, of whom 68% attended. Of these, 20 389 with systolic pressures in the range 160–209 mmHg, and a diastolic pressure below 115 mmHg, progressed to the run-in stage. In these latter subjects blood pressure was recorded again 1, 4, and 8 weeks after screening, and then, if still indicated, by their doctor on four further occasions. Those in whom the means of all four of the doctor's measurements were 160–209 mmHg systolic and less than 115 mmHg diastolic progressed to the main trial. Those already on treatment for hypertension, or with a recent history of cardiac disease or stroke, were excluded. A total of 4396 subjects eventually entered the trial proper.

Patients were randomly allocated, single-blind only, to one of four treatment categories: hydrochlorothiazide plus amiloride (or matching placebo); or atenolol (or matching placebo). The dose in each trial category could be increased as necessary. Later, the two active treatments might be combined, and nifedipine or other supplementary drugs could be added. Target blood pressure was a systolic pressure at or below 150 mmHg for those starting with a systolic pressure below 180 mmHg, or at or below 160 mmHg for those starting with a systolic pressure at or above 180 mmHg. Participants were followed fortnightly for 1 month, then monthly for 2 months, and every 3 months thereafter.

Declared trial endpoints were fatal or nonfatal stroke, coronary events (including sudden death), other major cardiovascular events, or death from any cause. Statistical analysis was primarily by intention to treat, although a limited supplementary on-treatment analysis was also presented. In all analyses the placebo groups were merged. The trial was monitored by an independent committee. The trial entry groups (diuretic n = 1081, beta-blocker n = 1102, placebo n = 2213) were well matched in all relevant aspects.

Both the systolic and diastolic pressure fell shortly after randomization in all groups, the greatest systolic fall being in the diuretic group at 3 months. From 2 years onwards, the average blood pressures in all groups changed little, settling at around 165/85 mmHg in controls and 150/80 mmHg in treated patients. These differences between actively treated patients and controls are probably significant, although this was not stated. From the data given for control subjects, it is evident that many patients had 'isolated systolic' hypertension.

More patients randomized to atenolol required supplementary drugs (52% at 5 years) than did those randomized to diuretic (38%). Of the initial atenolol group, 16% of the observation period included treatment supplementation with a diuretic, while in the initial diuretic group 11% of the period of observation included supplementation with a beta-blocker. Active treatment was started during the trial in 11% of those allocated to placebo.

Over the course of the trial 'about 25% of people' were stated to be lost to follow-up. However, as was pointed out in a later paper,[53] this was according to a more rigid criterion than was used in other trials.[35,50] Mortality was verified in all instances (*Tables 8.1* and *8.2*). The cumulative percentages of those who stopped taking their randomized treatment, including those withdrawn but continuing to be followed plus those lost to follow-up, were 48% in the initial diuretic group, 63% in the initial atenolol group, and 53% of those allocated to placebo.

The intention-to-treat analysis showed that the total of strokes, fatal plus nonfatal, was significantly reduced by 25% in patients randomized to active treatment (n = 101 versus total cardiovascular events (95% CI 0.25–0.64), for stroke (95% CI 0.24–0.77), and for severe arrhythmia (95% CI 0.03–0.66). While all-cause mortality was lower with nifedipine, considered alone this difference was not statistically significant. These broad conclusions were not altered when additional analyses were done according to the actual therapy received during the trial, as well as after exclusion of the 74 patients reallocated initially because of severe hypertension. There was no evidence that cancer was more frequent with nifedipine. As in two other trials in elderly hypertensive subjects,[6,44] the serum cholesterol level at entry was not a predictor of clinical cardiovascular events.

There are inevitable reservations concerning this trial, especially the assignment of patients to treatment groups alternately rather than at random, the licence afforded to physicians to switch some patients with severe hypertension from placebo to nifedipine at the outset, and the ambiguous description of the use of supplementary therapy in those allocated to placebo. Nevertheless, the data deserve attention because they deal with Chinese subjects, who comprise a large proportion of the world's population, and because active therapy was based on the calcium antagonist nifedipine, which figures infrequently, and then only as an additive drug, in other trials of antihypertensive treatment.

Summary of Trials in the Elderly

Treatment of hypertension in elderly subjects has provided clear benefits for a range of complications, namely stroke, congestive heart failure, major coronary events, cardiovascular mortality, and mortality from all causes. Women, as well as men, have profited from therapy. Drug therapy does not appear to affect cognitive function.

Trials with Multiple Risk Factor Interventions and Comparing Different Healthcare Systems

HDFP 1979

The US Hypertension Detection and Follow-up Program (HDFP)[57–63] was a very large multicenter study. Initial population screening identified a possible 178 000 male and female hypertensive participants aged 30–69 years. Of these, 89% completed a first screening procedure, when 22 978 were found to have a diastolic pressure of 95 mmHg or more. Rescreening was completed on 17 476, of whom 10 940 had a mean diastolic pressure of 90 mmHg or more and entered the definitive study. Trial entrants were allocated to one of three strata of severity: stratum I, entry diastolic pressure 90–104 mmHg, $n = 7825$; stratum II, entry diastolic pressure 105–114 mmHg, $n = 2052$; stratum III, entry diastolic pressure above 114 mmHg, $n = 1063$.

After initial clinical assessment, entrants were randomly assigned either to the special intervention group (stepped care; SC) or to the ostensible control group (referred care; RC). SC participants were offered a free preset program of antihypertensive therapy in special HDFP centers; the stepwise drug stages were first diuretic, to which were added progressively, as indicated: reserpine or methyldopa; then hydralazine; then guanethidine (with or without withdrawal of drugs previously added); finally, the addition or substitution of other (unnamed) drugs. Target diastolic pressure was 90 mmHg or less for those with initial pressures over 100 mmHg, or a fall of at least 10 mmHg if the initial diastolic pressure was 90–99 mmHg. Recruits were advised to avoid a high salt intake. The protocol further provided[57] that for SC patients 'who were markedly overweight (40% or more above desirable weight), frankly hypercholesterolemic (250 mg dl^{-1} or more), or heavy smokers (ten or more cigarettes per day), counseling was to be offered with regard to control of these risk factors'. SC subjects additionally received substantial financial and other material support: 'Economic barriers to adherence were removed as far as possible; drugs, visits at the centers, laboratory tests, and if necessary, transportation were provided at no cost to the participant. Waiting times were minimized ... Appointments were made at convenient hours ... A Program physician was on call at all times ...'. SC participants were seen 'at least every four months'. The persons assigned to the RC group 'were advised to consult their personal sources of medical care for treatment of their hypertension. If no such source was identified, RC participants were given a list of local physicians or other sources of medical care'. The trial was to proceed over 5 years, all patients (SC and RC) being seen at home at 1, 2, 4 and 5 years for examination, including blood-pressure measurement. However, when taking into account clinic attendances also, SC patients were seen more often than RC subjects.

The primary endpoint of the study was all-cause mortality; detailed reports were also made of cerebrovascular and coronary heart disease. Fatal myocardial infarctions were counted from death certificates. Nonfatal coronary events were diagnosed if indicated by any one of three approaches at follow-up: electrocardiographic Minnesota coding; Rose questionnaire; or an affirmative response to the question 'Have you been told by a doctor, nurse, therapist, or medical assistant that you have had a heart attack or a coronary (myocardial infarction, coronary thrombosis, or coronary occlusion)?'.[58,62] Reported events were subject to independent scrutiny.

The average age of trial entrants was 51 years; 54% were men and 56% were white. Comparability of subjects in the SC and RC groups in all three strata was similar at the outset in relevant characteristics. Over the 5 years of the study home visits were completed in some 90% of both the SC and the RC group.[60] At 5 years, 23 SC and 38 RC patients had been lost to follow-up.[57] The percentage of patients receiving antihypertensive drugs increased each year in both groups, being consistently higher for the SC subjects. Notably, however, 60% of the RC patients were receiving such treatment by the fifth year, while more than 20% of the SC patients were not.[60] Throughout, blood pressure was lower in the SC than the RC group.

All-cause mortality at 5 years was evidently less with SC than RC overall (349 versus 419; $P < 0.01$), being clearest in stratum I (I, 231 versus 291; II, 70 versus 77; III, 48 versus 51). However, a substantial number of deaths were attributable to noncardiovascular causes (154 versus 179). Whereas black men and women and white men did better in the SC group, white women suffered the same mortality rate in SC and RC groups.

The total number of strokes was also significantly lower with SC (102 versus 159; $P < 0.001$, 95% CI 0.05–0.16). By stratum of entry diastolic pressure, the figures were: I, 59 versus 88; II, 25 versus 36; III, 18 versus 35.[63]

The computation of coronary events is complicated, because slightly different figures appeared in various reports, and because different criteria were available for defining nonfatal myocardial infarction.[58,62,64] Fatal myocardial infarctions were given[64] as (SC versus RC): overall, 131 and 148 (stratum I, 86 and 107; stratum II, 29 and 22; stratum III, 16 and 19).

The 5-year incidence of nonfatal myocardial infarctions stepped care versus referred care according to differing diagnostic criteria, were (SC versus RC):[58] by electrocardiogram, 40 and 41; by history, 124 and 161 ($P < 0.03$); by Rose questionnaire, 320 and 379 ($P < 0.03$); overall, 346 and 413 ($P < 0.02$). The overall figures for nonfatal infarctions according to the entry diastolic pressure were: stratum I, 250 and 283; stratum II, 68 and 89; stratum III, 28 and 41 (all nonsignificant).

various cardiovascular causes (n = 32 versus 47; P = 0.017), fewer stroke deaths (n = 2 versus 9; P = 0.043), and fewer deaths from all cardiovascular causes combined (n = 42 versus 57; P = 0.012). Noncardiovascular deaths were similarly frequent in the two groups (n = 23 versus 26).

All first coronary events, including symptomless occurrences, were lower with metoprolol (n = 111 versus 144; P = 0.001, 95% CI 0.41–0.80 at median and 0.58–0.98 at the end of the trial). Nonfatal coronary events were also fewer with metoprolol (n = 82 versus 109; P = 0.0034). Nonfatal strokes were similarly frequent (metoprolol versus diuretic, n = 21 and 18). The evident advantage of metoprolol over diuretic in relation to coronary events was seen in both smokers and nonsmokers. There was also a clear benefit from metoprolol use concerning all-cause mortality in smokers, although this was less marked in nonsmokers.

The MAPHY reports have, despite their interest, and their obvious bearing on other studies, not been universally accepted, there being some vocal critics[98] as well as advocates.[99] The method of statistical analysis has attracted particular concern. Furthermore, a comparison with the HAPPHY data indicates a considerably higher mortality among smokers in MAPHY who took diuretic,[100] while atenolol failed to protect smokers, who seemed on that drug to have a higher mortality rate than did the smokers on diuretic. Undoubtedly, some commentators[101] have an aversion to a seemingly very positive trial which was closely associated with another, negative, study.

Summary

An interpretation of IPPPSH, HAPPHY, and MAPHY in the context of other trials is given in the following section.

Comparative Efficacy and Dangers of Various Drug Classes: Drugs used in Trials

Attempts to assess any differential capacity of various classes of drug to limit cardiovascular morbidity in hypertension have been, as has been seen, virtually confined in prospective trials to comparisons of thiazide diuretics with beta-blockers. Even that modest aim has provided inconsistent, sometimes conflicting, and generally unsatisfactory data. In large part, the problems have resulted from the usual need in trials to prescribe several drugs together in order to achieve control of blood pressure, thus hindering analysis.

Both the MRC trials[6,32] suggested that thiazide was superior to beta-blocker in preventing stroke, but this was not supported by other studies.[91,94–97]

One analysis[36] of the first MRC trial[32] indicated that patients allocated to propranolol had significantly fewer coronary events than those assigned to either placebo or bendrofluazide. In that trial, coronary events were notably less frequent in male nonsmokers on propranolol, and the rates of sudden death in men were markedly lower on propranolol than on bendrofluazide.[33] Those results were largely confirmed by the MAPHY trials[95–97] but not by the HAPPHY trial.[94]

The IPPPSH study[91] similarly showed substantially fewer critical cardiac events in male nonsmokers taking a beta-blocker. Conversely, the second MRC trial[6] found that initial allocation to a diuretic, but not to a beta-blocker, was associated with a reduction in coronary events.

In an analysis restricted to the first MRC trial, HAPPHY, and IPPPSH, an insignificant trend towards lower mortality was found with treatment based on a beta-blocker rather than alternatives.[101] In an evaluation of SHEP,[49] which was limited by small numbers, Kostis *et al.*[102] could not find evidence of additional benefit attributable to atenolol or reserpine when added to low-dose chlorthalidone.

There have been hints[79–81] that subjects with electrocardiographic abnormalities did worse on diuretic treatment, comparing intervention with control, in MRFIT,[73] HDFP,[57] and the Oslo trial.[29]

Deserving of re-emphasis is the fact that, especially in the MRC trials,[6,32] many patients did not continue on their initial drug alone, and that often comparisons were rather of overall treatment strategies.[53,54,64]

Case–control studies have well-recognized limitations. Accepting this caveat, it has been found that: (1) beta-blockers, when used to treat hypertension, might prevent first nonfatal myocardial infarctions;[103] and (2) that both beta-blockers and potassium-wasting diuretics could increase the risk of sudden death.[93,104] There is good evidence that with diuretic use potassium losses are best avoided, preferably by using potassium-conserving agents.[6,35,45,48–50,81,92]

A separate issue concerns the use of calcium antagonists. Although it has been stated that calcium antagonists have not been employed in clinical trials in hypertension, this is incorrect. Nifedipine was prescribed as initial therapy in one trial,[56] and as a supplementary drug in at least two studies,[6,46] while amlodipine was employed as initial therapy in one.[39] Some retrospective analyses have suggested that the use of calcium antagonists, particularly short-acting dihydropyridines, carries an increased risk of causing myocardial infarction. No evidence of this was seen in the Chinese STONE trial,[56] but there the incidence of myocardial infarction was very low. In a case–control study, Psaty *et al.*[105] found a dose-related enhanced likelihood of myocardial infarction in treating hypertension with a calcium antagonist. Furberg *et al.*,[106] reviewing 16 trials in the different context of ischemic heart disease, found that short-acting nifedipine was associated with a dose-related increased risk of mortality as compared with placebo. These matters have caused vigorous debate. Furberg and Psaty[107] have defended their findings, and have proposed that calcium antagonists are unsuitable for use as first- or second-step drugs in hypertension, that only low doses should be employed if they are considered necessary, and that dihydropyridines should in any event be avoided. Contrary opinions have been that newer, slow-acting dihydropyridines are safe for use as initial drugs in hypertension.[108,109] Prospective trials are needed to resolve these controversies.

Although it has been widely supposed that diuretics and beta-blockers are the only drugs that have been found to limit morbidity in hypertension, this is not correct. As indicated in *Table 8.1*, a wide range of drugs has been employed in the trials reviewed herein. Among 23 studies, diuretics (albeit in widely varying types and doses, and with very different attempts at potassium conservation) featured in 22,[6,15–17,19–21,25,28–30,32,35,39,40,46,48–50,56,57,73] methyldopa in 11,[15,17,19,20,29,30,32,40,41,46,57] rauwolfia in 10,[16,17,21,25,28,40,48,49,57,73] sundry beta-blockers in 9,[6,29,30,32,39,46,48–50] hydralazine in 6,[17,30,40,48,57,73] guanethidine in 5,[16,20,32,57,73] dihydropyridine calcium antagonists in 4,[6,39,46,56] an ACE inhibitor in two,[39,56] and bethanidine,[20] clonidine,[30] a ganglion blocker,[15] and an alpha-blocker,[39] in just one study each. Unspecified supplementary drugs were allowed in the protocols of at least six trials.[6,28,29,39,57,75] However, it is the case that diuretics and beta-blockers were favored as initial drugs in a World Health Organization (WHO) report in 1978,[110] and they have provided the basic therapy in several recent trials, while no angiotensin II antagonist has yet been evaluated.

Despite the above suggestions of differential drug benefit, the weight of evidence indicates that the undoubted clinical advantages derive from blood pressure reduction *per se*, largely independently of the agent or agents employed.

Thoroughness of Blood-pressure Reduction and Effect on Morbidity

Retrospective studies have shown that in both malignant[14] and nonmalignant hypertension[91,111,112] morbidity is less and the prognosis better the more thoroughly blood pressure is lowered with drugs, with the greater relative benefit being for stroke than coronary events. Nevertheless, in community surveys,[112–114] treated hypertensive patients have consistently been found still to fare worse than comparable control subjects drawn from the same population. At least in part,[115] this latter deficiency could reflect inadequate control of blood pressure in clinics.[112] Not surprisingly, blood-pressure reduction in trials is likely to be more thorough than in routine circumstances.[116] Even so, the finding in one meta-analysis[64] that antihypertensive therapy appeared quickly to abolish virtually all of the epidemiologically predicted risk of stroke was simultaneously unexpected and gratifying, and is so far unexplained. One tentative speculation[34] is that thiazides used in the trials surveyed may have conferred protection additional to that of blood-pressure reduction, although other studies[91,94–96] have not confirmed this. There is certainly considerable evidence to suggest that the reduction of blood pressure, both systolic and diastolic, should be as radical as possible.

A partly contrary hypothesis concerns hypertensive patients with coronary artery disease. In these, it has been suggested, the optimum range of diastolic pressure on treatment should be around 85–90 mmHg. Higher pressures are not desirable, while too marked a reduction will perhaps be accompanied by an increased risk of myocardial infarction. This is the concept of the J-curve, in support of which has been adduced epidemiological and therapeutic evidence.[117,118] The issue has aroused vehement and still unresolved controversy.[119]

The BBB trial[120] was directed at these matters, and compared two groups of patients, in one of which the diastolic pressure was sustained below that in the other by some 7–7.5 mmHg over 4 years. No differences in cardiovascular morbidity or mortality were found between the groups, possibly because the patients were too few.

Hypertension, Risk Factors, and Antihypertensive Therapy

The cardiovascular dangers of hypertension are increased in proportion to the height of the arterial pressure, and are compounded by the presence of other risk factors, prominent amongst which are cigarette smoking, a high serum concentration of total and/or LDL cholesterol, a low serum concentration of HDL cholesterol, diabetes mellitus, male gender, a history of vascular disease, and age.[1] It has been proposed that the absolute benefits to be derived from antihypertensive therapy should thus be greatest in those subjects at greatest risk, even where much of the excess risk is a consequence of factors other than hypertension. Browner and Hulley[80] formulated a model in which each additional risk factor multiplied the absolute benefit of treating hypertension. The concept has obvious clinical and economic attractions. Smith and Egger[121] pointed out that, if in antihypertensive treatment trials the risk of stroke, expressed in relative terms, was reduced by 40%, a tenfold variation in stroke rate in the different trials would mean that the number of patient-years of therapy needed to prevent one stroke could range from around 100 to

1000. This aspect is considered in more detail below. The balance between the benefits and side-effects of treatment should, moreover, be more favorable among patients at higher risk of vascular disease. A New Zealand group[122] has proposed, not without arousing dissent,[123] that decisions to treat raised blood pressure should be based primarily on the estimated absolute risk of cardiovascular disease rather than upon the blood-pressure level alone. It has been pointed out[121] that this concept runs directly counter to the notion advanced by some that antihypertensive drugs should be withheld in subjects who continue to smoke. One meta-analysis of treatment trials[27] has been specifically directed to the assessment of absolute benefit. Requiring emphasis, however, is the fact that, despite the greater quantitative benefit expected from treating hypertension in persons with additional risk factors, such persons retain the excess risk consequent upon those other factors.[80] Moreover, a person with hypertension as the sole discernable risk still carries the excess hazard of that hypertension. It will further be apparent that two aspects need to be distinguished: the risk of increasingly severe high blood pressure as such, and the compounding of that risk by other accompanying adverse influences.

There is little dispute regarding the need to lower markedly high blood pressure, and, as has already been shown, there is undoubted cardiovascular benefit from such action. With regard to more moderate hypertension, experience with antihypertensive treatment has, as we have also seen, been less consistent, although it seems generally to be worthwhile. It is rather the influence of additional cardiovascular risk factors on the absolute benefits of antihypertensive treatment that now concern centers. Browner and Hulley[80] illustrated their model with various supportive empirical examples drawn from the HDFP data.[57] However, since HDFP involved multiple risk factor interventions, not antihypertensive treatment alone, it was hardly an ideal or even appropriate source of confirmatory data. Some anomalies emerged, possibly by chance, in the analysis. In HDFP, the relative benefit of treatment on mortality, which was expected to be consistent irrespective of age, was found, for example, only in subjects aged over 50 years. Conversely, the Australian trial[30] showed that the relative therapeutic benefits were slightly greater in the younger age group. The Australian trial indeed produced several findings inconsistent with the model. In a detailed analysis of these aspects, Ramsay[72] pointed out that, while in the Australian trial complications were, predictably, more frequent in older subjects, men, cigarette smokers, leaner persons, and those with higher systolic pressures, the benefits of treatment were not related to these risk factors. The only variables to presage increased efficacy of treatment were, by univariate analysis, lower serum cholesterol and lower systolic blood pressure. None was significant by multivariate analysis. These data suggested to Ramsay that the decision to treat mild hypertension with drugs should not be influenced by the presence or absence of other risk factors, which rather merited direct attack.

Another inconsistency emerged in the first MRC trial.[32] In a paper emphasizing the importance of additional risk factors in affecting the absolute therapeutic benefit,[34] subgroup analysis indicated that male smokers allocated to initial treatment with propranolol did not show a reduction in stroke. As mentioned above, in the SHEP study[49] treatment benefit became less as the entry systolic pressure became higher.[52]

Data from trials conducted in hypertensive patients over the age of 60 years have, however, generally provided more consistent and supportive evidence for the model. In an evaluation of six such trials, Lever and Ramsay[53] showed that, despite wide variations in event rates with treatment, the proportionate reduction in fatal stroke was generally around 33% and that in fatal coronary events was 26%. Thus the absolute incidence of events, which they speculated could well have been governed by risk factors additional to hypertension, was lowered most in those elderly subjects at greatest hazard. These concepts were confirmed and extended in the meta-analysis by Gueyffier et al.,[27] which is considered in more detail below.

Hoes et al.[124] provided an analysis in which they raised the possibility that drug treatment in hypertensive patients at low risk not only had no benefit but might even increase mortality. Their paper was, however, criticised[125] because, inter alia, of the arbitrary exclusion of some trials from consideration plus the converse inclusion of multiple risk factor intervention studies such as HDFP[57] and MRFIT.[73]

Some commentators have cautioned against indiscriminate adherence to the concept of directing antihypertensive therapy to those at greatest overall cardiovascular risk.[123,126] Early treatment of mild, uncomplicated hypertension can effectively prevent the development of more severe blood-pressure elevation, with its attendant complications, which can then be more difficult to deal with. These cautionary notions become increasingly substantial with the progressive introduction of more effective and more acceptable antihypertensive drugs, and could additionally stimulate greater critical interest in the problematic area of nonpharmacological means of blood-pressure lowering.

Comments on Meta-analyses of Treatment Trials

It is neither intended, nor would it be appropriate, to review in detail the numerous meta-analyses that have been performed on the trials of drug treatment in hypertension. However, some observations are pertinent, in that they illustrate how the characteristics of the trials reviewed herein have affected their selection or omission in those meta-analyses and, of even greater importance, how such selectorial vagaries can lead to widely differing conclusions concerning the benefits attributable to therapy.

The trials by Hamilton et al.[15] and Kuramoto et al.[40] have usually, but not invariably,[127] been excluded from meta-analyses, because in these trials allocation to the actively treated and control groups was not randomized. Hampton[24] omitted the Oslo trial[29] on similar grounds, but this appears to have been an erroneous decision, as that study was appropriately randomized. The trial by Sprackling et al.[41] has been discarded by some reviewers[64] for the reason that only mortality results were made available. This again seems to be an error, because data on stroke, myocardial infarction, and heart failure were reported, although the intention to analyze them was not apparently declared beforehand.

In a meta-analysis of outcome trials in elderly hypertensives, Thijs et al.[127] excluded SHEP[49] on the grounds that it dealt exclusively with isolated systolic hypertension, which they regarded as a separate pathophysiological entity. They did, however, include data from two other trials[6,46] conducted in elderly patients, both of which included a substantial number of subjects with isolated systolic hypertension.

Almost certainly, most controversy has concerned the MRFIT[73] and HDFP[57] studies, neither of which involved a strict control group, while in both studies multiple risk factors, additional to hypertension, were addressed. HDFP[57] in particular has clouded meta-analyses, because it was a large study in which, in certain categories, the special intervention group showed a reduction in the frequency of adverse coronary events. Clearly, inclusion or exclusion of HDFP in meta-analyses can greatly affect the estimates of whether or not antihypertensive treatment benefits associated coronary artery disease. Several reviewers have indeed excluded both HDFP and MRFIT[24,26,27,125] on the specific grounds that these were confounded studies, and others have excluded them without comment.[66] Conversely, others have embraced both studies[77,82,124] although sometimes with reservations.[82,124] Some have rejected MRFIT but accepted HDFP.[64,128] Apparently, thus far no-one has included MRFIT while excluding HDFP.

Meta-analyses by MacMahon *et al.*

Particularly intriguing is a series of four meta-analyses performed over the years by largely the same group of authors (one appears as a coauthor of all four studies). In 1986, MacMahon *et al.*[82] analyzed seven controlled trials. They also considered separately, and with reservations concerning the lack of placebo control, HDFP[57] and MRFIT.[73] This analysis[82] showed that drug treatment in mild-to-moderate hypertension gave a substantial reduction, by some 40%, in both fatal and nonfatal stroke. Mortality from all causes was significantly lowered, but only if the data of HDFP were included. However, as described earlier, HDFP demonstrated that with intervention there was a reduction in deaths from a range of noncardiovascular causes, and this can hardly be taken to be a benefit of antihypertensive therapy. Neither in individual trials nor collectively was evidence found in this meta-analysis of a reduction in mortality or morbidity from coronary artery disease, unless the dubious inclusion of HDFP data obtained by Rose questionnaire or brief history[58] was allowed. As discussed below, the authors rejected the latter approach as probably distorting their analysis.[82]

In 1989, three of the four earlier authors presented a second meta-analysis,[77] comprising the same nine trials as were examined before,[82] again restricting the diagnosis of nonfatal myocardial infarction in HDFP[58] to evidence based on electrocardiography. Once more concern was voiced[77] that HDFP data obtained by Rose questionnaire or history included substantial numbers of 'false-positive' myocardial infarctions. However, their other previous reservations[82] concerning HDFP and MRFIT were no longer expressed, both studies being included with little comment. Indeed, the authors stated, incorrectly, that 'MRFIT is the only one of these trials with additional interventions by design (lipid-lowering diet and smoking cessation)'. They went on to claim that the exclusion of MRFIT 'would not materially affect the review findings'. While their results were, not surprisingly, much as they had obtained from somewhat similar data in 1986,[82] their conclusions were more buoyant. They now spoke of 'impressive ... results ... for stroke *and total mortality*' [my italics], and stated 'The results for coronary heart disease suggest that treatment is more likely than not to result in some benefit'.

In 1990, the third of this series of meta-analyses appeared,[64] surveying, in addition to those examined in 1986 and 1989, five other trials. HDFP was now elevated to the status of an unconfounded study, while MRFIT was discarded entirely 'because of the potential confounding likely to result from the concurrent interventions for smoking cessation and cholesterol lowering'.[129] No explanation was offered as to why HDFP, which also attempted these interventions, was not similarly rejected. A further aspect of concern, as noted above, was that in HDFP[58] coronary disease had been defined in three ways: on serial electrocardiographic criteria, by Rose questionnaire, or by medical history. In the first[82] and second[77] meta-analyses, electrocardiographic data only were used, the evidence from Rose questionnaires and annual medical enquiries being avoided as 'wholly subjective' and thus possibly biased. Specifically, it was concluded that self-reported data included many events apart from those considered as myocardial infarctions in other trials.[82] Notwithstanding these earlier reservations, in the third meta-analysis[64] coronary events were defined solely according to whether the patients had been medically informed that they had suffered a myocardial infarction; data from electrocardiography or Rose questionnaires were omitted. The 1990 meta-analysis,[64] with these important differences, concluded that on antihypertensive therapy there was a substantial reduction in stroke (by 42%; 95% CI 0.33–0.50), with a more marginal, but nevertheless nominally significant, reduction in coronary morbidity (by 14%; 95% CI 0.04–0.22). The latter significant finding

Only two trials dealt with recurrent stroke,[20,21] the number of patients was few, and the results heterogeneous. Although no result was significant, the data did not exclude the possibility of a beneficial effect of treatment on stroke recurrence or congestive heart failure.

Correction for bias because of withdrawals due to worsening hypertension in the control group[27,131] increased the estimate of treatment benefit in two of the groups. In elderly patients the absolute reduction in stroke incidence improved from five to nine, and that of major coronary events increased from three to four, both per 1000 patient-years. In mild-to-moderate hypertension in younger patients, the absolute risk reduction for stroke improved from one to two per 1000 patient-years, but coronary benefit remained insignificant.

Conclusions

This survey of the trials of drug treatment of hypertension that have been conducted over the past four decades has shown that there are definite, albeit circumscribed, benefits from such therapy. Treatment relieves overt hypertensive heart failure, and can correct the malignant phase. Short of these complications, treatment of what may broadly be defined as 'marked' hypertension (*Tables 8.1* and *8.2*) is effective, most obviously in preventing the onset of congestive heart failure.[27] With hypertension in a person who has suffered stroke, treatment started within 2–4 weeks can limit the chances of recurrence, and also possibly of developing congestive heart failure.[27] With mild-to-moderate hypertension in young to middle-aged subjects, treatment benefits are modest, concern only stroke obviously, and are even less clear in women. By contrast, in hypertensive subjects over 60 years of age, including those with isolated systolic hypertension, treatment limits congestive heart failure, stroke, and coronary events, and extends longevity, both in women and men. A curiosity of trials in the elderly[6,44,56] is that elevated serum total cholesterol concentration has thus far seemed beneficial rather than adverse, an aspect clearly needing further study. Antihypertensive drug therapy probably can, even short of malignant hypertension, slow a decline in renal function.

Antihypertensive drugs and their deployment have evolved in parallel with increasing expertise in clinical-trial methodology, a circumstance which has inevitably exposed the frailties of some early studies. Moreover, several large trials, which are expensive both in terms of time and financial cost, have spawned only modest, or even confusing results,[24,26] provoking the disparate reactions of nihilistic condemnation, defensive advocacy, or even evangelism, none of which appear to this commentator to be appropriate or productive. The achievements of antihypertensive drug therapy are considerable, although in some aspects limited. With regard to mild hypertension in particular,[132] more critical and creative research is required.

References

1. Robertson JIS, Ball SG. *Hypertension for the Clinician*. London: WB Saunders, 1994.
2. Ramsay LE, Waller PC. Strokes in mild hypertension: diastolic rules. *Lancet* 1986; ii: 854–6.
3. Wright BM. Diastolic versus systolic. *Lancet* 1986; ii: 1041–2.
4. Peart WS, Greenberg G. Diastolic versus systolic. *Lancet* 1986; ii: 1042.
5. Bullpitt CJ. Is systolic pressure more important than diastolic? *J Human Hypertens* 1990; 4: 471–6.
6. Medical Research Council Working Party. Medical Research Council trial of treatment in older adults: principal results. *Br Med J* 1992; 304: 405–12.

7. Alderman MH, Madhaven S, Cohen H, *et al.* Low urinary sodium is associated with greater risk of myocardial infarction among treated hypertensive men. *Hypertension* 1995; **25**: 1144–52.
8. Ramsay LE, Haq IU, Yeo WW, Jackson PR. Might non-pharmacological treatment disadvantage patients with hypertension? *J Human Hypertens* 1995; **9**: 653–7.
9. Robertson JIS. Guidelines for the treatment of hypertension: a critical review. *Cardiovasc Drugs Ther* 1994; **8**: 665–72.
10. Smirk FH. *High Arterial Pressure.* Oxford: Blackwell, 1957: 678–705.
11. Pickering GW. *High Blood Pressure*, 2nd edn. London: Churchill Livingstone, 1968: 414–25.
12. Leishman AWD. Hypertension – treated and untreated: a study of 400 cases. *Br Med J* 1959; **i**: 1361–8.
13. Leishman AWD. Merits of reducing high blood pressure. *Lancet* 1963; **i**: 1284–8.
14. Newman MJD, Robertson JIS. Some aspects of prognosis in treated hypertension. *Br Med J* 1959: **i**: 1368–73.
15. Hamilton M, Thompson EN, Wisniewski TKM. The role of blood pressure control in preventing complications of hypertension. *Lancet* 1964; **i**: 235–8.
16. Wolff FW, Lindeman RD. Effects of treatment in hypertension: results of a controlled study. *J Chron Dis* 1966; **19**: 227–40.
17. Veterans Administration Cooperative Study Group. Effects of treatment on morbidity in hypertension: results in patients with diastolic blood pressures averaging 115 through 129 mmHg. *J Am Med Assoc* 1967; **202**: 1028–34.
18. Freis ED. Reminiscences of the Veterans Administration Trial in the Treatment of Hypertension. *Hypertension* 1990; **16**: 472–5.
19. Barraclough MA, Joy MD, MacGregor GA, *et al.* Control of moderately raised blood pressure: report of a co-operative randomized controlled trial. *Br Med J* 1973; **3**: 434–6.
20. Carter AB. Hypotensive therapy in stroke survivors. *Lancet* 1970; **i**: 485–9.
21. Hypertension–Stroke Cooperative Study Group. Effect of antihypertensive treatment on stroke recurrence. *J Am Med Assoc* 1974; **229**: 409–18.
22. Veterans Administration Cooperative Study Group. Effects of treatment on morbidity in hypertension. II. Results in patients with diastolic blood pressure averaging 90 through 114 mmHg. *J Am Med Assoc* 1970; **213**: 1143–52.
23. Veterans Administration Cooperative Study Group. Effects of treatment on morbidity in hypertension. III. Influence of age, diastolic pressure, and prior cardiovascular disease. *Circulation* 1972; **45**: 991–1004.
24. Hampton JR. An appraisal of hypertension trials. *Medicographia* 1983; **5**(Suppl 2): 12–15.
25. McFate Smith W. Treatment of mild hypertension: results of a ten-year intervention trial. *Circ Res* 1977; **40**(Suppl 1): 98–105.
26. Hampton JR. Treating mild hypertension – an unnecessary luxury. *Cardiovasc Drugs Ther* 1989; **3**: 749–52.
27. Gueyffier F, Froment A, Gouton M. New meta-analysis of treatment trials of hypertension: improving the estimate of benefit. *J Human Hypertens* 1996; **10**: 1–8.
28. Perry HM, Goldman AI, Lavin MA, *et al.* Evaluation of drug treatment in mild hypertension: VA–NHLBI feasibility trial. *Ann NY Acad Sci* 1978; **304**: 267–88.
29. Helgeland A. Treatment of mild hypertension: a five year controlled drug trial: the Oslo study. *Am J Med* 1980; **69**: 725–32.
30. Australian Mild Hypertension Trial Management Committee. Australian therapeutic trial in mild hypertension. *Lancet* 1980; **i**: 1261–7.
31. Australian Mild Hypertension Trial Management Committee. Treatment of mild hypertension in the elderly. *Med J Aust* 1981; **2**: 398–402.
32. Medical Research Council Working Party. MRC trial of treatment of mild hypertension: principal results. *Br Med J* 1985; **291**: 97–104.
33. Medical Research Council Working Party. Coronary heart disease in the Medical Research Council trial of treatment of mild hypertension. *Br Heart J* 1988; **59**: 364–78.
34. Medical Research Council Working Party. Stroke and coronary heart disease in mild hypertension: risk factors and the value of treatment. *Br Med J* 1988; **296**: 1565–70.
35. Amery A, Birkenhäger W, Brixko P, *et al.* Mortality and morbidity results from the European Working Party on High Blood Pressure in the Elderly trial. *Lancet* 1985; **i**: 1349–54.
36. Green KG. British MRC trial of treatment for mild hypertension: a more favorable interpretation. *Am J Hypertens* 1991; **4**: 723–4.
37. Medical Research Council Working Party on Mild to Moderate Hypertension. Adverse reactions to bendrofluazide and propranolol for the treatment of mild hypertension. *Lancet* 1981; **ii**: 539–43.
38. Medical Research Council Working Party on Mild to Moderate Hypertension. Ventricular extrasystoles during thiazide treatment: substudy of the MRC mild hypertension trial. *Br Med J* 1983; **287**: 149–53.
39. Neaton JD, Grimm RH, Prineas RJ, *et al.* Treatment of Mild Hypertension Study: final results. *J Am Med Assoc* 1993; **270**: 713–24.
40. Kuramoto K, Matsushita S, Kuwajima I, Murakami M. Prospective study on the treatment of mild hypertension in the aged. *Jpn Heart J* 1981; **22**: 75–85.
41. Sprackling ME, Mitchell JRA, Short AH, Watt G. Blood pressure reduction in the elderly: a randomised controlled trial of methyldopa. *Br Med J* 1981; **283**: 1151–3.
42. Amery A, Birkenhäger W, Brixko R, *et al.* Efficiency of anti-hypertensive drug treatment according to age, sex, blood pressure, and previous cardiovascular disease in patients over the age of 60. *Lancet* 1986; **ii**: 589–92.

43. de Leeuw P. Renal function in the elderly: results from the European Working Party on High Blood Pressure in the Elderly trial. *Am J Med* 1991; **90**(3A): 45–9.
44. Staessen J, Amery A, Birkenhäger W, *et al*. Is a high serum cholesterol level associated with a longer survival in elderly hypertensives? *J Hypertens* 1990; **8**: 755–61.
45. Singh BN, Hollenberg NK, Poole-Wilson PA, Robertson JIS. Diuretic-induced potassium and magnesium deficiency: relation to drug-induced QT prolongation, cardiac arrhythmias, and sudden death. *J Hypertens* 1992; **10**: 301–16.
46. Coope J, Warrender TS. Randomised trial of treatment of hypertension in elderly patients in primary care. *Br Med J* 1986; **293**: 1145–51.
47. Coope J. Hypertension in the elderly. *J Hypertens* 1987; **5**(Suppl 3): 69–72.
48. Perry HM, Smith WM, McDonald RH, *et al*. Morbidity and mortality in the Systolic Hypertension in the Elderly Program (SHEP) pilot study. *Stroke* 1989; **20**: 4–13.
49. SHEP Cooperative Research Group. Prevention of stroke by antihypertensive drug treatment in older persons with isolated systolic hypertension: final results of the Systolic Hypertension in the Elderly Program (SHEP). *J Am Med Assoc* 1991; **265**: 3255–64.
50. Dahlöf B, Lindholm LH, Hansson L, *et al*. Morbidity and mortality in the Swedish Trial in Old Patients with Hypertension (STOP-Hypertension). *Lancet* 1991; **338**: 1281–5.
51. Staessen J, Fagard R, Amery A. Isolated systolic hypertension in the elderly: implications of SHEP for clinical practice and for ongoing trials. *J Human Hypertens* 1991; **5**: 469–74.
52. Staessen JA, Amery A, Birkenhäger W, *et al*. Inverse association between baseline pressure and benefit from treatment in isolated systolic hypertension. *Hypertension* 1994; **23**: 269–70.
53. Lever AF, Ramsay LE. Treatment of hypertension in the elderly. *J Hypertens* 1995; **13**: 571–9.
54. Robertson JIS. The case for antihypertensive drug treatment in subjects over the age of 60. *Cardiovasc Drugs Ther* 1992; **6**: 579–83.
55. Prince MJ, Bird AS, Blizard RA, Mann AH. Is the cognitive function of older patients affected by antihypertensive treatment? Results from 54 months of the Medical Research Council's treatment trial of hypertension in older adults. *Br Med J* 1996; **312**: 801–5.
56. Gong L, Zhang W, Zhu Y, *et al*. Shanghai trial of nifedipine in the elderly (STONE). *J Hypertens* 1996; **14**: 1237–45.
57. Hypertension Detection and Follow-up Program Cooperative Group. Five-year findings of the Hypertension Detection and Follow-up Program: I. Reduction in mortality in persons with high blood pressure, including mild hypertension. *J Am Med Assoc* 1979; **242**: 2562–71.
58. Hypertension Detection and Follow-up Program Cooperative Group. Effect of stepped care treatment on the incidence of myocardial infarction and angina pectoris: 5-year findings of the Hypertension Detection and Follow-up Program. *Hypertension* 1984; **6**(Suppl 1): 198–206.
59. Curb JD, Maxwell MH, Schneider KA, *et al*. Adverse effects of antihypertensive medications in the Hypertension Detection and Follow-up Program. *Prog Cardiovasc Dis* 1986; **29**(Suppl 1): 73–88.
60. Davis BR, Ford CE, Remington RD, *et al*. The Hypertension Detection and Follow-up Program design, methods, and baseline characteristics and blood pressure response of the study population. *Prog Cardiovasc Dis* 1986; **29**(Suppl 1): 11–28.
61. Langford HG, Stamler J, Wassertheil-Smoller S, Prineas RJ. All-cause mortality in the Hypertension Detection and Follow-up Program: findings for the whole cohort and for persons with less severe hypertension, with and without other traits related to risk of mortality. *Prog Cardiovasc Dis* 1986; **29**(Suppl 1): 29–54.
62. Borhani NO, Blaufox MD, Oberman A, Polk BF. Incidence of coronary heart disease and left ventricular hypertrophy in the Hypertension Detection and Follow-up Program. *Prog Cardiovasc Dis* 1986; **29**(Suppl 1): 55–62.
63. Daugherty S, Berman R, Entwisle G, Haerer AF. Cerebrovascular events in the Hypertension Detection and Follow-up Program. *Prog Cardiovasc Dis* 1986; **29**(Suppl 1): 63–72.
64. Collins R, Peto R, MacMahon S, *et al*. Blood pressure, stroke, and coronary heart disease. Part 2: Short-term reductions in blood pressure: overview of randomised drug trials in their epidemiological context. *Lancet* 1990; **335**: 827–38.
65. Swales JD, Ramsay LE, Coope JR, *et al*. Treating mild hypertension: report of the British Hypertension Society Working Party. *Br Med J* 1989; **298**: 694–8.
66. Isles CG, Brown JJ, Lever AF, Murray GD. What clinical trials have taught us. In: Bühler FR, Laragh JH (eds), *Handbook of Hypertension*, Vol. 13, *The Management of Hypertension*. Amsterdam: Elsevier, 1990: 18–32.
67. Holme I, Ekelund LG, Hjermann I, Leren P. Quality-adjusted meta-analysis of the hypertension/coronary dilemma. *Am J Hypertens* 1994; **7**: 703–12.
68. Freis ED. Should mild hypertension be treated? *New Engl J Med* 1982; **307**: 306–9.
69. Stamler J. In discussion. *Ann NY Acad Sci* 1978; **304**: 319.
70. Beevers DG. Comments on the Hypertension Detection and Follow-up Programme. *R Soc Med Int Congr Symp Ser* 1980; **26**: 9–11.
71. Stimmler WH, Plunkett M, McMillen M. Should mild hypertension be treated with drugs? *New Engl J Med* 1980; **302**: 1204.
72. Ramsay LE. Mild hypertension: treat patients, not populations. *J Hypertens* 1985; **3**: 449–55.
73. Multiple Risk Factor Intervention Trial Research Group. Multiple Risk Factor Intervention Trial: risk factor changes and mortality results. *J Am Med Assoc* 1982; **248**: 1465–77.
74. Multiple Risk Factor Intervention Trial Group. Statistical design considerations in the NHLI Multiple Risk Factor Intervention Trial (MRFIT). *J Chron Dis* 1977; **30**: 261–75.

75. Multiple Risk Factor Intervention Trial Group. The Multiple Risk Factor Intervention Trial. *Ann NY Acad Sci* 1978; **304**: 293–308.
76. Cohen JD, Grimm RH, Smith WM. Multiple Risk Factor Intervention Trial (MRFIT). VI: Intervention on blood pressure. *Prev Med* 1981; **10**: 501–18.
77. Cutler JA, MacMahon SW, Furberg CD. Controlled clinical trials of drug treatment for hypertension: a review. *Hypertension* 1989; **13**(Suppl 1): 36–44.
78. Multiple Risk Factor Intervention Trial Research Group. Baseline rest electrocardiographic abnormalities, antihypertensive treatment and mortality in the Multiple Risk Factor Intervention Trial. *Am J Cardiol* 1985; **55**: 1–15.
79. Holme I, Helgeland A, Hjermann I, *et al*. Treatment of mild hypertension with diuretics: the importance of ECG abnormalities in the Oslo study and in MRFIT. *J Am Med Assoc* 1984; **251**: 1298–9.
80. Browner WS, Hulley SB. Effect of risk status on treatment criteria: implications of hypertension trials. *Hypertension* 1989; **13**(Suppl 1): 51–6.
81. Grobbee DE, Hoes AW. Non-potassium-sparing diuretics and risk of sudden cardiac death. *J Hypertens* 1995; **13**: 1539–45.
82. MacMahon SW, Cutler JA, Furberg CD, Payne GH. The effects of drug treatment for hypertension on morbidity and mortality from cardiovascular disease: a review of randomized controlled trials. *Progr Cardiovasc Dis* 1986; **29**(Suppl 1): 99–118.
83. Epstein M. Effects of ACE inhibitors and calcium antagonists on progression of chronic renal disease. *Blood Pressure* 1995; **4**(Suppl 2): 108–12.
84. Swales J. Renal dysfunction in hypertension. *Lancet* 1995; **345**: 740–1.
85. Whelton PK, Perneger TV, Brancati FL, Klag MJ. Epidemiology and prevention of blood pressure-related renal disease. *J Hypertens* 1992; **10**(Suppl 7): 77–84.
86. Janssen WMT, de Zeeuw D, de Jong PE. Renal function during antihypertensive treatment. *Lancet* 1995; **346**: 193.
87. Zanchetti A, Sleight P, Birkenhäger WH. Evaluation of organ damage in hypertension. *J Hypertens* 1993; **11**: 875–82.
88. Tomson CRV, Petersen K, Heagerty AM. Does treated essential hypertension result in renal impairment? A cohort study. *J Human Hypertens* 1991; **5**: 189–92.
89. Ruilope L, Alcázar JM, Hernandez E, *et al*. Does an adequate control of blood pressure protect the kidney in essential hypertension? *J Hypertens* 1990; **8**: 525–31.
90. Kudo K. Renal function during antihypertensive treatment. *Lancet* 1995; **346**: 192–3.
91. The IPPPSH Collaborative Group. Cardiovascular risk and risk factors in a randomized trial of treatment based on the beta-blocker oxprenolol: the International Prospective Primary Prevention Study in Hypertension (IPPPSH). *J Hypertens* 1985; **3**: 379–92.
92. Hoes AW, Grobbee DE, Peet TM, Lubsen J. Do non-potassium-sparing diuretics increase the risk of sudden death in hypertensive patients? Recent evidence. *Drugs* 1994; **47**: 711–33.
93. Hoes AW, Grobbee DE, Lubsen J, *et al*. Diuretics, beta-blockers, and the risk of sudden cardiac death in hypertensive patients. *Ann Int Med* 1995; **123**: 481–7.
94. Wilhelmsen L, Berglund G, Elmfeldt D, *et al*. Beta-blockers versus diuretics in hypertensive men: main results from the HAPPHY trial. *J Hypertens* 1987; **5**: 561–72.
95. Wikstrand J, Warnold I, Olsson G, *et al*. Primary prevention with metoprolol in patients with hypertension: mortality results from the MAPHY study. *J Am Med Assoc* 1988; **259**: 1976–82.
96. Wikstrand J, Warnold I, Tuomilehto J, *et al*. Metoprolol versus thiazide diuretics in hypertension: morbidity results from the MAPHY study. *Hypertension* 1991; **17**: 579–88.
97. Olsson G, Tuomilehto J, Berglund G, *et al*. Primary preventiion of sudden cardiovascular death in hypertensive patients: mortality results from the MAPHY study. *Am J Hypertens* 1991; **4**: 151–8.
98. Moser M, Sheps S. Confusing messages from the newest of the beta-blocker/diuretic hypertension trials: the metoprolol atherosclerosis prevention in hypertensives trial. *Arch Int Med* 1989; **149**: 2174–5.
99. Kendall MJ. *Beta Blockade and Cardioprotection*. London: Science Press, 1991: 31–6.
100. Kaplan NM. Critical comments on recent literature. *Am J Hypertens* 1988; **1**: 428–30.
101. Shinton RA, Beevers DG. A meta-analysis of mortality and coronary prevention in hypertensive patients treated with beta-receptor blockers. *J Human Hypertens* 1990; **4**(Suppl 2): 31–4.
102. Kostis JB, Berge KG, Davis BR, *et al*. Effect of atenolol and reserpine on selected events in the Systolic Hypertension in the Elderly Program (SHEP). *Am J Hypertens* 1995; **8**: 1147–53.
103. Psaty BM, Koepsell TD, Logerfo JP, *et al*. Beta-blockers and primary prevention of coronary heart disease in patients with high blood pressure. *J Am Med Assoc* 1989; **261**: 2087–94.
104. Siscovick DS, Raghunathan TE, Psaty BM, *et al*. Diuretic therapy and the risk of primary cardiac arrest. *New Engl J Med* 1994; **330**: 1852–7.
105. Psaty BN, Heckbert SR, Koepsall TD, *et al*. The risk of myocardial infarction associated with antihypertensive drug therapies. *J Am Med Assoc* 1995; **274**: 620–5.
106. Furberg CD, Psaty BM, Meyer JV. Nifedipine: dose-related increase in mortality in patients with coronary heart disease. *Circulation* 1995; **92**: 1326–31.
107. Furberg CD, Psaty BM. Calcium antagonists: not appropriate as first line antihypertensive agents. *Am J Hypertens* 1996; **9**: 122–5.
108. Epstein M. Calcium antagonists: still appropriate as first line antihypertensive agents. *Am J Hypertens* 1996; **9**: 110–21.

109. Mancia G, van Zwieten PA. How safe are calcium antagonists in hypertension and coronary heart disease? *J Hypertens* 1996; **14**: 13–17.

110. Report of a WHO Expert Committee. *Arterial hypertension.* Technical Report Series No. 628. Geneva: WHO, 1978: 35–7.

111. Bulpitt CJ, Beevers DG, Butler A, *et al.* Treated blood pressure, rather than pretreatment, predicts survival in hypertensive patients. *J Hypertens* 1988; **6**: 627–32.

112. Hansson L. Shortcomings of current antihypertensive therapy. *Am J Hypertens* 1991; **4**(Suppl): 84–7.

113. Lindholm LH, Ejlertsson G, Schersten B. High risks of cerebrovascular morbidity in well treated male hypertensives: a retrospective study of 40–59 year old hypertensives in a Swedish primary care district. *Acta Med Scand* 1984; **216**: 251–9.

114. Isles CG, Walker LM, Beevers DG, *et al.* Mortality in patients of the Glasgow Blood Pressure Clinic. *J Hypertens* 1986; **4**: 141–56.

115. Robertson JIS. Should the costs of development inhibit research into new antihypertensive drugs? *Cardiovasc Drugs Ther* 1989; **3**: 757–9.

116. Ruilope LM. The hidden truth: what do the clinical trials really tell us about BP control? *J Human Hypertens* 1995; **9**(Suppl): 3–7.

117. Cruickshank JM. Coronary flow reserve and the J curve relation between diastolic blood pressure and myocardial infarction. *Br Med J* 1988; **297**: 1227–30.

118. D'Agostino RB, Belanger AJ, Kannel WB, Cruickshank JM. Relation of low diastolic pressure to coronary heart disease death in presence of myocardial infarction: the Framingham study. *Br Med J* 1991; **303**: 385–9.

119. Zanchetti A, Amery A, Berglund G, *et al.* How much should blood pressure be lowered? The problem of the J-shaped curve. *J Hypertens* 1989: **7**(Suppl 6): 338–48.

120. Hansson L. The BBB Study: the effect of intensified antihypertensive treatment on the level of blood pressure, side-effects, morbidity and mortality in 'well-treated' hypertensive patients. *Blood Pressure* 1994; **3**: 248–54.

121. Smith GD, Egger M. Who benefits from medical interventions? *Br Med J* 1994; **308**: 72–4.

122. Jackson R, Barham P, Bills J, *et al.* Management of raised blood pressure in New Zealand: a discussion document. *Br Med J* 1993; **307**: 107–10.

123. Nicholls MG, Richards AM. New Zealand core services committee repeats mistakes of JNC-V. *Am J Hypertens* 1995; **8**: 542.

124. Hoes AW, Grobbee DE, Lubsen J. Does drug treatment improve survival? Reconciling the trials in mild-to-moderate hypertension. *J Hypertens* 1995; **13**: 805–11.

125. Egger M, Smith GD. Risks and benefits of treating mild hypertension: a misleading meta-analysis? *J Hypertens* 1995; **13**: 813–15.

126. Zanchetti A. Antihypertensive therapy: pride and prejudice. *J Hypertens* 1995; **13**: 1522–8.

127. Thijs L, Fagard R, Lijnen P, *et al.* A meta-analysis of outcome trials in elderly hypertensives. *J Hypertens* 1992; **10**: 1103–9.

128. Collins R, MacMahon S. Blood pressure, antihypertensive drug treatment and the risks of stroke and of coronary heart disease. *Br Med Bull* 1994; **50**: 272–98.

129. MacMahon S. The effects of antihypertensive drug treatment on the incidence of stroke and of coronary heart disease. *Clin Exp Hypertens, Ser A* 1989; **11**: 807–23.

130. Alderman MH. Meta-analysis of hypertension treatment trials. *Lancet* 1990; **335**: 1092–3.

131. Murray GD, Findlay JG. Correcting for bias caused by drop-outs in hypertension trials. *Stat Med* 1988; **7**: 941–6.

132. Ménard J, Chatellier G. Mild hypertension: the mysterious viability of a faulty concept. *J Hypertens* 1995; **134**: 1071–7.

9

Aspirin, Heparin, and Fibrinolytic Therapy for Acute Coronary Syndromes without ST Elevation

Marcus Flather and Julian Collinson

Introduction

This chapter discusses the important randomized controlled trials of antiplatelet (aspirin, ticlopidine, and sulphinpyrazone), anticoagulant (heparin and warfarin), and fibrinolytic (tissue plasminogen activator, streptokinase, urokinase, and anistreplase) therapy in patients with acute coronary syndromes without ST elevation. Newer antithrombotic strategies for these syndromes are also discussed.

A clinically useful separation can be made between patients with ST elevation, and those without ST elevation on the electrocardiogram (ECG), at presentation. Patients with acute coronary syndromes and significant ST segment elevation have a high likelihood of acute myocardial infarction (MI), and most go on to receive treatment with thrombolytic therapy.[1] Patients without ST elevation are more likely to have unstable angina, or less severe MI. The measurement of sensitive enzyme markers such as CKMB, or muscle proteins such as troponin, may help to differentiate between unstable angina and MI during the early stages, but even so there may be a 'grey zone' where the diagnosis is still uncertain. Non-Q-wave MI is usually a *post hoc* diagnosis, which can be made on the basis of serial ECGs and cardiac enzymes 24–48 hours following presentation.[2] Subendocardial MI is a pathological diagnosis that can only be made with certainty at post mortem.[3] The term 'myocardial infarction without ST elevation' may be a more useful clinical description of non-Q-wave or subendocardial MI.

Acute coronary syndromes are usually triggered by rupture of an existing atheromatous plaque causing local exposure of thrombogenic material, which activates the coagulation system and platelets resulting in thrombus formation.[4] This results in a dynamic obstruction to coronary flow by the physical presence of thrombus and coronary spasm. The speed of onset of the acute coronary syndrome, degree of occlusion, presence of collateral circulation, and ability of local mechanisms to control the problem all influence the severity of the process and the clinical presentation. Thus rapid onset of a total coronary occlusion in a large epicardial artery may typically present as acute MI with ST segment

patients were actually randomized, but data were only presented for 214 patients. The results showed that the frequency of new transmural MI in the combined heparin groups at 7 days was 3% compared to 15% in the other groups (risk reduction 80%; $P < 0.01$). This result is difficult to interpret, since it could be biased by not including data from the 186 patients excluded for various reasons (including noncardiac pain, transmural MI, not eligible) after randomization.

Trials of Antiplatelet and Anticoagulant Therapy (Table 9.1)

Théroux et al.[18] randomized 479 patients with unstable angina with ECG changes compatible with myocardial ischemia to heparin ($n = 118$; 5000 units bolus followed by 1000 units per hour), aspirin ($n = 121$; 650 mg initial dose followed by 325 mg twice daily), both ($n = 122$), or neither ($n = 118$). The main outcomes were death, MI, or refractory angina (recurrent angina with ECG changes on optimal medical therapy, or need for an urgent intervention) assessed at a mean of 6 days. There were no deaths in any of the three treatment groups (aspirin, heparin, or the combination) compared to two deaths (1.7%) in the control group. The rates of new MI were 3.3%, 0.8%, 1.7%, and 12% for the aspirin, heparin, combination, and control groups, respectively ($P = 0.012$, <0.001, and 0.001 compared to control). The rates of any event (death, new MI, or refractory angina) were 16.5%, 9.3%, 11.4%, and 26.2% ($P = 0.66$, <0.001, 0.003), respectively. Major bleeds occurred in 1.7% in the aspirin alone group, 1.7% in heparin alone, 3.4% in the combination, and 1.7% in placebo. About half of these bleeds were related to a puncture-site bleed following cardiac catheterization. In a follow-up study, patients who had an outcome event in the first study were censored from the analysis and events were recorded during a 96-hour period after cessation of the study heparin infusion.[19] Events (mostly refractory angina, but MI and death were also documented) were recorded more frequently in the heparin group (13.1%) compared to aspirin alone, aspirin plus heparin or placebo (5.0%, 4.6%, 9.2%, respectively; $P < 0.01$ for comparison of heparin with the other groups). This observation generated the hypothesis of reactivation of the thrombotic process, particularly when heparin is discontinued. Event-free survival over the 90 days after randomization was reported to be significantly better in the aspirin plus heparin group compared to the aspirin alone and heparin alone groups, and all treatment groups had a better outlook than placebo. Thus administration of aspirin helped to reduce the rate of ischemic events over the longer term.

The RISC group[20] from Sweden randomized 796 men with acute myocardial ischemia without ST elevation to control ($n = 199$), heparin ($n = 198$; 5000 units 6 hourly for 24 hours, then 3750 units 6 hourly for 4 days), aspirin ($n = 189$; 75 mg daily), or aspirin plus heparin ($n = 210$). The rates of death or MI for patients receiving aspirin compared to controls at 5, 30 and 90 days were 2.5% versus 5.8% ($P = 0.33$), 4.3% versus 13.4% ($P < 0.001$), and 6.5% versus 17.1% ($P < 0.0001$), respectively. There was no apparent benefit observed in the group treated with heparin compared to placebo heparin. Analysis of the four groups separately showed benefit only in the groups tested with aspirin (i.e. aspirin alone or aspirin plus heparin), and the combination treatment did not demonstrate any clear advantage of adding heparin to aspirin, although the event rate was slightly lower (3.7% in the aspirin alone group versus 1.4% in the aspirin plus heparin group) in the first 5 days when heparin was given. Only one major bleed was recorded in the heparin-treated group (0.25%).

The ATACS (Antithrombotic Therapy in Acute Coronary Syndromes) research group[21] studied the effects of aspirin alone (162.5 mg daily; $n = 109$) compared to aspirin plus

Table 9.1 Results for death or MI in randomized controlled trials of antiplatelet and/or anticoagulant therapy compared to controls for acute coronary syndromes without ST elevation (one trial by Telford and Wilson[17] evaluating intravenous heparin reported on only 50% of randomized patients and has been excluded from the table)

Trial	Treatment	Eligibility	Follow-up	Death or MI events/patients (%)			
				AP	Control	Hep	Control
Lewis *et al.* 1983[14]	1. ASA 324 mg daily 2. Placebo	Men with UA screened <48 h after hospital admission	12 weeks	31/625 (5.0)**	65/641 (10.1)	—	—
Cairns *et al.* 1985[15]	1. ASA 325 mg 4 times daily 2. Sulfinpyrazone 200 mg 4 times daily 3. ASA plus sulfinpyrazone 4. Control	UA <70 years randomized within 8 days of admission to CCU	18 months (mean)	29/276 (10.5)†	41/279 (14.6)	—	—
Balsano *et al.* 1990[16]	1. Ticlopidine 250 mg twice daily for 6 months 2. Control	UA within 48 h of admission to CCU, ST depression on ECG	6 months	23/314 (7.3)**	46/338 (13.9)	—	—
Théroux *et al.* 1988[18,19]	1. ASA 650 mg first dose then 325 mg twice daily for 6 days 2. i.v. Hep initial bolus 5000 iu, then 1000 iu h^{-1} target aPTT 1.5–2.0 3. ASA plus Hep 4. Placebo	UA with most recent pain <24 h, CK <2 × normal, ECG changes of ischemia	6 days	6/243 (2.5)**	15/236 (6.4)	3/240 (1.2)**	18/239 (7.5)
RISC 1990[20]	1. ASA 75 mg daily for 3 months 2. i.v. Hep intermittent bolus 5000 iu every 6 h for first 24 h, then 3750 iu every 6 h for 4 days 3. ASA plus Hep 4. Placebo	Men <70 years with UA or suspected non-Q-wave MI onset within previous 4 weeks and randomized within 72 h of admission to CCU	12 weeks	26/399 (6.5)**	68/397 (17)	45/408 (11.0)	49/388 (12.6)
ATACS 1994[21]	1. ASA 162.5 mg + Hep 100 iu kg^{-1} bolus + infusion for 3 days (target aPTT 2 × normal), then ASA + warfarin (target INR 2–3 × normal) for 12 weeks 2. ASA 162.5 mg daily	UA or suspected non-Q-wave MI <48 h from last attack of pain. No prior ASA use	12 weeks	—	—	8/105 (7.6)	11/109 (10)
FRISC 1996[22]	1. ASA + LMWH 120 iu kg^{-1} s.c. twice daily for 6 days, then 7500 iu daily for 35–45 days 2. ASA first dose 300 mg, then 75 mg daily	Men >40 years UA or suspected MI with ECG changes but no ST↑ or Q-waves. Pain onset <72 h	6 days 40 days	—	—	13/741 (1.8)** 59/738† (8.0)	36/757 (4.8) 81/755 (10.7)

AP, antiplatelet therapy; aPTT, activated partial thromboplastin time; ASA, aspirin; CCU, coronary care unit; ECG, electrocardiogram; Hep, heparin; INR, international normalized ratio; i.v., intravenous; LMWH, low-molecular-weight heparin; MI, myocardial infarction; s.c., subcutaneously.
†$P = 0.07$, **$P < 0.01$, for comparison of treatment with control.

heparin followed by aspirin plus warfarin after 3–4 days (heparin 100 iu kg^{-1} bolus and infusion to maintain activated partial thromboplastin time (aPTT) at two times control, and warfarin to maintain an international normalized ratio (INR) between 2 and 3; $n = 105$) in patients with acute myocardial ischemia without ST elevation who were not prior aspirin users. The main outcomes were recurrent angina, defined as rest pain with associated ECG changes in spite of maximal medical therapy, new MI, and death. At 14 days the rate of the primary outcome (recurrent angina, new MI, or death) was 27% in the aspirin group compared to 10% in the aspirin plus anticoagulant group ($P = 0.004$), and after 12 weeks the rate of the primary outcome was 28% in the aspirin alone group compared to 19% in the combination group ($P = 0.09$). There were no major bleeds recorded in the aspirin alone group compared to 2.9% in the aspirin plus warfarin group. These results help to support the hypothesis that the combination of an antiplatelet agent plus an anticoagulant may be more effective than an antiplatelet agent alone, especially if anticoagulant therapy is continued longer term.

The Fragmin during Instability in Coronary Artery Disease (FRISC) study[22] group evaluated subcutaneous low-molecular-weight heparin (LMWH) (dalteparin 120 iu kg^{-1} for 6 days, followed by 7500 iu daily for 35–45 days) plus aspirin (initial dose 300 mg, then 75 mg daily) compared with aspirin alone. LMWH acts mainly by AT III-mediated inhibition of factor Xa. A total of 1506 patients with acute myocardial ischemia with ECG changes (excluding established Q-waves or ST segment elevation) were randomized. The rate of death or MI at 6 days of follow-up (the primary outcome) was 1.8% in the LMWH group compared to 4.8% in the control group ($P = 0.001$). After 40 days the rate of death or MI was 8.0% versus 10.7% ($P = 0.07$) and after 150 days it was 14.0% versus 15.5% ($P = 0.41$), respectively. The secondary outcome of death, MI, or need for revascularization was significantly lower in the LMWH group compared to controls, at both 6 and 40 days of follow-up, and a nonsignificant trend was maintained at 150 days. Major bleeds occurred in 8 patients (1.1%) in the LMWH group compared to 6 patients in the control group (0.8%).

Two other studies were primarily concerned with the effects of heparin and aspirin on recurrent ischemic events detected by Holter monitoring. The study by Serneri et al.[23] randomized 97 patients to either heparin infusion, heparin by intermittent intravenous injection, or aspirin. The main outcome of recurrent ischemic episodes was less frequent in the heparin infusion group compared to the intermittent heparin bolus group or the aspirin group ($P < 0.001$). Statistical comparisons were also presented as the number of episodes of recurrent ischemia in the 3 days after compared to the 2 days prior to randomization (for heparin infusion, heparin bolus, and aspirin groups the numbers of events were 5 versus 55 ($P < 0.001$), 61 versus 51 (NS), and 54 versus 40 (NS), respectively). Holdright et al.[24] randomized patients with acute myocardial ischemia to aspirin alone, or aspirin plus intravenous heparin (the latter given for 48 hours). No statistical differences in the number or duration of ischemic episodes during the 48 hours after randomization were detected, although total duration of ischemia (sum of all patients in each group) was lower in the combination group compared to aspirin alone (2911 versus 4908 minutes, respectively). The rate of death or MI in hospital was reported as 27.0% in the heparin plus aspirin group compared to 30.5% in the aspirin alone group (NS).

Trials of Thrombolytic Therapy (Table 9.2)

Eight randomized trials of thrombolytic therapy versus control in patients with acute coronary syndromes without ST elevation have been identified with information about rates of death and MI.[25–32] In the seven smaller trials (200 patients or less each), a variety of

Table 9.2 Results for death or MI in randomized controlled trials of thrombolytic therapy compared to controls for acute coronary syndromes without ST elevation

Trial	Treatment	Eligibility	Outcome in table	Follow-up	Outcome (events/patients (%)) Treatment	Control	Relative risk	P
TIMI IIIB 1994[25]	1. t-PA 0.8 mg kg⁻¹, ⅓ as bolus, rest of dose over 90 min 2. Placebo control	Ischemic chest pain, lasting >5 min and <6 h with evidence of IHD and enrollment <24 h	Death or MI	42 days	65/729 (8.9)	51/774 (6.9)	1.29	0.05
Bar et al. 1992[26]	1. Anistreplase 30 units over 5 min 2. Placebo control	Unstable angina with ECG changes and onset of pain <12 h	Death or MI	In-hospital	32/80 (40.0)	22/79 (27.8)	1.44	NS
Schreiber et al. 1992[27]	1. UK 3 MU over 90 min + Hep 2. UK 3 MU + ASA 3. Placebo control	Angina lasting longer than 10 min at rest with ischemic ECG changes and enrollment <24 h	Death or MI	4 days	8/96 (8.3)	2/53 (3.8)	2.18	NS
Freeman et al. 1992[28]	1. t-PA 0.49 MU kg⁻¹ over 1 h then 0.07 MU kg⁻¹ h⁻¹ for 9 h 2. Placebo control	Pain lasting longer than 20 min and <12 h prior to admission. Age <75 years	Death or MI	Inpatient	3/35 (8.6)	2/35 (5.7)	1.50	NS
Karlsson et al. 1992[29]	1. t-PA 1 mg kg⁻¹ over 4 h 2. Placebo control	Ongoing unstable angina <48 h with ECG changes. Men aged 40–70 years	Death and MI	45 days	11/105 (10.4)	12/100 (12.0)	0.92	NS
Saran et al. 1990[30]	3. SK 1.5 million units over 30 min 4. Placebo control	Prolonged chest pain with repeated episodes lasting >20 min	Death or MI	6 months	4/24 (17)	7/24 (29)	0.71	NS
Williams et al 1990[31]	1. t-PA 0.75 mg kg⁻¹ over 1 h 2. t-PA 0.75 mg kg⁻¹ over 1 h (total of 100 mg over 6 h) 3. Placebo control	Chest pain at rest. Ischemic ECG changes or angiography demonstrating at least 80% stenosis in an epicardial artery	MI	48 h	3/44 (6.8)	1/22 (4.5)	1.51	NS
Nicklas et al. 1989[32]	1. t-PA 150 mg/8 h 2. Placebo control	Unstable angina, angiographic evidence of CAD, ECG changes. Age 18–80 years	Death or MI	In-hospital	2/20 (10)	0/20 (0)		

ASA, aspirin; CAD, coronary artery disease; ECG, electrocardiogram; Hep, heparin; IHD, ischemic heart disease; MI, myocardial infarction; MU, mega units;

primary outcome measures were reported, including death, MI, recurrent ischemia, need for revascularization, ischemic pacing threshold, and percentage change in lumen diameter. The majority of these trials had a short follow-up period of 48–96 hours; but one reported a 6-month follow-up[30] and another a 1-year follow-up.[29] All allowed conventional antianginal treatment. Only one trial demonstrated a significant reduction in the rate of death, MI or need for revascularization with the use of SK (1.5 million units over 30 minutes) after 6 months follow-up (20.8% in the SK group versus 50.0% in the placebo group; $P < 0.05$).[30]

Four trials evaluated an angiographic outcome.[26,28,29,32] One trial found a reduced rate of coronary thrombi (52% for the t-PA group versus 92% in the control group; $P = 0.002$)[28] and another found a significant decrease in diameter stenosis with anistreplase (11% in the t-PA group versus 3% in the control group; $P = 0.008$.[26] However, in these studies there were no significant differences in clinical outcomes in terms of death, MI, or the need for urgent revascularization.

The TIMI IIIB (Thrombolysis in Myocardial Infarction) trial[25] enrolled 1473 patients with acute coronary syndromes and objective evidence of coronary artery disease. Patients were randomized to t-PA (dose 0.8 mg kg^{-1}; one-third given as a bolus dose, the rest as an infusion over 90 minutes) or placebo. Patients were also treated with conventional therapy (aspirin, heparin, and beta-blockers). At 6 weeks follow-up, the rate of death or nonfatal MI was 8.8% in the t-PA group versus 6.2% in the placebo group ($P = 0.05$, Kaplan–Meier method). The study also compared an early invasive approach (cardiac catheterization with subsequent angioplasty or coronary artery bypass grafting) with a conservative strategy (medical therapy, proceeding to cardiac catheterization only if initial treatment failed). There was no significant difference in the rates of death, or nonfatal MI in the two groups (7.5% for the early invasive strategy versus 8.2% for the conservative strategy). However, the readmission rate for the invasive strategy group was significantly lower than for the conservative group (7.8% for invasive, 14.1% for conservative; $P < 0.001$). The rate of intracranial hemorrhage (confirmed with computed tomography) in TIMI IIIB was 0.55% in the t-PA group (4 patients) versus none in the control group at the 42-day follow-up ($P = 0.06$).

Discussion

All of the five randomized trials that evaluated antiplatelet therapy versus control presented above have shown reductions in the rate of death or nonfatal MI in patients with acute coronary syndromes without ST elevation.[14–16,18,20] Benefit was observed with aspirin or ticlopidine, but not sulfinpyrazone, The relative risk reduction ranged from 30% to 60%. The trials also show that the amount of benefit is related to the length of treatment, with greater benefit accruing with more prolonged treatment. The systematic overview of randomized controlled trials by the Antiplatelet Trialists' (APT) Collaboration has clearly demonstrated that prolonged antiplatelet therapy reduces the rate of death, MI, or stroke by about 25% in high-risk patients with a wide range of cardiovascular syndromes.[33] The amount of benefit of prolonged antiplatelet therapy observed in patients with stable angina in the APT overview was similar to that of patients with other acute coronary syndromes, but the number of patients studied in these trials was about 500, with a total of just 69 events. However, there is clear evidence of benefit of antiplatelet therapy in patients with acute and nonacute coronary syndromes.

Four trials have reported on the effects of intravenous heparin on rates of death or MI in patients with unstable angina or MI without ST elevation.[17,18,20,22] The studies by Telford and Théroux[17–19] showed clear early benefits of heparin in the absence of aspirin. In the RISC study,[20] intravenous heparin was administered by intermittent injection, and there was no apparent early benefit of heparin alone compared to controls in this setting. The FRISC study compared LMWH plus aspirin to aspirin alone.[22] At 6 days of follow-up there was a reduction of about 60% in the relative risk of death or MI, and at 5 weeks (with subcutaneous injections of LMWH continuing up to this point) there was a 30% reduction in the rate of death or MI ($P = 0.07$). A similar nonsignificant benefit for LMWH was observed in the ATACS study at 12 weeks of follow-up when heparin was followed by oral anticoagulation with warfarin.[21] The more recently reported FRIC[34] and ESSENCE[35] trials have compared LMWH plus aspirin to unfractionated heparin plus aspirin in the setting of acute coronary syndromes without ST elevation. Promising benefits for LMWH were observed on the outcomes of death, MI or recurrent ischemia in the ESSENCE trial, but the full reports are awaited before it can be determined whether LMWH should replace conventional heparin as the anticoagulant of choice. Overall, the trials consistently show an early benefit of heparin, particularly in the absence of aspirin, but also in combination with aspirin. The beneficial effects of heparin appear to wear off fairly rapidly after stopping treatment, and there is growing evidence of reactivation of coagulation and recurrence of ischemic events around the time of stopping heparin infusions. LMWH may be more effective than conventional heparin, requires minimal anticoagulant monitoring, and can be given subcutaneously for longer treatment periods.

Studies evaluating thrombolytic therapy for acute coronary syndromes without ST elevation have shown improvements in angiographic or anatomical measures, but no overall benefit on clinical outcomes. The reason for this lack of clinical benefit, despite angiographic improvements, is not clear. It is known that thrombolytic agents have prothrombotic effects[36,37] and also activate platelets.[38] Thrombolytic therapy is also associated with higher rates of bleeding. The available evidence suggests that there is no indication for giving routine thrombolytic therapy to patients with acute myocardial ischemia without ST elevation.

Newer antithrombotic strategies are also being evaluated. Hirudin is a potent direct antithrombin agent which has shown promising benefits over conventional heparin in the GUSTO-IIb (Global Use of Strategies to Open Occluded Coronary Arteries) study,[5] which included 12 142 patients with acute coronary syndromes, with about one-third having ST elevation at study entry. During the infusion period hirudin showed about a 40% reduction in the risk of death or MI compared to heparin ($P = 0.001$), but the proportional benefits were reduced at 30 days of follow-up (8.9% in the hirudin group versus 9.8% in the heparin group; $P = 0.06$). Interestingly, the absolute benefit of about 1% remained throughout. The OASIS (Organization to Assess Strategies for Ischemic Syndromes) investigators[39] are undertaking a study of 10 000 patients to evaluate a higher dose of hirudin in patients with acute coronary syndromes without ST elevation, as well as a 5-month course of warfarin. Other direct antithrombin agents such as hirulog are also being evaluated.[40,41] The management of acute coronary syndromes is also likely to be influenced by studies evaluating the potent platelet surface glycoprotein IIb/IIIa receptor antagonists.[42] These agents act in a different way to aspirin and have already been shown to improve outcome after percutaneous coronary revascularization procedures.[43] Whether newer antiplatelet agents, direct antithrombin agents, LMWH, and longer term anti-coagulation will be useful in the routine management of acute coronary syndromes remains to be determined by the results of recently reported and ongoing trials. In the meantime, early intravenous heparin given for a few days and early aspirin continued indefinitely remain the cornerstone of antithrombotic treatment for acute coronary syndromes without ST elevation.

10

Coronary Bypass Surgery

Thomas Killip and Kumar Ravi

Introduction

Three decades ago, Favaloro[1] described the application of coronary bypass grafting (CABG) to patients with symptomatic coronary artery disease. Early in the experience with the procedure, it became evident that symptoms of angina pectoris were relieved and exercise capacity increased in 80% or more of patients undergoing a successful procedure.[2] Such results had never before been observed with medical therapy. Whether CABG improved prognosis, however, remained highly controversial. Chalmers, who championed the concept 'randomize the first patient' for new forms of therapy,[3] suggested as early as 1972 that the effects of treatment with coronary artery bypass compared to medical care could only be evaluated by randomized trials.[4] Many argued, however, that such trials were unneeded and perhaps unethical in view of improved symptoms and, presumably, quality of life. Publications utilizing 'historical' controls argued that bypass surgery markedly improved prognosis.

Randomized trials for CABG are fraught with difficulty. Blinding is not possible and utilizing a sham operation as a control is unacceptable. Despite lack of scientifically valid information, many physicians and surgeons have been convinced of the necessity of surgical treatment in symptomatic patients, thus limiting the pool of potentially randomizable subjects. Lack of selection from a representative group limits the generalizability of results from a randomized trial. Furthermore, since bypass surgery improves symptoms, crossover from medical to surgical therapy cannot be denied if the clinical status of the medical control group deteriorates. Indeed, experience with randomized trials for CABG confirms that crossover is a serious confounding problem. Additionally, accepting a random allocation to surgery or no surgery requires a compliant, trusting subject. This is not for everyone.

Despite these difficulties a number of randomized clinical trials comparing CABG with medical therapy in patients with coronary artery disease have been carried out.[5–21] In addition, Yusuf et al.[22] recently presented an overview of seven trials evaluating CABG compared to medical therapy in symptomatic patients with coronary artery disease. A series of smaller trials will be discussed first, followed by an analysis of the three large trials, and finally comments on the recent meta-analysis are given.

prevents definitive conclusions about ... long term mortality', they recommended 'intensive medical management in unstable angina pectoris with later elective surgery as required'. Another randomized trial in a small number of patients (40) with unstable angina followed for a mean of 21 months, reached similar conclusions.[9]

A third randomized study comparing medical and surgical treatment in unstable angina was reported by Luchi et al.[12] A total of 468 subjects were randomized, 273 to medical treatment and 231 to CABG. Measured clinical and angiographic variables were similar in the two groups. Analysis was by intention to treat. Entry criteria required onset of unstable angina with progressive, severe exertional symptoms or pain at rest with ischemic ECG changes. Randomization was by computer random number allocation at the coordinating center. Eleven patients (5%) did not have initial surgery. Seventy-eight medical patients (34%) crossed over to surgical therapy. After 1 year, 75% of the bypass grafts were patent. After 2 years of follow-up, mortality for the two treatment groups was not significantly different. The rates of nonfatal myocardial infarction were similar. Analysis by logistic regression strongly suggested a negative effect on survival of poor ventricular function in medically treated patients. This predictive effect was not present in those who underwent CABG. The authors concluded that in unstable angina 'patients with reduced left ventricular ejection fraction may have a better 2-year survival rate after coronary bypass surgery.'

Norris et al.[10] evaluated 205 patients for randomization after recurrent myocardial infarction. One-hundred subjects had few or no symptoms, one or more coronary arteries suitable for bypass grafting and were randomized 50:50 between 1972 and 1979. Clinical descriptors on entry were similar in the two groups. The ejection fraction was $\leqslant 0.50$ in about half of each group. After 5.5 years, 9 patients (18%) crossed over from medical to surgical treatment. At a mean follow-up of 3 years, 65% of the bypass grafts studied were patent. After a follow-up of 7 years (mean 4.5 years) there were 6 deaths in the surgical group and 5 in the medical group, a nonsignificant difference. After 10 years there were 15 deaths in the CABG group and 16 deaths in the medical group. (Yusuf et al.[22] contacted the authors to obtain unpublished follow-up data.) With an annual mortality rate of 3–4%, which was lower than anticipated, this study lacked power to discriminate a possible significant difference. However, the authors commented: 'Our results do not give strong support for the use of surgery in relatively asymptomatic patients with three-vessel disease who have survived more than one infarction.'

Lorimer et al., for the European Coronary Surgery Bypass Group,[11] have reported a randomized trial of medical versus surgical therapy after myocardial infarction. Prior to hospital discharge, 3334 patients had a modified exercise test, 728 were positive, 598 had coronary arteriography, and 348 were randomized. The angiographic criteria are described in Table 10.1. Medical morality during follow-up was considerably lower than predicted, thus limiting the power of the study. After 5 years there were no significant differences in survival rate or other variables measured between the medical and surgical groups.

Comment

Many details currently accepted as standard in reporting a clinical trial[23] are not available in the published reports of these early studies. Few of the subjects randomized were women. Randomization techniques, although most probably carried out properly, were not foolproof. Medical therapy was generally not controlled by protocol. Surgical mortality was acceptable, reflecting a high standard of care. However, in most of the studies the medical mortality was much lower than anticipated. This, together with the small number of patients randomized per trial, followed in many studies for only a few years, could easily have caused type II statistical errors. Furthermore, both medical treatment and surgical techniques have advanced greatly in the more than 20 years since these trials began, making generalizability of the results to patients under current clinical management debatable.

Large Trials

Three large clinical trials designed to evaluate coronary arterial bypass procedures have been reported: the US Veteran Administration Trial (VA),[13,14] the European Cooperative Surgical Study (ECSS),[15–17] and the Coronary Artery Surgical Study (CASS).[18–20] The characteristics of these trials are summarized in *Table 10.2*.

Randomization occurred from December 1971 until late 1984. Statistical power was probably adequate to reasonably discriminate a difference from no difference. Subjects for study were mostly male, exclusively so in the VA and ECSS trials, there being only 11% female subjects in CASS. Randomization techniques were excellent in two and probably adequate in another (ECSS), although in the latter trial there were inexplicably 21 more patients assigned to surgery, mostly with three-vessel disease, than to medical treatment. All patients had angina, aside from a small subgroup in CASS who was asymptomatic following myocardial infarction. In each study, a few patients did not receive timely surgical treatment, but the numbers are too small to influence outcome. Follow-up was essentially complete in all three studies. Baseline clinical descriptors were similar between the two matched treatment groups in each of the three studies. The ejection fraction was <0.45 in 26% of subjects in the VA study, >0.50 in ECSS, and <0.50 in 22% but $\leqslant 0.35$ of those randomized in CASS. The number of grafts placed was similar in the three studies, ranging from 2.0 to 2.3 per patient. Internal mammary grafts were placed in 16% of the surgical patients in CASS, but in almost none in VA or ECSS. Surgical mortality, which decreased progressively from the earliest to the latest study, probably reflected both the degree of surgical risk (the VA patients appear to be at highest risk) and improvement in the state of the art. Few patients were lost to follow-up.

A confounding aspect of all randomized trials of medical versus surgical therapy in coronary artery disease is the crossover rate to CABG. In the vast majority of cases, the reason recorded was worsening ischemic symptoms, usually the development of unstable angina. The rates were remarkably similar and generally linear, averaging 3% per year in VA, 3.5% per year in ECSS, and 4% per year in CASS. Because this problem could not be controlled, it has been argued that the trials were of initial surgery versus medical therapy with later surgery if clinically indicated.

Results

In the VA trial, a significant difference in mortality in patients without left main disease was found at 7 years (medical mortality 30%, surgical mortality 23%; $P < 0.045$). Subjects were categorized as high risk based on angiographic (three-vessel disease, poor left ventricular function) and clinical (ECG abnormality, history of myocardial infarction, history of hypertension) criteria. Statistically high significant differences were observed in these high risk groups after 7 years and 10 years of follow-up in subgroup analysis. The reduction in surgical mortality showed maximum advantage at about 7 years, and diminished over time with continued follow-up. In patients who were not at high risk by

Table 10.2 Summary of three large randomized trials of medical compared to surgical treatment in symptomatic coronary artery disease

	VA[13,14]	ECSS[15–17]	CASS[18–20]
Enrollment period	Jan. 1972–Dec. 1974	Sep. 1973–Mar. 1976	Aug. 1975–May 1979
Eligible randomized (%)	73	31–100, by center	37
No. randomized	686: med. 354, surg. 332	768: med. 373, surg 395	780: med. 390, surg. 390
Follow-up (years)	11	12	10
Age (years)	44% <50	<65, mean 50	≤65, mean 51
Sex	Male	Male	10% female
Entry criteria:			
Inclusion	Angina >6 months with resting or exercise ECG change, CHC 2, 3, 4	Angina >3 years, no data on post-MI status	Angina CHC 0, 1, 2; post-MI no angina, 21%
Exclusion	MI <6 months, marked cardiomegaly, significant valvular disease, aneurysm	'Unreasonable surgical risk', LM > 50% excluded variably	MI <3 weeks, CHC 3, 4, valvular disease, CHF, aneurysm, diabetics on insulin, diastolic BP > 105, LM ≥ 70% stenosis, EF < 0.35
Angiographic criteria	≥50% stenosis of at least one graftable vessel, LM stenosis included	≥50% stenosis of 2 vessels with at least one graftable vessel, LVEF ≥ 0.50, LM stenosis could be included	≥70% stenosis of at least one vessel or 50–69% LM stenosis
Randomization	Call to coordination center	100 envelopes of 1 : 1 ratio at each site	Call to randomization center
Intention to treat	Yes	Yes	Yes
Ejection fraction	<0.45 in 28% med., 24% surg.	0.65 ± 0.10	22% had EF <0.50
Time to CABG	94% within 2 months	Mean 3.9 ± 3.5 months	Mean 54 days
No. grafts per patient	2.0	2.2	2.3, 16% IMA
Operative mortality (%)	5.6	3.3	1.4
Graft patency	12–18 months, 70%; 60 months, 67%	12–18 months, 75%; 60 months, 69%	12–18 months, 90%; 60 months, 82%
Compliance (No. (%)):			
Refused surgery	–	27 (5.8)	43 (11)
Medical to surgical	135 (38)	133 (36)	156 (40)

BP, blood pressure; CABG, coronary artery bypass graft; CHC, Canadian Heart Class; CHF, congestive heart failure; ECG, electrocardiogram; EF, ejection fraction; IMA, internal mammary artery; LM, left main coronary artery; LVEF, left ventricular ejection fraction; med., medical; MI, myocardial infarction; surg., surgical.

angiographic or clinical criteria, no significant differences in mortality between the medical and surgical groups were observed.

ECSS reported a significantly higher survival rate in patients assigned to CABG (92.4 ± 2.7%) compared to medical therapy (83.1 ± 3.9%) ($P < 0.0001$) after 5 years. By 12 years of observation, the advantage of surgery had gradually decreased (70.6 ± 5.8% surgical, 66.7 ± 5.3% medical), but remained statistically significant ($P < 0.04$). Trends in surgical benefit were noted in patients who were older, had an abnormal ECG, a positive exercise test, peripheral arterial disease, or proximal obstruction of the left anterior descending coronary artery.

After 10 years of follow-up, CASS reported no difference in cumulative survival, or percentage alive and free of myocardial infarction, between the initial strategy of randomization to CABG and medical therapy with late surgery if clinical conditions changed. However, patients with an ejection fraction of <0.50, the majority of whom also had three-vessel disease, had improved survival after assignment to CABG (79% surgical versus 61% medical; $P = 0.01$). CASS concluded that patients with mild angina and good ventricular function do not have a survival advantage with selection of early surgical bypass, but that early surgical treatment improves survival in patients with three-vessel disease and reduced ventricular function.

Left main disease. In the VA trial, a subgroup of 113 patients with left main disease (luminal restriction ⩾50% estimated diameter) were randomized, 53 to medical treatment and 60 to CABG.[21] This group of patients was originally included in the larger randomized trial. Thirty-day operative mortality declined from 25% during the first 2 years to 7% in the last 3 years of the trial. The distribution of measured clinical variables, including angiographic findings, was similar in the two groups. The average age was 53 years. Six medical patients (11%) underwent bypass subsequent to randomization. Analysis was by intention to treat. After a mean follow-up of 30 months (maximum 60 months), survival was significantly better with CABG than medical treatment between 18 and 30 months.

That CABG improves longevity in patients with high-grade obstruction of the left main coronary artery is an axiom that has achieved the status of dogma among cardiovascular physicians. Surprisingly, the VA report, an analysis of a subset of a larger trial, is the only randomized study of the subject. Some patients with left main disease were randomized in ECSS, but the number was too small to be meaningful. In the pooled analysis done by Yusuf et al.,[22] 150 patients had left main disease. After 10 years of follow-up, CABG was associated with increased survival of 19.3 months (13.7 ± 1.96 SE). In addition, a large number of nonrandomized reports confirm the advantage of CABG in left main disease. For example, Caracciolo et al.[24] recently reported 16 years of follow-up of 1484 patients with ⩾50% left main coronary artery stenosis. Median survival in the surgical group was 13.3 years (range 12.8–13.8 years; 95% CI) compared to 6.6 years (range 5.4–7.9 years; 95% CI) ($P < 0.0001$). However, survival was not prolonged with normal left ventricular function, even with ⩾70% left main obstruction. Thus there is little doubt, based on a wide variety of observations, both randomized and nonrandomized, that CABG improves survival in selected patients with left main coronary artery obstruction.

Utilizing the tool of meta-analysis, Yusuf et al.[22] have attempted to extend the conclusions drawn by the authors of earlier studies. In the seven combined reports totaling 1325 medical and 1324 CABG patients, bypass surgery increased survival by 1.8 months (3.0 ± 1.96 SE) in patients with one- or two-vessel disease, a conclusion not reached in the individual trials. In three-vessel disease, the gain post-CABG was 5.7 months (3.6 ± 1.96 SE). For left main ventricle involvement the advantage was 19.3 months (13.7 ± 1.96 SE). In the trials analyzed, 93.7% of patients assigned to CABG underwent surgery. However, after 10 years 41% of the medical patients had undergone bypass. Thus, the benefits of surgery are probably underestimated by analysis based on intention to treat. The application of meta-analysis to these trials with different entry criteria, varying indices of clinical severity, and uncontrolled but different medical treatment protocols is troublesome to many investigators.

Other outcomes. A revascularization procedure that improves exercise tolerance and relieves ischemia might be anticipated to reduce the incidence of myocardial infarction during subsequent follow-up. VA, ECSS, and CASS tabulated the incidence of myocardial infarction after randomization, with explicit criteria for diagnosis.[14,16,25] Unfortunately, in none of the three studies was the incidence of myocardial infarction reduced after surgery. After 5 years of follow-up there was no difference in the frequency of myocardial infarction in patients randomized to medical or surgical treatment. Interestingly, the mode of death appears to change after CABG. CASS reported a reduction in sudden death in the subjects assigned to surgical treatment and an increase an death due to congestive heart failure.

Effect of bypass surgery on quality of life is of great interest. In CASS, investigators found a reduction in the occurrence of angina pectoris, improved exercise tolerance, and a decrease in intake of the anti-ischemic medications in patients randomized to CABG.[26] Disappointingly, bypass surgery did not improve work status or the physical extent of recreational activity. Although indices of quality of life were initially superior with surgical treatment, by 10 years of follow-up the differences were less evident, due in part to the crossover to surgery by a large proportion of the medical group.[27] Others have made similar observations.[28]

Generalizability. Frederickson has termed the randomized clinical trial the 'indispensable ordeal'. The climate of clinical opinion existing when the three trials were initiated made them difficult to carry out. Many clinicians were convinced that the results of bypass surgery were so obvious that trials were unnecessary. The investigators who initiated the VA study, for example, had to repeatedly defend themselves against vociferous criticism at public presentations. Persuading a patient with symptomatic ischemic heart disease that is potentially life-threatening to voluntarily enter a trial in which therapy is determined by chance can truly be an ordeal, as the author (T.K.) can personally attest.

Hidden selection bias is a component in every healthcare system. The VA trial randomized patients, generally at high risk, who chose to seek medical care in the US Veterans Administration health system, a choice suggesting that other avenues were less attractive or not available. The randomized patients in CASS were selected from a registry of over 24 000 patients.[18] However, the criteria for entry were highly restrictive, and only about 10% of the registry qualified. Of the patients meeting entry criteria, less than half chose to participate. Several groups in ECSS did not inform its subjects they were entering a randomized trial. The denominator from which the randomized fraction was chosen in ECSS has not been described.

Strictly speaking, the generalizability of conclusions for these trials is clearly limited because of the narrowly defined entry criteria and the selection from limited populations. However, a large number of well-executed observational studies involving a wide variety of clinical situations have generally confirmed the results of the randomized trials, suggesting that the findings may be applied in a broad range of clinical situations involving symptomatic patients, extensive coronary involvement, and reduced ventricular function.

A unique feature of CASS, however, was the parallel analysis of 'randomizable patients', i.e. those subjects who could have been randomized but chose not to enter the study.[29] In the overwhelming number of instances, the decision not to enter the randomized trial was based on a personal physician's recommendation about treatment. Of the 1319 randomizable patients, 570 received early surgical treatment (within 90 days), with the remaining 745 being treated medically. More patients undergoing early bypass had three-vessel disease and poor ventricular function compared to the medical group. The study is, of course, observational and, although many of the clinical descriptors were similar in the medical and surgical groups, some were not. After 10 years of follow-up, the results in the randomizable group paralleled those in the randomized study.[30] Mortality was essentially the same in the randomized and randomizable medical patients (79% and 80%, respectively) and in the randomized and randomizable surgical patients (82% and 81%, respectively). Patients with three-vessel disease and an ejection fraction <0.50 and those with a proximal left anterior descending coronary artery stenosis of ≥70% had improved survival after CABG. The general comparability of the follow-up results in the CASS randomized and randomizable patients support the view that the results of the randomized trial can be generalized to similar subjects who meet the CASS entry criteria.

Critique and Unresolved Problems

It is unlikely that further randomized trials of bypass surgery will be carried out, except perhaps in comparison to angioplasty. This is unfortunate, because there are many unanswered questions. Very few women were included in the randomized trials, yet the risk and outcome for women continues to be debated.[31] Bypass mortality is said to be higher in women, possibly due to the smaller size of the coronary vessels. The average age randomized in all three trials was less than 60 years; few patients over 65 years were entered into any trial. Bypass surgery in patients in their 7th, 8th, and even 9th decade is increasingly common, yet a critical comparison of medical compared to surgical therapy in this important population is not available.[32] Similarly, no randomization of patients with a truly low ejection fraction has been done. The average ejection fraction in the trials was normal. Few patients were randomized with an ejection fraction of <0.35. It is now clear that the greatest absolute benefit from bypass surgery may occur in the patient at highest risk, i.e. those with the worst left ventricular function. Successful bypass surgery is now frequently carried out in patients with exceedingly poor ventricular function and ejection fractions of <0.35. However, again, no critical comparison of outcome in this important group is likely to become available.

The influence of comorbidity in the selection and outcome of patients considered for bypass surgery remains unresolved. This is especially a challenge for those with diabetes mellitus or with renal failure, including patients on dialysis. Coronary artery disease is the leading cause of mortality in these two groups of patients, and the role of bypass surgery is not clear. Diabetic patients tend to have more hypertension, left ventricular hypertrophy, more 'diffuse' vascular disease, require more grafts, and have a higher operative mortality than do nondiabetics.[33] Although it seems likely that bypass surgery improves outcome in the high-risk diabetic, comparison studies with nondiabetics undergoing surgery and medically treated diabetics are not available. Owen *et al.*[34] in a retrospective analysis noted improved functional status and symptomatic relief in a small group of patients on dialysis undergoing CABG. They commented, however, that 'limited long-term survival suggests that the relative costs and benefits of surgical revascularization need further examination in this patient population.'

The deterioration of the venous bypass graft with time is another unresolved problem.[35] Obstruction may occur because of inadequate anastomosis at the bypass site, with thrombus formation during the first postoperative year, and secondary to progressive atherosclerosis during longer term follow-up. Arterial conduits fare much better than venous grafts, with patency rates above 90% after 10 years.[36] For reasons not fully explained, the internal mammary artery is generally resistant to the ravages of athero-sclerosis. Current surgical recommendations include at least one arterial graft to a major diseased vessel, usually the left internal mammary artery to the left anterior descending coronary artery. Fear of mediastinal infection if both internal mammary arteries are utilized appears to be waning.[37] Use of both vessels during bypass surgery appears to be on the increase. Experience is growing also with the use of harvested radial arteries,[38] thus permitting three, four, or more arterial bypasses. It is likely that these aggressive surgical techniques have a favorable influence on long-term outcome.

Twenty years ago, Mundth and Austen[39] commented: 'There is considerable difference of opinion concerning the effectiveness of myocardial revascularization in improving left ventricular function and symptoms of cardiac failure associated with coronary artery disease.' Early after the introduction of bypass surgery there was hope for major improvement in global left ventricular function in selected patients after a successful procedure. But this effect is not commonly observed. Anecdotal reports suggest improve-ment in left ventricular function in highly selected patients with presumed hibernating myocardium.[40] Reports of remarkable recovery after bypass surgery in patients with cardiogenic shock due to poor myocardial contractile state are impressive,[41] but clearly are subject to selective bias. Poor results are seldom reported. Utilizing [^{18}F]deoxyglucose uptake assayed by positron emission tomography as a measure of myocardial viability despite decreased left ventricular wall motion, Grandin et al.[42] reported improved wall-motion scores in areas of viable myocardium detected preoperatively, after revasculariza-tion. These results suggest that patients with ischemic but metabolically functioning myocardium may have improved left ventricular function after CABG. Effect on long-term outcome is not known.

Medical and surgical therapy have vastly improved since the randomized trials were completed. Use of intravenous nitroglycerin, a variety of beta-adrenergic blockers, calcium channel blockers, aspirin, angiotensin converting enzyme inhibitors, and lipid-lowering agents, to name a few drugs, has been a valuable addition to medical therapy. Operative techniques have similarly improved with shorter cardiopulmonary pump times, more grafts per patient, the use of arterial conduits, limitation of transfusion, and early extubation and mobilization. Postoperative morbidity and mortality have progressively declined. Although precision in diagnosis is difficult, the perioperative myocardial infarction rate has fallen to about 5% nationally in the US. Recognition of the role of atherosclerotic emboli in postoperative stroke and organic mental impairment has led to improved bypass and aortic cross-clamping techniques to reduce the risk of atherosclerotic emboli. Whether the balance of improvement has tipped slightly toward medicine or surgery does not really matter: outcomes are better all around.

Conclusion

Taken in the aggregate, published randomized trials comparing medical therapy with bypass surgery have made an invaluable contribution of our understanding of the selection of proper treatment for patients with symptomatic coronary artery disease. That the patients are 'symptomatic' is emphasized, since there are no data from randomized trials on outcomes in asymptomatic patients. Yet the trials have imperfections, including restricted entry selection, randomization of mostly men, subjects that are too young with regard to today's aggressive treatment of older patients, the use of nonprotocol medical and postoperative care, venous bypass grafts only, the completion of randomization on average 20 years ago, and limited statistical trial, in many instances. The results, however, are basically consistent. Reasonable generalizability is supported by a wide range of nonrandomized reports reaching conclusions similar to those of the randomized trials.

In patients at acceptable risk, properly performed bypass surgery improves survival and quality of life, especially in those with multivessel disease and reduced left ventricular function. The greatest benefit occurs in subjects with the greatest risk. Benefits in single- and double-vessel disease appear to be marginal. Selection for surgery must ultimately depend on the clinical characteristics of the individual case. In view of the improvements in both medical and surgical treatment, and the recognition that aggressive medical treatment following bypass surgery is both warranted and necessary, it is likely that the outcome from patients undergoing bypass is better currently than those reported in the trials.

There is no doubt that CABG surgery is one of the important contributions of modern medicine. What further advances the future holds cannot be foretold. Hopefully, the proper role of medical therapy, bypass surgery, and angioplasty (currently in a rapid technical growth phase) in the management of coronary artery disease will be revealed by well-designed and executed randomized trials. But that is a story for another chapter in another book some time in the future.

References

1. Favaloro RG. Saphenous vein graft in the surgical treatment of coronary artery disease. *J Thorac Cardiovasc Surg* 1969; **58**: 178–185.
2. Alderman EL, Matlof HJ, Wexler I, *et al*. Results of direct coronary artery surgery for the treatment of angina pectoris. *N Engl J Med* 1973; **288**: 535–539.
3. Chalmers TC. When should randomization begin? *Lancet* 1968; **1**: 858 (letter).
4. Chalmers TC. Randomization and coronary artery surgery. *Ann Thorac Surg* 1972; **42**: 323–7.
5. Kloster FE, Kremkau EL, Ritzmann LW, *et al*. Coronary bypass for stable angina. A prospective randomized study. *N Engl J Med* 1979; **300**: 149–57.
6. Mathur VS, Guinn GA, Anastassiades LC, *et al*. Surgical treatment for stable angina pectoris. *N Engl J Med* 1975; **292**: 709–13.
7. Mathur VS, Guinn GA. Prospective randomized study of coronary bypass surgery in stable angina. The first 100 patients. *Circulation* 1975; **51/52**: I-33–140.
8. National Cooperative Study Group. Unstable angina pectoris: to compare surgical and medical therapy. *Am J Cardiol* 1978; **42**: 839–48.
9. Selden R, Neill WA, Ritzmann W, *et al*. Medical versus surgical therapy for acute coronary insufficiency. *N Engl J Med* 1975; **293**: 1329–33.
10. Norris RM, Agnew TM, Brandt PWT, *et al*. Coronary surgery after recurrent myocardial infarction: progress of a trial comparing surgical with nonsurgical management for asymptomatic patients with advanced coronary disease. *Circulation* 1981; **4**: 785–92.
11. Lorimer AR, Karlsson T, Varnauskas E, for the European Coronary Surgery Bypass Group. The role of early surgery following myocardial infarction. *Br J Clin Pract* 1992; **46**: 238–42.
12. Luchi RJ, Scott SM, Deupree RH, and the Principal Investigators and their Associates of Veterans Administration Cooperative Study No. 28. Comparison of medical and surgical treatment for unstable angina pectoris. *N Engl J Med* 1987; **316**: 977–84.
13. Murphy ML, Hultgren HN, Detre K, *et al*. Participants of the VA Cooperative Study: treatment of chronic stable angina: a preliminary report of survival data of the randomized VA Cooperative Study. *N Engl J Med* 1977; **297**: 621–627.
14. Detre KM, Takaro T, Hultgren H, *et al*. Long-term mortality and morbidity results of the Veterans Administration randomized trial of coronary artery bypass surgery. *Circulation* 1985; **72**(Suppl V): V-84–9.
15. European Coronary Surgery Study Group. Coronary artery bypass surgery in stable angina pectoris: survival at two years. *Lancet* 1979; **ii**: 889–893.

16. Varnauskas E, European Coronary Surgery Study Group. Survival, myocardial infarction, and employment status in a prospective randomized study of coronary bypass surgery. *Circulation* 1985; **72**(Suppl V): V-90–101.

17. Varnauskas E, The European Coronary Surgery Study Group. Twelve-year follow-up of survival in the randomized European coronary surgery study. *N Engl J Med* 1988; **319**: 332–7.

18. CASS Principal Investigators and their associates. Coronary Artery Surgery Study (CASS): a randomized trial of coronary artery bypass surgery. Survival data. *Circulation* 1983; **68**: 939–950.

19. Alderman EL, Bourassa MG, Cohen LS, *et al*. Ten-year follow-up of survival and myocardial infarction in the Randomized Coronary Artery Surgery Study. *Circulation* 1990; **82**: 1629–46.

20. Passamani E, Davis KB, Gillespie MJ, Killip T. A randomized trial of coronary artery bypass surgery. *N Engl J Med* 1985; **312**: 1665–71.

21. Takaro T, Hultgren HN, Lipton MJ, *et al*. The VA Cooperative Randomized Study of Surgery for Coronary Arterial Occlusive Disease. II: Subgroup with significant left main lesions. *Circulation* 1976; **54**: III-107–116.

22. Yusuf S, Zucker D, Peduzzi P, *et al*. Effect of coronary artery bypass graft surgery on survival: overview of 10-year results from randomised trials by the Coronary Artery Bypass Graft Surgery Trialists Collaboration. *Lancet* 1994; **344**: 563–70.

23. Begg C, Cho M, Eastwood S, *et al*. Improving the quality of reporting of randomized controlled trials. *JAMA* 1996; **276**: 637–9.

24. Caracciolo EA, Davis KB, Sopko G, *et al*. Comparison of surgical and medical group survival in patients with left main coronary artery disease. *Circulation* 1995; **91**: 2325–34.

25. CASS Principal Investigators and their Associates. Myocardial infarction and mortality in the Coronary Artery Surgery Study (CASS) randomized trial. *N Engl J Med* 1984; **310**: 750–8.

26. CASS Principal Investigators and their Associates. Coronary Artery Surgery (CASS): a randomized trial of coronary artery bypass surgery. Quality of life in patients randomly assigned to treatment groups. *Circulation* 1983; **68**: 951–60.

27. Rogers WJ, Coggin J, Gersh BJ, *et al*. Ten-year follow-up of quality of life in patients randomized to receive medical therapy or coronary artery bypass graft surgery. The Coronary Artery Surgery Study (CASS). *Circulation* 1990; **82**: 1647–58.

28. Booth DC, Deupree RH, Hultgren HN, *et al*. Quality of life after bypass surgery for unstable angina. 5-year follow-up results of a Veterans Affairs Cooperative Study. *Circulation* 1991; **83**: 87–95.

29. CASS Principal Investigators and their Associates. Coronary Artery Surgery Study (CASS): a randomized trial of coronary artery bypass surgery: comparability of entry characteristics and survival in randomized patients and non-randomized patients meeting randomization criteria. *J Am Coll Cardiol* 1984; **3**: 114–28.

30. Chaitman BR, Ryan TJ, Kronmal RA, *et al*. Coronary Artery Surgery Study (CASS): comparability of 10 year survival in randomized and randomizable patients. *J Am Coll Cardiol* 1990; **16**: 1071–8.

31. Becker RC, Corrao JM, Alpert JS. Coronary artery bypass surgery in women. *Clin Cardiol* 1988; **11**: 443–8.

32. Gersh BJ, Kronmal RA, Schaff HV, *et al*. Comparison of coronary artery bypass surgery and medical therapy in patients 65 years of age or older. A nonrandomized study for the Coronary Artery Surgery Study (CASS) Registry. *N Engl J Med* 1985; **313**: 217–24.

33. Salomon NW, Page US, Okies JE, *et al*. Diabetes mellitus and coronary artery bypass. Short-term risk and long-term prognosis. *J Thorac Cardiovasc Surg* 1983; **85**: 264–71.

34. Owen CH, Cummings RG, Sell TL, *et al*. Coronary artery bypass grafting in patients with dialysis-dependent renal failure. *Ann Thorac Surg* 1994; **58**: 1729–33.

35. Bourassa MG. Fate of venous grafts: the past, the present and the future. *J Am Coll Cardiol* 1991; **17**: 1081–3.

36. Cameron A, Davis KB, Green G, Schaff HV. Coronary bypass surgery with internal-thoracic-artery grafts – effects on survival over a 15-year period. *N Engl J Med* 1996; **334**: 216–19.

37. Kouchoukos NT, Wareing TH, Murphy SE, *et al*. Risks of bilateral internal mammary artery bypass grafting. *Ann Thorac Surg* 1990; **49**: 210–19.

38. Calafiore AM, Teodori G, Di Giammarco G, *et al*. Coronary revascularization with the radial artery: new interest for an old conduit. *J Card Surg* 1995; **10**: 140–6.

39. Mundth ED, Austen WG. Surgical measures for coronary heart disease. *N Engl J Med* 1975; **293**: 13–19, 75–9, 124–30.

40. Ballantyne CM, Verani MS, Short DH, *et al*. Delayed recovery of severely 'stunned' myocardium with the support of a left ventricular assist device after coronary artery bypass graft surgery. *J Am Coll Cardiol* 1987; **10**: 710–12.

41. Moosvi AR, Khaja F, Villanueva L, *et al*. Early revascularization improves survival in cardiogenic shock complicating acute myocardial infarction. *J Am Coll Cardiol* 1992; **19**: 907–14.

42. Grandin C, Wijns W, Melin JA, *et al*. Delineation of myocardial viability with PET. *J Nucl Med* 1995; **36**: 1543–52.

11

Interventional Cardiology

Pim J. de Feyter

Introduction

In 1977, Grüntzig introduced percutaneous transluminal balloon coronary angioplasty (PTCA) in the treatment of coronary atherosclerosis in man. As is often the case with new surgical or diagnostic procedures, very unlike the introduction of new pharmacological agents, the initiation of PTCA was not performed in the setting of a randomized trial. It was almost 10 years before the first randomized trial in interventional cardiology took place comparing the efficacy of medical treatment to coronary angioplasty in the treatment of single-vessel coronary artery disease.

Since then other randomized trials have been performed comparing established surgical treatment with percutaneous revascularization techniques, with comparisons of various modes of percutaneous revascularization techniques such as directional coronary atherectomy, coronary stenting, or excimer laser with coronary angioplasty. Several randomized trials have been performed to establish the role of balloon angioplasty in acute myocardial infarction. In addition, very recently, the efficacy of adjunctive thrombolytic or antiplatelet treatment during balloon angioplasty has been tested in randomized trials. This chapter critically reviews these trials.

PTCA versus Medical Treatment for Symptomatic Single-vessel Coronary Artery Disease

The ACME investigators were the first, and so far the only ones, to compare the efficacy of PTCA versus medical treatment on angina and exercise tolerance in patients with single-vessel disease.[1] The patients qualified for the study if they had any of the following clinical requirements: stable angina, a positive exercise test, or a previous myocardial infarction (<3 months). Angiography should reveal a single 70–99% stenosis and the exercise-stress test requirement was a horizontal or down-sloping ST-segment depression $\geqslant 1.0$ mm in at least one lead. A positive thallium scan could be included if a patient had a negative electrocardiogram (ECG) exercise test.

Six months after randomization, each patient underwent repeat exercise testing and coronary angiography. The primary endpoints of the study were the changes in exercise tolerance between baseline and follow-up, and the frequency of anginal attacks and the use of nitroglycerin. The exercise-test changes in the PTCA group were determined after

Table 11.1   Exercise test and clinical outcome of PTCA versus medical treatment at 6 months

	Medical (n = 107)	PTCA (n = 105)	P
Exercise test changes			
Total duration (min)	$+0.5 \pm 2.2$	$+2.1 \pm 3.1$	<0.0001
Time to onset of angina (min)	$+0.8 \pm 3.8$	$+2.6 \pm 4.1$	<0.01
Time to onset of ST segment decrease (min)	$+1.1 \pm 2.7$	$+2.2 \pm 4.4$	0.26
Max. ST-segment decrease (mm)	-0.3 ± 1.1	-0.1 ± 1.2	0.36
Max. HR–BP ($\times 10^{-3}$)	-2.8 ± 5.8	$+1.8 \pm 6.0$	<0.0001
Clinical angina pectoris changes			
Mean change in No. episodes per month	-7 ± 22	-15 ± 39	0.06
Per cent angina-free in 6th month	46	64	<0.01
Nitroglycerin use			
Mean change in tablets per month	-5 ± 25	-9 ± 30	0.25

HR–BP, Heart rate–blood pressure product; PTCA, percutaneous transluminal coronary angioplasty.

discontinuing medical treatment for 24 hours, whereas the medical group exercised under continued medical treatment.

The study was a multicenter study. A total of 9573 patients were screened, of which 371 satisfied the entry criteria. Of these, 212 (57%) were randomly assigned: 105 to PTCA and 107 to medical therapy. The patients on medical treatment were managed in a 'stepped care approach' designed to eliminate angina. Treatment consisted of isosorbide dinitrate, a beta-blocking drug, and calcium-channel blocking agents, either alone or in combination. PTCA was successful in 80 patients (80%, because 100 of the 105 actually underwent the procedure). Two patients underwent emergency bypass surgery and 4 had an acute myocardial infarction. There were no deaths at 6 months in the PTCA group. Repeat PTCA was performed in 16 patients; 5 patients had late bypass surgery and 1 patient had a myocardial infarction. None of the patients in the medical group underwent bypass surgery, but 11 underwent PTCA. Three patients had a myocardial infarction and one of these died.

The results of the study are summarized in *Table 11.1*. The increase in the total duration of exercise and time to onset of angina was significantly larger, and the maximal heart rate–blood pressure product was higher in the PTCA group compared to the medical group. Patients in the PTCA group had less angina and less use of nitroglycerin than the medical group.

The investigators also compared quality-of-life scores in both groups. Patients assigned to PTCA demonstrated a significantly greater improvement in both physical and psychological measures. This improvement was particularly noted in patients with improved exercise performance and a reduction of lesion severity.[2]

During a median follow-up of 4 years, the occurrence of death and nonfatal myocardial infarction in both groups was similar. However, the frequency of unstable angina and need for PTCA or coronary artery bypass graft (CABG) surgery was significantly higher in the medical group (*Figure 11.1*). It is of note that this study was a comparison between two treatment strategies: PTCA (including repeat PTCA if necessary) and a multiple-drug antianginal regimen. However, about one-third of PTCA patients used antianginal treatment.

In conclusion, PTCA offers earlier and more complete relief of angina and better exercise

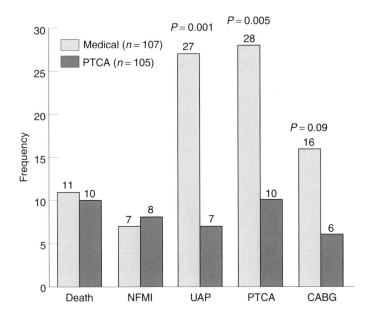

Figure 11.1 Late coronary events (median follow-up 4 years) in the ACME trial. CABG, coronary artery bypass grafting; NFMI, nonfatal myocardial infarction; PTCA, percutaneous transluminal coronary angioplasty; UAP, unstable angina pectoris.

tolerance than does medical treatment, leading to an improved quality of life. This beneficial effect persisted throughout the 4-year follow-up.

Early Invasive Strategy or Early Conservative Strategy for Patients with Unstable Angina or Non-Q-wave Myocardial Infarction

The TIMI-IIIB trial randomized 1473 patients with unstable angina or non-Q-wave myocardial infarction admitted within 24 hours of chest pain. The trial used a 2 × 2 factorial design comparing tissue plasminogen activator (t-PA) versus placebo, and an early invasive versus an early conservative strategy. The TIMI-IIIB trial tested the hypothesis that an early invasive strategy (early coronary angiography followed by revascularization) versus an early conservative strategy (coronary angiography followed by revascularization if initial medical therapy failed) was beneficial in terms of a composite endpoint consisting of death, myocardial infarction, or an unsatisfactory symptom-limited exercise stress test at 6 weeks.[4] The cumulative revascularization rate at 6 weeks was 61% for the early invasive strategy and 48% for the early conservative strategy (about 25% of the patients underwent CABG in both strategies).

There was no difference in the primary endpoint (*Figure 11.2*), but the average length of initial hospitalization, and the incidence and days of rehospitalization were lower in the early invasive strategy. An early invasive strategy offers no benefit over an early conservative strategy. The fact that there was no difference in the outcome of the two strategies was not surprising, because there was only a 13% absolute difference in the revascularization rate between the two strategies.

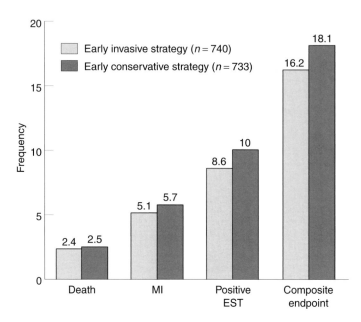

Figure 11.2   TIMI-IIIB trial: outcome at 6 weeks of early invasive and early conservative strategy. The composite endpoint comprises data on death, myocardial infarction, and a positive exercise stress test. EST, exercise stress test; MI, myocardial infarction.

Coronary Angioplasty in the Setting of Acute Myocardial Infarction

In patients with acute myocardial infarction, balloon angioplasty may be used to restore immediate coronary flow without adjunctive thrombolytic treatment (primary PTCA), to restore coronary flow after failed thrombolysis (rescue PTCA), or to reduce the severity of the 'infarct obstruction' after successful thrombolysis.

Various randomized trials testing the efficacy of PTCA performed either immediately (as soon as possible), early (within several hours or within a few days), or delayed (4 or more days) after successful thrombolysis, have shown no additional benefit of PTCA over thrombolytic and conservative treatment. Furthermore, no benefit was obtained with rescue PTCA compared to conservative treatments.[5,6] However, primary PTCA in acute myocardial infarction appears to improve prognosis. In the primary PTCA trials comparing the efficacy of PTCA versus thrombolytic treatment,[7–13] angioplasty was performed as soon as possible after the patient was admitted to the hospital, and thrombolytic treatment was given as soon as possible. The patients were randomized within 6–12 hours of onset of symptoms. Various thrombolytic treatment strategies were used: intracoronary or intravenous streptokinase, or t-PA. Pooling the data of the seven trials, 571 patients were randomly treated with PTCA and 574 received thrombolytic treatment. The intervention rate in the PTCA group was 93% compared with 29% in the thrombolytic group, who underwent PTCA during hospitalization or within the first 6 weeks after infarction.

Compared with thrombolytic treatment, primary PTCA was associated with a lower mortality and reinfarction rate at 6 weeks (*Figure 11.3*). Long-term data (i.e. beyond 6 weeks) are not yet available from a sufficiently large number of patients to convincingly show a sustained long-term benefit of PTCA.

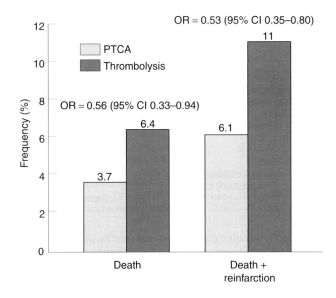

Figure 11.3 Primary PTCA versus thrombolysis: death and reinfarction at 6 weeks (pooled data on 1175 patients). OR, Odds ratio, with 95% confidence intervals. (Adapted from Michels and Yusuf.[6])

The dramatic beneficial efficacy of PTCA over thrombolytic treatment is achieved by the rapid restoration of a thrombolysis in myocardial ischemia (TIMI) flow of 3 (normal) with PTCA in over 90% of patients. Complete reperfusion (TIMI 3) is associated with an improved survival rate. Even with the most aggressive thrombolytic regimen currently available, complete reperfusion can only be obtained in about 50% of patients.

Primary PTCA is more effective than thrombolysis, but the limited availability of PTCA facilities and the inevitable logistic problems involved are serious limitations that prevent widespread implementation of direct PTCA in acute myocardial infarction. Innovative thrombolytic approaches that can establish more rapid and complete reperfusion are needed (notwithstanding the fact that adjunctive new thrombolytic approaches after successful primary PTCA may further increase its efficacy).

Directional Coronary Atherectomy versus Coronary Balloon Angioplasty for *de novo* Coronary Lesions

Directional atherectomy was devised as a debulking tool that would be able to completely remove coronary plaques in a safe, effective, and predictable way. This is different from balloon angioplasty which, although safe, is not always predictable and is only relatively effective because it often only reduces the culprit lesion to a remaining lesion of about 30% diameter stenosis. It was hypothesized that directional coronary atherectomy would have a better clinical outcome and a lesser restenosis rate. This was tested in two randomized trials comparing the efficacy of directional coronary atherectomy versus balloon angioplasty for *de novo* coronary artery lesions.[14-16]

The Caveat-I trial was a multicenter trial conducted at 35 sites in the USA and Europe.[14] A total of 1012 patients were randomly assigned to either atherectomy (512 patients) or angioplasty (500 patients). The CCAT trial was a multicenter trial conducted at nine

Table 11.5   Rate of adverse clinical events at 1 year in Caveat-I

	DCA ($n = 512$)		PTCA ($n = 500$)		
	No. of patients	%	No. of patients	%	*P*
Death	11	2.2	3	0.6	0.035
MI:					
Q-wave	15	2.9	6	1.2	0.053
Non-Q-wave	30	5.9	16	3.2	0.041
Total	45	8.9	22	4.4	0.005
CABG	47	9.3	45	9.1	0.862
Repeat target lesion PTCA	123	24.4	129	25.9	0.467

CABG, coronary artery bypass graft; DCA, directional coronary atherectomy; MI, myocardial infarction; PTCA, percutaneous transluminal coronary angioplasty.

Directional Atherectomy for *de novo* Venous Bypass Obstructions

Balloon angioplasty of an obstruction in saphenous venous bypass graft is often associated with embolization of graft material, leading to a non-Q-wave infarction in 5% of patients. In addition, there is a high restenosis rate (over 50%). The Caveat-II study compared the immediate and 6-month outcome after directional atherectomy or balloon angioplasty in patients with *de novo* bypass graft stenoses.[20]

The study was a multicenter study performed in 54 sites in North America and Europe. Study subjects were patients with prior coronary bypass surgery and a *de novo* obstruction in the vein graft suitable for treatment with either directional atherectomy or balloon angioplasty. The angiographic inclusion criteria were: (a) a vein graft suitable for a $\geqslant 6$ French atherectomy catheter ($\geqslant 3.0$ mm); (b) a stenosis diameter $\geqslant 60\%$ and $< 100\%$; and (c) a lesion length $\leqslant 12$ mm. Patients with a recent (< 5 days) myocardial infarction were excluded. The acute endpoints were procedural success and major complications (death, myocardial infarction, emergency bypass surgery, or abrupt closure). The 6-month endpoints were restenosis (minimum luminal diameter) or major late adverse clinical events (death, myocardial infarction, CABG).

A total of 305 patients were randomized: 149 to atherectomy and 156 to PTCA. The majority of the patients had unstable angina. The baseline clinical and angiographic characteristics were similar in both groups. There were more acute complications in the atherectomy group than the PTCA group owing to the more frequent occurrence of distal embolization and the associated occurrence of non-Q-wave myocardial infarction in the atherectomy group (*Table 11.6*).

The 6-month survival was 95.3% for atherectomy and 92.3% for PTCA. The occurrence of late Q-wave infarction was rare (2.7% for atherectomy, 4% for PTCA). Repeat surgery was rare in both groups. The survival rate without repeat balloon angioplasty was 86.8% for atherectomy patients and 77.6% for PTCA patients ($P = 0.041$). The initial lumenal gain was higher for atherectomy than PTCA (1.45 versus 1.12 mm; $P < 0.001$). Angiographic

Table 11.6 Caveat-II: in-hospital acute complications

	Directional atherectomy (%)	PTCA (%)	P
Death	2.0	1.9	
Emergency CABG	0.67	0.64	
Nonfatal MI	17.4	11.5	
Non-Q-wave	16.1	9.6	0.09
Q-wave	1.3	1.9	
Acute closure	4.7	2.6	
Distal embolization	13.4	5.1	0.012
Composite endpoint[a]	20.1	12.2	0.059

CABG, coronary artery bypass grafting; MI, myocardial infarction; PTCA, percutaneous transluminal coronary angioplasty.
[a]Death, nonfatal myocardial infarction, acute closure, emergency bypass surgery.

restenosis ($>50\%$) occurred less often after atherectomy (45.6%) than after PTCA (50.5%); however, this was not statistically significant. At 6 months the net lumenal gain with atherectomy was larger (0.68 versus 0.50 mm; NS).

In conclusion, atherectomy is able to accomplish a better initial widening of the lumen, but this is offset by a higher rate of distal embolization and non-Q-wave myocardial infarction. The restenosis rate is a little less for atherectomy patients and they require fewer target-vessel revascularization procedures. There is no clear advantage of atherectomy over PTCA for the treatment of obstructions in venous bypass grafts. It is suggested that a more aggressive atherectomy or postatherectomy dilatation may have resulted in a better immediate and 6-month outcome. Ongoing trials (BOAT, OARS, and EUROCARE) must answer this question.

Stent Implantation versus Coronary Balloon Angioplasty for *de novo* Coronary Lesions

Owing to the scaffolding properties of stents it was thought that, by decreasing the elastic recoil of the vessel and by sealing intimal flaps, thus providing a wider and smoother coronary lumen, stent implantation might reduce the restenosis rate. Two multicenter randomized trials have compared the efficacy of stent implantation with balloon angioplasty for *de novo* coronary lesions.[21,22] The Benestent trial,[21] conducted in Europe, randomly assigned a total of 520 patients to either Palmaz–Schatz stent implantation (262 patients) or balloon angioplasty (258 patients). The STRESS trial[22] randomly assigned patients to either elective placement of a Palmaz–Schatz stent (205 patients) or balloon angioplasty (202 patients). The inclusion and exclusion criteria and endpoints of both trials are given in *Table 11.7*.

The early and late clinical outcomes of the trials are shown in *Table 11.8*. At 6 months the adverse clinical event rate in the Benestent trial was lower in the stent group than in the balloon group. This was mainly caused by the lower frequency of repeat angioplasty in stented patients (20.6% versus 10.0%, respectively). After 1 year there were no significant differences in mortality (1.2% versus 0.8%), stroke (0.0% versus 0.8%), myocardial infarction (5.0% versus 4.2%) or coronary bypass grafting (6.9% versus 5.1%) between the stent and angioplasty groups, respectively.[23] The clinical success rate in the STRESS trial

Table 11.7   Inclusion and exclusion criteria and endpoints for the Benestent and STRESS trials

Benestent	STRESS
Inclusion criteria	
Stable angina	Stable, unstable angina
Single native lesion <15 mm long; vessel >3 mm	Single native lesion <15 mm long; vessel >3 mm
Normal myocardium	
Exclusion criteria	
Ostial lesion	Myocardial infarction <7 days
Bifurcation lesion	Contraindication on anticoagulation or aspirin
Intracoronary thrombus	Left ventricular ejection fraction <40%
	Coronary thrombus
	Multilesions, diffuse disease
	Left main disease, ostial lesion
	Severe tortuosity
Primary endpoints at 6 months	
Clinical	
Death	Clinically successful procedure
Cerebrovascular accident	
Myocardial infarction	
Bypass surgery	
Repeat balloon angioplasty	
Angiographic	
Minimum luminal diameter at follow-up	Restenosis >50% at follow-up
Secondary endpoints	
Clinical	
Clinical success	Death
Angina	Myocardial infarction
Stress test at 6 months	Bypass surgery
	Repeat PTCA
Angiographic	
Restenosis >50%	Minimal luminal diameter: immediate and at follow-up
Procedural success	Procedural success

PTCA, Percutaneous transluminal coronary angioplasty.

was higher in the stent group than in the balloon angioplasty group (96.1% versus 89.6%; $P = 0.011$) and the target vessel revascularization rate was lower in the stent group than the balloon angioplasty group (10.2% versus 15.4%; $P = 0.06$). The subacute thrombosis rate in the Benestent trial was 3.5% in the stent group and 2.7% in the balloon group; in the STRESS trial the corresponding values were 3.4% and 1.5%, respectively.

The angiographic outcomes of both trials are summarized in *Table 11.9*. In the Benestent trial the net gain at follow-up was larger in the stent group than in the balloon group, which resulted in a slightly larger minimal luminal diameter at follow-up in the stented group. However, this difference was not statistically significant. The restenosis rate was lower in the stented group than the balloon group (22% versus 32%; $P = 0.02$). In the STRESS trial, the favorable changes in the minimum luminal diameter were greater in the stented group than the balloon angioplasty group. The net gain at follow-up was larger in the stented group, and this resulted in a lower restenosis rate in the stent patients (31% versus 42% in the balloon patients; $P = 0.05$).

From the results of both trials it may be concluded that, overall, stents produce better

Table 11.8 In-hospital and 6-month clinical outcomes in the Benestent and STRESS trials

	Benestent			STRESS		
	Angioplasty (%)	Stent (%)	Relative risk (95% CI)	Angioplasty (%)	Stent (%)	P
Clinical success	91.1	92.7		89.6	96.1	0.011
Early events[a]						
Death	0	0		1.5	0	
CVA	0.8	0		0.5	1.0	
MI/Q-wave	3.1/0.8	3.4/1.9		5.0/3.0	5.4/2.9	
Bypass surgery	1.6	3.1		4.0	2.4	
Repeat angioplasty	1.2	0.4		1.0	2.0	
Any event	6.2	6.9		7.9	5.9	
Late events:						
Death	0.4	0.8		0	1.5	
Total MI/Q-wave	3.9/1.6	4.2/2.7		2.0/2.5	1.5/1.0	
Bypass surgery	3.9	5.0		4.5	2.4	
Repeat angioplasty	20.6	10.0	0.49 (0.32–0.75)	11.4	9.8	
Any late event	–	–		15.8	15.1	
All events:						
Death	0.4	0.8		1.5	1.5	
CVA	0.8	0		0.5	1.0	
Total MI/Q-wave	4.6/1.9	4.2/2.7		6.9/3.5	6.3/3.4	
Bypass surgery	4.2	6.2		8.4	4.9	
Repeat angioplasty	23.3	13.5	0.58 (0.40–0.85)	12.4	11.2	
Any event	29.6	20.1	0.68 (0.50–0.92)	23.8	19.5	

CVA, Cerebrovascular accident; MI, myocardial infarction.
[a]Benestent: in-hospital events. STRESS: 0–14 days events.

Table 11.9 Angiographic results in the Benestent and STRESS trials

	Benestent		STRESS	
	Angioplasty	Stent	Angioplasty	Stent
Before the procedure				
Minimum lumen diameter (mm)	1.08 ± 0.31	1.07 ± 0.33	0.75 ± 0.25	0.77 ± 0.27
At follow-up:				
Minimum lumen diameter (mm)	1.73 ± 0.55	1.82 ± 0.64	1.56 ± 0.65	1.74 ± 0.60*
Restenosis (% of patients)	32	22**	42	31**
Change in minimum lumen diameter				
Immediate gain (mm)	0.97 ± 0.39	1.40 ± 0.44*	1.23 ± 0.48	1.72 ± 0.46*
Late loss (mm)	0.32 ± 0.47	0.65 ± 0.57*	0.38 ± 0.66	0.74 ± 0.58*
Net gain (mm)	0.65 ± 0.59	0.75 ± 0.66	0.80 ± 0.63	0.98 ± 0.80**

*P < 0.001; **P < 0.05.

immediate and late angiographic outcomes, resulting in a lower need for repeat target vessel revascularization. The stent-implantation procedure is relatively safe, with acceptable low subacute thrombosis rates. It should be emphasized that the beneficial results obtained in the Benestent trial and the STRESS trial were obtained in a highly selected

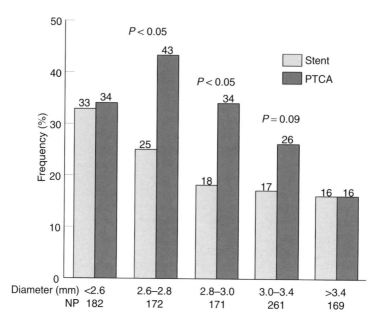

Figure 11.4 Meta-analysis: adverse clinical event rates in the Benestent and STRESS trials at 6 months in relation to vessel diameter. NP, Number of patients. (Adapted from Azar et al.[24])

patient population: a short, discrete lesion (<15 mm) in a relatively large vessel (>3 mm). Thus similar results should not be expected in more general coronary intervention patient groups with longer lesions, smaller vessels, restenosed lesions, or obstructions in venous bypass grafts.

A recent meta-analysis of the clinical and angiographic outcomes in patients recruited in the Benestent and STRESS trials indicated that stenting reduced the restenosis and clinical event rate in vessels with a diameter of 2.6–3.4 mm, but not in those less than 2.6 mm or more than 3.4 mm in diameter (*Figures 11.4* and *11.5*).[24]

A significant problem with stent implantation is the question of how to treat patients after the procedure in order to prevent the occurrence of subacute thrombotic occlusion. Antiplatelet (ticlopidine plus aspirin) and anticoagulant (intravenous heparin, phenprocoumon, and aspirin) therapy were compared in a randomized trial.[25] After successful placement of a Palmaz–Schatz stent, 257 patients were allocated to antiplatelet treatment and 260 to anticoagulant treatment. The primary cardiac composite endpoint at 30 days after coronary stenting consisted of cardiac death, nonfatal myocardial infarction, and early revascularization. The primary noncardiac endpoint comprised noncardial death, cerebrovascular accident, severe hemorrhage, and peripheral vascular events. Antiplatelet therapy after stent implantation significantly reduced cardiac complications (1.6% versus 6.2%; relative risk (RR) 0.25, CI 0.06–0.77) and noncardiac complications (1.2% versus 12.3%; RR 0.09, CI 0.07–0.31). Stent occlusion occurred in 0.8% of the patients of the antiplatelet treated group and in 5.4% in the anticoagulant group, whereas severe hemorraghic complications only occurred in the anticoagulant group (12.3%).

The downside of stent implantation in both the STRESS and Benestent trials was the rather high rate of bleeding complications occurring as a side-effect of the strict anti-

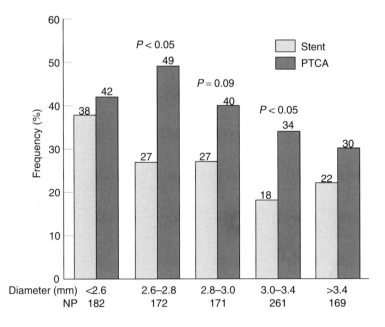

Figure 11.5 Meta-analysis: restenosis rates in the Benestent and STRESS trials at 6 months in relation to vessel diameter. NP, number of patients. (Adapted from Azar *et al.*[24])

coagulation regimens. However, this problem seems to have now been resolved by the use of improved anticoagulation treatment (aspirin and ticlopidine), improved stent-implantation techniques (high-pressure balloons and intracoronary ultrasound guidance), and the use of a less thrombogenic stent (the heparin coated Palmaz–Schatz stent).

The results of both trials were obtained with implantation of a Palmaz–Schatz stent. Although it may seem reasonable to believe that other stents may produce similar results, this needs to be proven in further randomized studies.

Excimer Laser Angioplasty versus Balloon Angioplasty

Excimer laser coronary angioplasty has been introduced as an attractive, sophisticated ablative technique for the treatment of stable, long, or complex coronary lesions. Although laser-based techniques in intervention cardiology have been around for many years, only one randomized study has been performed recently. The AMRO trial[26] randomly assigned 151 patients to excimer laser angioplasty and 157 patients to balloon angioplasty. All patients had stable angina and culprit lesions longer than 10 mm. The primary clinical endpoints were death, nonfatal myocardial infarction, and repeat target vessel revascularization at 6 months. The primary angiographic endpoint was the net gain in the minimum lumen diameter at follow-up relative to baseline. The laser procedure was followed by balloon angioplasty in 98% of patients. There were no significant differences in clinical endpoints between the two study groups (*Table 11.10*). The laser procedure resulted in an immediate larger minimum luminal diameter than did balloon angioplasty. However, the late loss was also larger, so that the minimum lumen diameter at follow-up was almost

Table 11.10   Primary clinical and angiographic endpoints of the AMRO trial

Endpoint at 6 months follow-up	Excimer laser ($n = 151$) (%)	Balloon ($n = 157$) (%)	
Clinical endpoints			
Death	0	0	–
Nonfatal MI	4.6	5.7	NS
Repeat revascularization	31.8	29.3	NS
Combined clinical endpoint	33.1	29.9	NS
Angiographic endpoints			
Minimum luminal diameter (mm):			
Before procedure	0.77 ± 0.5	0.77 ± 0.5	–
After procedure	1.69 ± 0.4	1.59 ± 0.4	0.05
At follow-up	1.17 ± 0.7	1.25 ± 0.7	NS
Net gain	0.40 ± 0.7	0.48 ± 0.7	NS
Late loss	0.52 ± 0.7	0.34 ± 0.6	0.04
Restenosis ($>50\%$)	52	41	NS

MI, myocardial infarction.

identical (1.17 ± 0.7 mm versus 1.25 ± 0.7 mm for laser and balloon angioplasty, respectively) (see *Table 11.10*).

It is noteworthy that excimer laser angioplasty was followed by balloon angioplasty in 98% of the procedures. This added significantly to the already costly laser procedure (due to the large investment in laser equipment), making the cost–benefit analysis for laser treatment even more unfavorable. Two important new adjustments in laser technique, not included in the AMRO trial, may improve future excimer laser angioplasty results. First, saline flushing during the laser procedure has been shown to reduce the formation of fast expanding and imploding vapor bubbles, which is associated with fewer procedural complications.[27] Secondly, the development of a new laser catheter design, which provides homogeneous light distribution, allows the use of lower energy fluence without loss of ablative power. This may be expected to be associated with less laser damage to the vessel wall.

The AMRO trial demonstrated that excimer laser angioplasty followed by balloon angioplasty provides no benefit over balloon angioplasty alone.

Adjunctive Thrombolytic Treatment during Balloon Angioplasty in Patients with Unstable Angina or Non-Q-wave Infarction

Balloon angioplasty in patients with acute coronary syndromes is associated with a high risk of major complications owing to the occurrence of an abrupt thrombotic occlusion during the procedure. Two trials, TIMI-IIIB and TAUSA, have addressed the issue of whether adjunctive thrombolytic treatment would reduce the thrombotic major complication rate.[4,28] In the TIMI-IIIB trial, 1473 patients seen within 24 hours of ischemic chest pain at rest who were thought to represent unstable angina or non-Q-wave myocardial infarction were randomized. The trial used a 2×2 factorial design comparing t-PA versus placebo as initial therapy, and an early invasive strategy versus an early conservative strategy. All patients were treated with bed rest, anti-ischemic medication,

Table 11.11 Primary endpoints of the TAUSA and TIMI-IIIB trials

	TAUSA		TIMI-IIIB		
	UK (n = 232)	Placebo (n = 237)	t-PA (n = 729)	Placebo (n = 744)	P
Death (%)	0	0	2.3	2.0	
MI (%)	2.6	2.1	7.4	4.9[a]	0.04
Death or MI (%)	2.6	2.1	8.8	6.2[a]	0.05
Ischemia, MI, or CABG (%)	12.9	6.3*	–	–	0.018

CABG, Coronary artery bypass graft; MI, myocardial infarction; t-PA, tissue plasminogen activator; UK, urokinase.
[a] Placebo versus treatment.

aspirin, and heparin. The primary endpoint consisted of a combination of death, myocardial infarction, and failure of initial therapy at 6 weeks. There was no difference in the outcome between the t-PA and placebo patients (54.2% versus 55.5%, respectively). However, fatal and nonfatal myocardial infarction occurred more frequently in the t-PA-treated group: 8.8% versus 6.2%; P = 0.05) (*Table 11.11*).

The TAUSA trial randomized 469 patients with ischemic pain at rest, with or without a recent (<1 month) infarction, to intracoronary urokinase or placebo. The clinical endpoints of the trial were in-hospital death, nonfatal myocardial infarction, recurrent ischemia, or CABG. The incidence of acute closure was increased with urokinase (10.2%) versus placebo (4.3%). Adverse in-hospital clinical endpoints occurred more frequently in the urokinase patients than in the placebo patients (12.9% versus 6.3%, respectively) (see *Table 11.11*).

The results of both trials indicated that adjunctive thrombolytic treatment is, contrary to what one may expect, not beneficial, and in fact may even be harmful.

Adjunctive Glycoprotein IIb/IIIa Receptor Antagonist in High-risk Coronary Angioplasty

Patients with an evolving infarction, severe unstable angina or high-risk coronary morphologic characteristics (such as complex, ulcerated, thrombotic, or long lesions) are at increased risk of abrupt coronary occlusion, and thus have a high major complication rate during coronary angioplasty or atherectomy. Platelets are believed to play a role in the cause of abrupt occlusion. The EPIC trial tested the hypothesis that adjunctive treatment with a glycoprotein (GP) IIb/IIIa receptor antagonist may reduce the major complication rate in high-risk coronary angioplasty.[29,30] GP IIb/IIIa receptor antagonists are potent platelet inhibitors, because they affect the final common pathway for platelet aggregation. A total of 2099 patients undergoing balloon angioplasty or atherectomy were randomly assigned to a bolus and an infusion of placebo, a bolus of c7E3 Fab and an infusion of placebo, or a bolus and an infusion of c7E3 Fab. The primary endpoint of the trial was a composite endpoint consisting of death, nonfatal myocardial infarction, revascularization for acute ischemia (including stent implantation), and the insertion of an intra-aortic balloon pump during the first 30 days after randomization.

There was a 35% reduction in the rate of the primary endpoint of the c7E3 Fab bolus and infusion compared to placebo (12.8 versus 8.3%; P = 0.008). The reduction was less with the

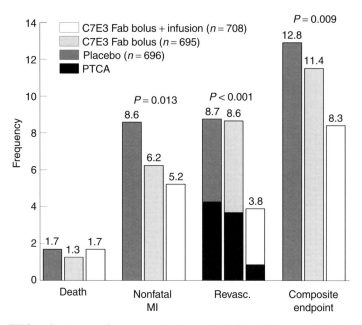

Figure 11.6 EPIC trial: primary adverse-event outcome at 30 days. MI, myocardial infarction; Revasc, revascularization (coronary angioplasty or bypass surgery). Composite endpoint: death, nonfatal MI, and revascularization.

c7E3 bolus alone (11.5%). The reduction was mainly achieved in the rate of nonfatal myocardial infarction and repeat revascularization procedures (*Figure 11.6*).

The major bleeding complications associated with the use of these potent platelet aggregation blockers were highest in the bolus and infusion group, less high in the bolus group, and lowest in the placebo group (14%, 11%, and 7%, respectively). At 6 months this beneficial effect continued, with a major ischemic event or elective revascularization occurring in 35.1% of patients on the placebo bolus plus placebo infusion, in 32.6% on bolus plus placebo infusion, and 27.0% on bolus plus infusion. This beneficial long-term effect was statistically significant and mainly due to a diminished need for subsequent coronary revascularization procedures.

Preliminary results of the Epilog and Capture trials have confirmed the EPIC trial findings, showing that adjunctive treatment with rheopro in patients undergoing elective or urgent PTCA (Epilog) or in patients with refractory unstable angina (Capture) is highly effective[31] in reducing major procedural complications, particularly in patients with acute unstable coronary syndromes. However, the overall beneficial efficacy of GP IIb/IIIa antagonists appears not to be universal, since preliminary data from the IMPACT-II trial (investigating the efficacy of another GP IIb/IIIa antagonist, integrelin) and the RESTORE trial (investigating tirofiban) did not demonstrate a beneficial effect at 30 days, possibly suggesting a lack of specificity of rheopro (i.e. it may antagonize not only the fibrinogen receptor, but also, unlike integrelin and tirofiban, the vitronectin receptor), or an inappropriate dose of integrelin or tirofiban.

It is concluded that 7E3 Fab reduces the major complications in high-risk patients undergoing percutaneous intervention. In addition, there is a reduced need for subsequent coronary revascularization procedures. The downside is the high frequency of major bleedings, mainly occurring at the puncture site, and the relatively high cost of the treatment with 7E3 Fab, as has been shown in EPIC and CAPTURE. However, bleeding complications can be reduced by adjusting the heparin dose according to preliminary data from Epilog.

References

1. Parisi AF, Folland ED, Hartigan P. A comparison of angioplasty with medical therapy in the treatment of single vessel coronary artery disease. *N Engl J Med* 1992; **326**: 10–16.
2. Strauss WE, Fortin T, Hartigan P, Folland ED, Parisi AF. A comparison of quality of life scores in patients with angina pectoris after angioplasty compared with after medical therapy. *Circulation* 1995; **92**: 1710–19.
3. Morris KG, Folland ED, Hartigan PM, Parisi A. Unstable angina in late follow-up of the ACME trial. *Circulation* 1995; **92**(Suppl I): 1–725.
4. TIMI-III B Investigators. Effects of tissue plasminogen activator and a comparison of early invasive and conservative strategies in unstable angina and non-Q-wave myocardial infarction. *Circulation* 1994; **89**: 1545–56.
5. Landau C, Glamenn B, Willard JE, Hillis D, Lange RA. Coronary angioplasty in the patient with acute myocardial infarction. *Am J Med* 1994; **96**: 536–43.
6. Michels KB, Yusuf S. Does PTCA in acute myocardial infarction affect mortality and reinfarction rate? A quantitative overview (meta-analysis) of the randomized clinical trials. *Circulation* 1995; **91**: 476–85.
7. O'Neill W, Timmis GC, Bourdillon PD, *et al*. A prospective randomized clinical trial of intracoronary streptokinase versus coronary angioplasty for acute myocardial infarction. *N Engl J Med* 1986; **314**: 812–18.
8. De Wood MA, Fisher MJ, for the Spokane Heart Research Group. Direct PTCA versus intravenous rtPA in acute myocardial infarction: preliminary results from a prospective randomized trial. *Circulation* 1989; **80**(Suppl II): II-418 (abstract).
9. Grines CL, Browne KF, Marco J, *et al*., for the Primary Angioplasty in Myocardial Infarction Study Group. A comparison of immediate angioplasty with thrombolytic therapy for acute myocardial infarction. *N Engl J Med* 1993; **328**: 673–9.
10. Zijlstra F, Jan de Boer M, Hoorntje JAC, Reiffers S, Reiber JHC, Suryapranata H. A comparison of immediate coronary angioplasty with intravenous streptokinase in acute myocardial infarction. *N Engl J Med* 1993; **328**: 680–4.
11. Gibbons RJ, Holmes DR, Reeder GS, *et al*., for the Mayo Coronary Care Unit and Catheterization Laboratory Groups. Immediate angioplasty compared with the administration of a thrombolytic agent followed by conservative treatment for myocardial infarction. *N Engl J Med* 1993; **328**: 685–91.
12. Ribeiro EE, Silva LA, Carneiro R, *et al*. Randomized trial of direct coronary angioplasty versus intravenous streptokinase in acute myocardial infarction. *J Am Coll Cardiol* 1993; **22**: 376–80.
13. Elizaga J, Garcia EJ, Delcan JL, *et al*. Primary coronary angioplasty versus systemic thrombolysis in acute anterior myocardial infarction: in-hospital results from a prospective randomized trial. *Circulation* 1993; **88**(Suppl I): I-411 (abstract).
14. Topol EJ, Leya F, Pinkerton CA, *et al*., for the Caveat Study Group. A comparison of directional atherectomy with coronary angioplasty in patients with coronary artery disease. *N Engl J Med* 1993; **329**: 221–7.
15. Adelman AG, Cohen EA, Kimball BP, *et al*. A comparison of directional atherectomy with balloon angioplasty for lesions of the left anterior descending coronary artery. *N Engl J Med* 1993; **329**: 228–33.
16. Holmes DR, Topol EJ, Adelman AG, Cohen EA, Califf RM. Randomized trials of directional coronary atherectomy: implications for clinical practice and future investigators. *J Am Coll Cardiol* 1994; **24**: 431–9.
17. Boehrer JD, Ellis SG, Pieper K, *et al*., for the Caveat-I Investigators. Directional atherectomy versus balloon angioplasty for coronary ostial and nonostial left anterior descending coronary artery lesions: results from a randomized multicenter trial. *J Am Coll Cardiol* 1995; **25**: 1380–6.
18. Elliot JM, Berdan LG, Holmes DR, *et al*., for the Caveat Study Investigators. One-year follow-up in the coronary angioplasty versus excisional atherectomy trial (CAVEAT-I). *Circulation* 1995; **91**: 2158–66.
19. Omoigui NA, Califf RM, Pieper K, *et al*. Peripheral vascular complications in coronary angioplasty versus excisional atherectomy trial (CAVEAT-I). *J Am Coll Cardiol* 1995; **26**: 922–30.
20. Holmes DR, Topol EJ, Califf RM, *et al*., for Caveat II Investigators. A multicenter, randomized trial of coronary angioplasty versus directional atherectomy for patients with saphenous vein bypass graft lesions. *Circulation* 1995; **91**: 1966–74.
21. Serruys PW, de Jaegere P, Kiemeneij F, *et al*., for the Benestent Study Group. A comparison of balloon expandable stent implantation with balloon angioplasty in patients with coronary artery disease. *N Engl J Med* 1994; **331**: 489–95.
22. Fischman DL, Leon MB, Baim DS, *et al*., for the Stent Restenosis Study Investigators. A randomized comparison of coronary stent placement and balloon angioplasty in the treatment of coronary artery disease. *N Engl J Med* 1994; **331**: 496–501.
23. Macaya C, Serruys PW, Ruygrok P, *et al*. Continued benefit of coronary stenting compared to balloon angioplasty: one year clinical follow-up of the Benestent trial. *J Am Coll Cardiol* 1996; **27**: 255–61.
24. Azar AJ, Detre K, Goldberg S, Kiemeneij F, Leon MB, Serruys PW. A meta-analysis on the clinical and angiographic

outcomes of stents versus PTCA in the different coronary vessel sizes in the Benestent-I and STRESS-II trials. *Circulation* 1995; **92**(Suppl I): I-475 (abstract).

25. Schömig A, Neumann FJ, Kastrati A, *et al*. A randomized comparison of antiplatelet and anticoagulant therapy after the placement of coronary artery stents. *N Engl J Med* 1996; **334**: 1084–9.

26. Appelman YEA, Piek JJ, Strikwerda S, *et al*. Excimer laser coronary angioplasty versus balloon angioplasty in the treatment of obstructive coronary artery disease: a randomized clinical trial. *Lancet* 1996; **347**: 79–84.

27. Deckelbaum LT, Natarajan MK, Bittl JA, *et al*. Effect of intracoronary saline infusion on dissection during excimer laser coronary angioplasty: a randomized trial. *J Am Coll Cardiol* 1995; **26**: 1264–9.

28. Ambrose JA, Almeida OD, Sharma SK, *et al*. Adjunctive thrombolytic therapy during angioplasty for ischemic rest angina. *Circulation* 1994; **90**: 69–77.

29. EPIC Investigators. Use of a monoclonal antibody directed against the platelet glycoprotein IIb/IIIa receptor in high-risk coronary angioplasty. *N Engl J Med* 1994; **330**: 956–61.

30. Topol EJ, Califf RM, Weisman HF, *et al*. Randomised trial of coronary intervention with antibody against platelet IIb/IIIa integrin for reduction of clinical restenosis: results at six months. *Lancet* 1994; **343**: 881–6.

31. Ferguson III JJ. Epilog and Capture trials halted because of positive interim results. *Circulation* 1996; **93**: 637.

12

Coronary Angioplasty and Coronary Artery Bypass Surgery

Robert A. Henderson

Introduction

Patients with angina can be treated with antianginal medication, or myocardial revascularization with coronary artery bypass graft (CABG) surgery or percutaneous transluminal coronary angioplasty (PTCA). CABG was first carried out in the 1960s[1,2] and rapidly became a routine operation for patients with coronary artery disease. Since then, advances in surgical technique have led to reductions in operative mortality, and the widespread use of internal mammary artery grafts has resulted in improved long-term clinical outcome.[3] Moreover, several randomized clinical trials have compared CABG with medical therapy, and in subsets of patients with left main stem disease or triple-vessel disease surgery improves long-term survival.[4]

Andreas Grüntzig introduced PTCA into clinical practice in 1977, as an alternative to CABG for selected patients with angina.[5,6] The procedure was initially considered appropriate for patients with a discrete proximal stenosis in a single coronary artery,[7] but with increasing experience the indications for PTCA expanded to include patients with complex coronary stenoses and multivessel disease.[8]

Early experience with PTCA demonstrated that in selected cases balloon dilatation of coronary artery stenoses improves subjective and objective measures of myocardial ischemia.[5,9] However, enthusiasm for PTCA was tempered by the recognition that not all coronary lesions can be safely treated, and in about 30% of successful cases the dilated stenosis recurs within 6 months (restenosis).[10,11] Moreover, for many years information about the late results of PTCA was confined to registry studies, which cannot reliably compare PTCA with other treatment options.[12,13] As a result, many clinicians remained sceptical about the benefits of the procedure, and there have been frequent calls for randomized clinical trials to compare PTCA with alternative medical and surgical treatment strategies.[14,15]

In the late 1980s several randomized trials designed to compare an initial treatment strategy of PTCA with an initial treatment strategy of CABG were begun.[16] These trials differed in design and execution, but they all enrolled patients who were clinically and angiographically suitable for either method of myocardial revascularization. Nine such trials involving cardiac centers around the world have reported preliminary results, and are the subject of this chapter.

The Trials

Bypass Angioplasty Revascularization Investigation (BARI)

The largest of the trials of PTCA versus CABG is the Bypass Angioplasty Revascularization Investigation (BARI), which enrolled patients at 14 centers across North America. BARI was designed to test the hypothesis that in patients with multivessel disease an initial treatment strategy of PTCA does not compromise clinical outcome over 5 years, when compared with an initial treatment strategy of CABG.[17] The main trial endpoint was 5-year mortality and the initial recruitment target of 2400 patients was calculated by assuming that this outcome would affect 5% in both treatment groups. In a trial of this size, the upper 95% confidence interval for the true difference in 5-year mortality between the two revascularization procedures is unlikely to exceed 2.5%.[17]

From August 1988 to July 1991 the BARI investigators screened 25 200 patients with multivessel disease but no previous myocardial revascularization, of whom 4100 with severe angina or objective evidence of myocardial ischemia were clinically and angiographically suitable for randomization.[18] Patients aged over 80 years, or patients with single-vessel or left main stem disease were ineligible.[17] Trial recruitment was slower than anticipated and was terminated after 1829 (7.2%) patients had been randomized. The baseline clinical and angiographic characteristics of the randomized patients have been reported in detail[19,20] and are summarized in *Table 12.1*.

In BARI the objective of revascularization was relief of myocardial ischemia, and the protocol did not require a specific revascularization strategy. Of the 914 patients assigned to CABG, 892 underwent surgery as the initial revascularization procedure, but 15 were treated by PTCA, and seven were treated medically. The majority of patients (87%) were operated within 2 weeks of randomization, with a mean of 2.8 grafts per patient. At least one internal mammary graft was used in 82% of cases.[21,22]

Of the 915 patients assigned to PTCA, 904 underwent the assigned PTCA procedure, nine were treated by CABG, and two patients were treated medically. On average PTCA was attempted in 2.4 lesions per patient, with multivessel PTCA in 70%, and staged procedures in 17%.[23]

The in-hospital mortality was 1.3% among the CABG patients, and 1.2% among the PTCA patients. Procedure-related Q-wave myocardial infarction occurred in 4.6% of the CABG group and 2.1% of the PTCA group, and emergency bypass surgery was required in 6.3% of the PTCA patients.[22]

Table 12.1   Baseline clinical and angiographic characteristics of trial subjects

	BARI	CABRI	RITA	EAST	GABI	MASS	Lausanne	ERACI	Toulouse
No. of patients	1829	1054	1011	392	359	142	134	127	152
Mean age (years)	61	60	57	62	?	56	55	58	?
Female (%)	27	22	19	26	20	18	20	15	?
Previous MI (%)	55	43	43	41	46	?	?	50	?
Diabetes mellitus (%)	25	12	6	23	12	16	12	11	?
Grade 3/4 angina (%)	16	62	59	80	81	?	79	?	?
Single-vessel disease (%)	2	1	45	–	–	100	100	–	–
Two-vessel disease (%)	57	57	43	60	81	–	–	55	78
Three-vessel disease (%)	41	42	12	40	19	–	–	45	22
Ejection fraction (%)	57	63	56	61	?	75	?	60	?

MI, Myocardial infarction.

After 5 years, mortality was 10.7% in the CABG group and 13.7% in the PTCA group, but this difference of 2.9% was not statistically significant (95% CI -0.2 to 6, $P = 0.19$). Moreover, there were no treatment differences in subgroups of patients with three-vessel disease or impaired left ventricular function, in whom CABG might be expected to confer a survival advantage. However, in a retrospective subgroup analysis involving 353 patients with treated diabetes mellitus, 5-year mortality was 34.5% among 173 patients assigned to PTCA, and 19.4% among 180 patients assigned to CABG ($P < 0.003$).[22,24]

The combined 5-year rate of death and Q-wave myocardial infarction was 19.6% in the CABG group and 21.3% in the PTCA group, and this 1.6% difference was not statistically significant (95% Cl -2.2 to 5.4, $P = 0.84$). Within 5 years of randomization, 8% of the CABG patients and 54% of PTCA patients required an additional revascularization procedure. Nevertheless, 69% of patients assigned to PTCA avoided CABG during this period, and 45% required only one angioplasty procedure.[23] Both treatment strategies relieved angina, but antianginal drug use was lower amongst CABG patients during follow-up. Physical functioning also improved in both groups, with a significantly greater improvement in the CABG group at 1 and 3 years, but not at 5 years, after randomization. PTCA patients returned to work an average of 6 weeks after the initial revascularization procedure, compared to 11 weeks for CABG patients, but there was no difference in long-term employment status.[25,26]

An economic analysis involving 934 patients at seven participating sites calculated costs of the two revascularization strategies. The mean costs of the initial revascularization strategy were US$32 347 for the CABG group and US$21 113 for the PTCA group. Over 5 years the costs increased to US$58 889 for patients assigned to CABG and US$56 225 for patients assigned to PTCA.[26]

Coronary Artery Bypass Revascularization Investigation (CABRI)

The Coronary Artery Bypass Revascularization Investigation (CABRI) is a multinational European study involving 26 centers, and was designed to compare initial strategies of PTCA and CABG in patients with multivessel coronary artery disease.[27] Patients with angina or inducible ischemia on stress testing were considered for randomization if coronary arteriography demonstrated stenoses in two or more major (>2 mm diameter) epicardial arteries. Before randomization, the participating surgeon and cardiologist had to agree that either method of revascularization would be likely to result in clinical improvement. There was no requirement for all coronary lesions to be treated, and patients with occluded coronary arteries were eligible for randomization. Patients with an ejection fraction less than 35%, or with 'high risk' coronary anatomy (including left main stem disease and occlusion of two major epicardial arteries) were excluded.[27]

Between July 1988 and December 1992 a total of 42 850 interventions for coronary artery disease were carried out at the participating centers, including 20 977 CABG and 21 603 PTCA procedures. Overall, 19 633 patients were ineligible for randomization because of single-vessel disease, recent acute myocardial infarction, or previous myocardial revascularization. Of the remaining 23 047 patients, 1054 were randomized, representing 2.4% of all revascularization procedures.[27] The baseline characteristics of the randomized patients are shown in *Table 12.1*.

The main trial endpoints were mortality and angina status at 5 years. The CABRI investigators estimated that the 5-year mortality in the CABG patients would be 5%, and a trial of 1054 patients has 80% power at the 5% significance level to detect a 60% reduction in 5-year mortality in the PTCA patients.[27] A trial of this size has greater power to detect clinically important treatment differences in the 5-year prevalence of angina.

Of the 513 patients assigned to CABG, 498 (97.1%) underwent a revascularization procedure (CABG in 478 and PTCA in 20) within a mean of 53 days of randomization. Among the surgically treated patients, 1318 of 1601 diseased coronary segments were grafted, with an average of 2.8 grafts per patient and at least one arterial graft in 81% of cases. Of 541 patients assigned to PTCA, 537 (99%) underwent a revascularization procedure (PTCA in 522, and CABG in 15) within a mean of 27 days. Among patients treated by PTCA, dilatation was attempted in 1072 of 1815 diseased coronary segments, with procedural success in 983 (91.7%) segments, or an average of 2.1 successfully dilated stenoses per patient.

Follow-up data have been reported on 1050 patients. One year after randomization there were 14 (2.7%) deaths among patients assigned to CABG and 21 (3.9%) deaths among patients assigned to PTCA, but this difference was not statistically significant (relative risk (RR) 1.42, 95% CI 0.73–2.76). In addition, nonfatal myocardial infarction occurred in 18 CABG patients and 27 PTCA patients (RR 1.42, 95% CI 0.80–2.54). Symptoms improved in both treatment groups, but at 1 year PTCA patients were more likely to have angina (grade 2 or worse) (13.9% versus 10.1%; $P = 0.012$), and to be taking antianginal medication (70% versus 53%; $P < 0.001$) than CABG patients.[27]

Additional revascularization procedures were carried out more frequently among PTCA patients than among CABG patients. Overall, 85 patients randomized to PTCA, but 4 patients randomized to CABG, underwent a nonassigned bypass operation. In addition, 113 PTCA patients and 14 CABG patients underwent a nonassigned coronary angioplasty procedure. During the first year, 93% of CABG patients, but 66% of PTCA patients, were managed by a single revascularization procedure.

In a subgroup analysis involving 147 patients randomized at centers in Belgium, the costs of the initial revascularization procedure (based on hospital charges) were estimated at 11 870 ECU for patients assigned to CABG and 5624 ECU for patients assigned to PTCA. During follow-up over 20 months, costs increased in both treatment groups, to 11 966 ECU in the CABG group, and 10 326 ECU in the PTCA group.[28]

Longer term follow-up results of the CABRI trial are awaited: in a preliminary report there were 17 deaths among the CABG patients and 37 deaths among the PTCA patients after a mean follow-up of 2 years. In a subgroup analysis involving 120 patients with diabetes there were 10 deaths among 64 PTCA patients and 2 deaths among 56 CABG patients.[29]

Randomized Intervention Treatment of Angina Trial (RITA)

The Randomized Intervention Treatment of Angina (RITA) trial, based at 16 centers in the UK, was designed to compare the effects of initial treatment strategies of PTCA and CABG on the 5-year risk of death or nonfatal myocardial infarction.[30] Patients with arteriographically proven coronary artery disease were considered for the study if the participating cardiologist and cardiothoracic surgeon agreed that equivalent revascularization could be achieved by either procedure. Patients were prospectively stratified into groups with one, two, or three vessels requiring treatment; patients with more than three vessels requiring treatment were ineligible for randomization. Patients with left main stem disease or previous myocardial revascularization were also excluded from the study.

The trial size of 1000 patients was calculated by assuming that the 5-year incidence of death or myocardial infarction would be 20% in one group, and that a one-third reduction in this event rate in the other group would be clinically important (80% power, 5% significance). During the first 34 months of the recruitment phase of the RITA trial the participating centers collected data on over 33 000 coronary arteriograms: of 28 400 patients with coronary artery disease, 62% were referred for revascularization, of whom 16% were eligible for the trial and 5% were randomized.[31] From March 1988 to November 1991, 1011 patients were randomized (of whom 45% had single-vessel disease); the baseline characteristics are shown in *Table 12.1*.

Of 501 patients randomized to CABG, 490 underwent the assigned revascularization procedure. In 97% of these patients all treatment vessels were grafted, and in 74% at least one internal mammary artery graft was used. Of 510 patients assigned to PTCA, coronary angioplasty was carried out in at least one vessel in 493 patients. In total, dilatation was attempted in 779 vessels (mean 1.6 vessels per patient), with an angiographic success rate of 87% (90% excluding occluded vessels). In 7% of PTCA patients the angioplasty procedure was staged over more than one hospital admission.[32]

The trial patients have been followed for a mean of 4.7 years, during which time there have been 26 deaths among the CABG patients and 24 among the PTCA patients. The primary endpoint of death or definite myocardial infarction occurred in 53 CABG and 64 PTCA patients (RR 1.22, 95% CI 0.83–1.79).[33] In an earlier analysis of 2.5-year follow-up data, 38% of the PTCA patients and 11% of the CABG patients had experienced a primary event (death or myocardial infarction) or underwent at least one additional revascularization procedure (*Figure 12.1*). Repeat coronary arteriography during follow-up was only carried out for clinical reasons, and was four times more frequent among PTCA patients than among CABG patients (31% versus 7%).[32]

The prevalence of angina during follow-up was greater among PTCA patients than among CABG patients (32% versus 11% at 6 months), but this difference decreased over time because of angina recurrence among the CABG patients. One month after revascularization the CABG patients were less physically active, with greater coronary related unemployment and lower mean exercise times than the PTCA patients. Thereafter, physical activity, employment status, and exercise treadmill times improved among the CABG patients, with no significant long-term differences between the two treatment groups. Perceived health status was assessed using the Nottingham Health Profile: over 2 years follow-up there were only small differences in perceived health status between the two treatment groups, reflecting the slightly greater prevalence of angina amongst the PTCA patients.[34] In the RITA trial there was no evidence of a difference in treatment effect between patients with single-vessel disease and those with multivessel disease.[32]

In a detailed economic analysis the initial cost of treating a patient assigned to PTCA was estimated at £3389, compared with an initial cost of treating a patient assigned to CABG of £6520. This initial cost advantage of PTCA was offset by the higher rate of coronary arteriograms and revascularization procedures during subsequent follow-up: over 2 years the mean costs increased to £6186 for the PTCA patients and £7619 for the CABG patients.[35]

Emory Angioplasty Surgery Trial (EAST)

The Emory Angioplasty Surgery Trial, based at Emory University in Atlanta, was designed to compare initial policies of CABG and PTCA in patients with multivessel disease.[36] Patients were required to have a clinical indication for revascularization (angina or objective signs of myocardial ischemia), and coronary lesions angiographically suitable for coronary angioplasty. Patients with totally occluded coronary arteries greater than 1.5

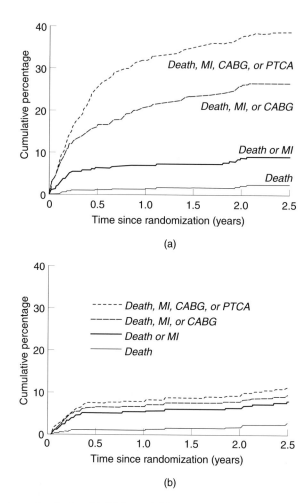

Figure 12.1 Patients randomized to (a) PTCA and (b) CABG in the RITA trial: cumulative risk of later PTCA, CABG, myocardial infarction, or death. (Reproduced with permission from Ref. 32.)

mm in diameter and supplying viable myocardium, or patients within 5 days of acute myocardial infarction were ineligible. Patients with previous myocardial revascularization, left main stem disease, occlusion of two major coronary vessels, or an ejection fraction of less than 25% were also excluded.

From July 1987 to April 1990, a total of 16 499 patients with coronary artery disease were screened for the trial, of whom 842 with multivessel disease were considered eligible for randomization. Consent to randomization was refused in 450 cases; the baseline characteristics of the 392 randomized patients (2.4% of screened patients) are shown in *Table 12.1.*[36]

Of 194 patients assigned to CABG, 193 were treated surgically (with an internal mammary artery graft in 86%) and one patient was treated by PTCA. Of 198 patients assigned to PTCA, 196 were treated by balloon dilatation and two by CABG. In 88% of the PTCA patients at least one lesion was dilated without major complication, but in 40% the procedure was staged over several days. Two patients (1%) in both treatment groups died

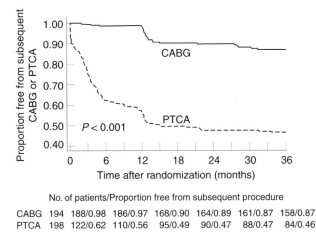

No. of patients/Proportion free from subsequent procedure

CABG	194	188/0.98	186/0.97	168/0.90	164/0.89	161/0.87	158/0.87
PTCA	198	122/0.62	110/0.56	95/0.49	90/0.47	88/0.47	84/0.46

Figure 12.2 Patients remaining free from additional revascularization procedures in EAST. (Reproduced with permission from Ref. 37.)

in hospital, and procedure-related Q-wave myocardial infarction occurred in 20 (10.3%) of the CABG patients and 6 (3.0%) of the PTCA patients. The initial assigned PTCA procedure was complicated by CABG in 20 patients (10.1%).[37]

Over 3 years follow-up there were 12 deaths among the CABG patients and 14 deaths among the PTCA patients. Q-wave myocardial infarction was diagnosed in 38 (19.6%) of the CABG group and 29 (14.6%) of the PTCA group, but no 3-year electrocardiogram was available for 13 patients in both treatment groups. A large ischemic defect on a thallium myocardial perfusion scan was detected at 3 years in 11 (5.7%) of the CABG group and 19 (9.6%) of the PTCA group (thallium scans were obtained in 77% of patients and were interpreted by two investigators, blinded to the patients' treatment assignment). Thus the combined main trial endpoint of death (from all causes), nonfatal Q-wave myocardial infarction, and detection of a large ischemic defect on a stress thallium scan occurred in 27.3% of the surgical group and 28.8% of the angioplasty group ($P = 0.81$).[37] In a subsequent report, 5-year mortality was 8.8% in the CABG group and 12.1% in the PTCA group, but this difference was not statistically significant.[38]

At randomization, the EAST trialists identified index myocardial segments that were supplied by the diseased coronary arteries judged suitable for treatment by PTCA or CABG. All index segments were revascularized by the initial procedure in 96% of the CABG group and 71% of the PTCA group.[39] Repeat coronary arteriography was performed in 87% of eligible patients 1 year after randomization and in 76% of eligible patients 3 years after. At 1 year, 88% of the index segments were revascularized in the CABG group compared with 59% in the PTCA group, but by 3 years this difference had narrowed (87% versus 70%).[37,39]

The follow-up coronary arteriograms were required by protocol but influenced clinical management, as evidenced by clustering of additional revascularization procedures around 1 year follow-up (*Figure 12.2*). Over 3 years 1% of the CABG group and 22% of the PTCA group underwent additional (nonrandomized) bypass surgery, and 13% of the CABG group but 41% of the PTCA group underwent additional angioplasty. At least one additional revascularization procedure was required in 13% of the CABG patients, but in 54% of the PTCA patients.[37]

At 3 years 20% of PTCA patients had angina (grade 2 or higher) compared with 12% of CABG patients (P = 0.039). PTCA patients were also more likely to be taking antianginal medication (66% versus 51%; P = 0.005), and were readmitted to hospital with chest pain more frequently than CABG patients (36% versus 16%; P < 0.0001). At 3 years, 38% of CABG and 36% of PTCA patients were in gainful employment.[40]

The estimated mean costs of the initial revascularization procedures per patient (inflated to 1993 US dollars) were US$24 821 for the PTCA group and US$36 728 for the CABG group. At 3 years treatment costs had increased in both groups, to US$36 313 for patients assigned to PTCA and US$38 724 for patients assigned to CABG.[40]

German Angioplasty Bypass Investigation (GABI)

The German Angioplasty Bypass Investigation (GABI) is a multicenter study designed to compare the effects of PTCA and CABG in patients with stable angina and multivessel coronary artery disease. Patients aged under 75 years were considered for randomization if revascularization of at least two major coronary vessels (with at least 70% diameter stenosis) was judged clinically necessary and technically feasible. Patients with previous myocardial revascularization, recent acute myocardial infarction, complete coronary occlusion, left main stem disease, or other high-risk coronary anatomy were excluded. Other specific arteriographic exclusion criteria included long (>2 cm) coronary lesions, diffuse distal disease, and coronary aneurysms.[41]

GABI was designed to show that the two revascularization procedures were equally effective at relieving angina. The trialists assumed that 65% of patients would be free from angina 1 year after CABG, and that clinical equivalence would be demonstrated if the prevalence of angina in the two treatment groups did not differ by more than 15% at 1 year after randomization. The trialists screened 8981 patients with multivessel disease, and aimed to recruit 400 patients. However, recruitment was terminated prematurely after 359 patients had been randomized, because an interim analysis showed no difference in angina rates between the two treatment groups.[41]

Between randomization and revascularization (median 53 days for CABG and 19 days for PTCA) there were 4 deaths among 177 patients assigned to CABG and 1 death among 182 patients assigned to PTCA. In addition, 17 patients withdrew their consent to participation (12 in the CABG group and 5 in the PTCA group). Among the 176 patients treated by PTCA, an average of 1.9 vessels were dilated per patient, with complete revascularization in 86%. PTCA was performed as a staged procedure in 30%, and emergency CABG was required in 5 patients (2.8%). In the 161 patients treated by CABG, an average of 2.2 vessels were grafted per patient, with an internal mammary graft in 37%.[41]

One-year follow-up data have been reported for 155 PTCA and 139 CABG patients (82% of the randomized patients). The cumulative 1-year rate of death and Q-wave myocardial infarction was 13.6% for the CABG patients and 6.0% for the PTCA patients (P = 0.017), and this difference was mainly due to an excess of procedure-related myocardial infarctions in the CABG group. During the first year, 44% of the PTCA patients underwent an additional revascularization procedure (CABG in 21%, and repeat PTCA in 26%). By contrast, in the CABG group only 6% underwent additional revascularization procedures (PTCA in 5% and repeat CABG in 1%).[41]

At 3 months, 84% of the CABG patients, but 60% of the PTCA patients, were free from major anginal symptoms. This difference attenuated with further follow-up, and by 12 months 74% of the CABG patients and 71% of the PTCA patients were angina free. In a subgroup of patients the symptomatic improvement was matched by an increase in exercise treadmill time, but 78% of the CABG patients and 88% of the PTCA patients continued to take antianginal medication.[41]

In an economic analysis the costs of an initial policy of PTCA were 51% of the costs of an initial policy of CABG. Because of the subsequent higher rate of repeat interventions in the PTCA group this increased to 75% after 2 years of follow-up.[42]

Medicine Angioplasty or Surgery Study (MASS)

The Medicine Angioplasty or Surgery Study (MASS) is a single-center Brazilian trial, in which 214 patients with isolated left anterior descending artery disease were randomized to treatment with internal mammary bypass grafting, coronary angioplasty, or medical therapy. All patients had at least 80% diameter stenosis in the anterior descending artery, before the first major diagonal branch. Patients with unstable angina, previous myocardial infarction, left ventricular dysfunction, or previous myocardial revascularization were excluded.[43]

The primary endpoint of the trial was the combined incidence of cardiac death, myocardial infarction, or refractory angina requiring an additional (non-randomized) revascularization procedure. After 3 years of follow-up this endpoint had occurred in 2 patients assigned to CABG (3%), 17 patients assigned to PTCA (24%), and 12 patients assigned to medical therapy (17%). There was no difference in mortality or myocardial infarction between the treatment groups, but 8 PTCA patients and 7 medical patients underwent additional (nonrandomized) interventions. Both revascularization techniques resulted in symptomatic improvement: after a mean of 3 years, 32% of the medically assigned patients but 82% of PTCA patients and 98% of CABG patients were asymptomatic. Nevertheless, during follow-up, 78% of medical, 64% of PTCA, and 80% of CABG patients remained in regular work.[43]

Lausanne Trial

The Lausanne trial is a single-center study, designed to compare coronary angioplasty and internal mammary artery grafting in patients with single-vessel proximal left anterior descending artery disease and normal left ventricular function. Patients were required to have evidence of myocardial ischemia (on exercise testing, or electrocardiographic abnormalities during angina), but patients with unstable angina or previous Q-wave myocardial infarction were excluded.[44]

From October 1989 to May 1993 a total of 5119 patients underwent coronary arteriography, of whom 1786 had single-vessel disease, and 134 were randomized. Of 66 patients assigned to CABG, 59 were managed surgically, 6 were treated by PTCA, and 1 was managed medically following a preoperative myocardial infarction. All 68 patients assigned to PTCA underwent balloon dilatation, but two patients required emergency CABG.[44]

The primary trial endpoint was the combined rate of cardiac death, myocardial infarction, and the need for repeat (nonrandomized) revascularization procedures. After a median of 24 months this endpoint had occurred in 25 patients assigned to PTCA and 5 patients assigned to CABG. This difference was mainly due to an excess of additional revascularization procedures among the PTCA patients. Both treatments resulted in sustained symptomatic improvement, but at 2 years the prevalence of angina was lower among the surgically assigned patients (11% versus 23%). In addition, patients in the CABG group required less antianginal medication.[44]

Argentine Trial (ERACI)

The Argentinean ERACI trial compared initial treatment strategies of PTCA and CABG in patients with multivessel disease in whom complete functional revascularization could be achieved by either treatment method. Complete functional revascularization was defined as no residual stenosis greater than 50% in any major epicardial vessel supplying viable myocardium. Patients were eligible for randomization if they had stable or unstable angina in spite of antianginal medication, or were judged to be at risk on the basis of an exercise treadmill test. Exclusion criteria included impaired left ventricular function, left main stem disease, severe three-vessel disease, and evolving acute myocardial infarction.[45]

From June 1988 to December 1990, a total of 1409 patients investigated by coronary arteriography were considered for randomization. Revascularization was judged necessary in 748 patients, of whom 302 met the entry criteria. The trial was designed with a recruitment target of 160 patients, but randomization was terminated for undisclosed reasons after 127 patients had been randomized.

Of 64 patients assigned to CABG, 56 were treated surgically (with an internal mammary artery graft in 76.5%), and 8 were treated by angioplasty. Of the 63 patients assigned to PTCA, 55 underwent balloon dilatation and 8 were treated by CABG. Complete anatomical revascularization was achieved in 88% of the CABG patients and 55% of the PTCA patients, but revascularization was functionally complete in 89% of the PTCA group.

During follow-up over 3 years there was no difference in risk of death or myocardial infarction between the two treatment groups. However, patients assigned to PTCA were more likely to complain of angina (43% versus 21%) or require repeat revascularization (37% versus 6%) than were patients assigned to CABG. The 3-year costs of an initial strategy of PTCA were estimated at US$7500 per patient, compared with US$13 000 per patient for an initial strategy of CABG.[46]

Toulouse Trial

The single-center Toulouse trial was designed to compare the two revascularization procedures in patients in whom treatment of at least two major coronary vessels was deemed clinically necessary and technically feasible. From June 1989 to June 1993, the trialists screened 1939 patients with multivessel disease and randomly assigned 152 patients to PTCA or CABG.[47,48] In-hospital mortality was 1.3% in both groups and after 5-years mortality had increased to 11.6% in the CABG group and 13.2% in the PTCA group ($P = 0.69$). Nonassigned CABG procedures were required in 14.5% of the PTCA group; nonassigned PTCA procedures were carried out in 7.9% of the CABG group and 14.5% of the PTCA group. At five years, event-free survival (myocardial infarction, angina) was 82.9% in the CABG group and 68.4% in the PTCA group.[47]

Discussion

The nine trials described above were designed to compare two revascularization policies for patients with coronary artery disease. In all the trials patients who were suitable for either method of revascularization were randomly assigned to initial treatment by PTCA or CABG. Treatment crossovers occurred in both treatment groups at the time of the initial revascularization procedure and during subsequent follow-up, but in all the trials the main results were analyzed by initial treatment assignment.

The individual trials differed in objectives, inclusion criteria, and follow-up. For instance, most of the trials were restricted to patients with multivessel disease, but two of the trials only recruited patients with single-vessel proximal left anterior descending artery disease. Some of the trials also excluded patients with completely occluded coronary arteries or impaired left ventricular function, but in other trials these patients were eligible for randomization. Nevertheless, the results of the individual trials are remarkably consistent and provide valuable information on which clinicians can base decisions about the choice of revascularization procedure for patients with angina.

Limitations

During recruitment, the trials of PTCA versus CABG screened a total of over 130 000 patients with coronary artery disease. However, in several trials recruitment was slower than anticipated, and in some trials (BARI, GABI, and ERACI) recruitment was terminated before the target number of patients had been randomized. In total, only 5200 patients were randomized, and these highly selected patients may not be typical of the general population of patients undergoing myocardial revascularization. Nevertheless, the randomized patients may be more representative of patients considered clinically and angiographically suitable for either revascularization strategy. Data from the BARI and RITA trial registries suggest that about 16% of all patients undergoing myocardial revascularization may be suitable for treatment by either PTCA or CABG.[18,31]

Randomized trials of CABG conducted in the 1970s suggested that some patients, including those with three-vessel coronary disease and impaired left ventricular function, gain a long-term survival advantage from surgical revascularization.[4] However, the trials of PTCA versus CABG generally excluded such high-risk patients and a substantial proportion of the randomized patients had two-vessel disease and good left ventricular function (*Table 12.1*). Overall, the trial patients were at only moderate cardiovascular risk, with a mortality of approximately 7% over 3–4 years. On the basis of previous evidence, such patients would not be expected to gain a major prognostic advantage from CABG.[4]

Some of the trial protocols required complete anatomical (GABI), complete functional (ERACI), or equivalent (RITA) myocardial revascularization, but in other trials (BARI, EAST, and CABRI) the revascularization strategy was directed towards effective symptom relief. Nevertheless, in most of the trials the extent of revascularization achieved by an initial strategy of PTCA was less than that achieved by an initial strategy of CABG. This difference between the two treatment strategies reflects routine clinical practice, where most PTCA procedures involve dilatation of a limited number of coronary stenoses. By contrast, during CABG all major diseased vessels will usually be grafted during a single operation.

Registry studies provide conflicting information about the influence of the extent of revascularization on long-term clinical outcome. Some studies suggest that the extent of revascularization achieved by CABG may be of prognostic importance,[49,50] although prognosis may be more dependent on the number of vessels suitable for grafting.[51] Several small studies also suggest that clinical outcome after PTCA may be more favorable in those patients with complete revascularization,[52–54] but this has not been confirmed in all reports.[55] These conflicting results reflect the fact that coronary artery disease is a diffuse process, and balloon dilatation or placement of a bypass graft may not revascularize all myocardial territories supplied by a single epicardial artery. Moreover, the concept of complete myocardial revascularization neglects early graft occlusion in surgically treated patients or restenosis in angioplasty patients. When applying the results of the trials of PTCA versus CABG to clinical practice the revascularization strategy and extent of revascularization achieved in individual trials may therefore be of limited relevance.

Mortality and Meta-analysis

The BARI trial was designed to compare the effects of the two revascularization strategies on mortality in 2400 patients, but recruitment was terminated after only 1829 patients had been randomized. The other smaller trials were designed to compare the effects of the two procedures on composite endpoints. All the trials, therefore, have limited statistical power to detect small, but potentially important, differences in mortality between the two treatment strategies.

In an attempt to overcome this problem the results of the trials have been combined in meta-analyses. Sim et al.[56] carried out an analysis of the published results of five trials involving 1449 patients with multivessel disease. In this study, mortality did not differ significantly between the two revascularization strategies.

In a more comprehensive overview, Pocock and colleagues reported an analysis of updated summary results from eight trials of angioplasty versus bypass surgery. In an analysis involving 3371 patients, there were 73 deaths in the CABG group and 79 in the PTCA group, with no overall evidence of a treatment difference (RR 1.08, 95% CI 0.79–1.50). About half of all deaths occurred at the time of the initial revascularization procedure and thereafter mortality was low in both treatment groups.[48]

Since the publication of these meta-analyses the results of the BARI trial have been released, and mortality data on 5200 patients randomized in nine trials of PTCA versus CABG are now available. During a mean follow-up of around 3.6 years there were 184 deaths (7.1%) among 2575 patients assigned to an initial strategy of CABG, and 210 deaths (8.0%) among 2625 patients assigned to an initial strategy of PTCA (fixed-effects estimate of RR 1.13, 95% CI 0.94–1.37; heterogeneity test χ^2 6.52, $P = 0.59$). Although this difference is not statistically significant, the data do not exclude the possibility that over 3–4 years an initial strategy of PTCA is associated with a 13% relative increase in the risk of death (equivalent to an absolute excess of 9 deaths per 1000 patients). The clinical significance of such a difference in mortality is a matter for debate, but in other areas of cardiology trialists claim that mortality differences of similar magnitude are clinically important.[57–59] The effects of the two revascularization procedures on long-term mortality could only be fully elucidated by much larger randomized trials, which would be expensive and difficult to conduct, and as yet there are no plans for such trials anywhere in the world.

In the BARI trial a subgroup analysis suggested that diabetic patients treated by an initial policy of PTCA were at higher risk of mortality, compared with diabetic patients treated by an initial policy of CABG.[23] The relevance of this finding is uncertain, but a similar statistically nonsignificant effect was reported in 122 patients with diabetes in CABRI.[29] Numerous studies have demonstrated that diabetes increases the risk of restenosis after successful PTCA, and the difference in mortality between the two groups of diabetic patients may be due to a real biological difference.[60] Nevertheless, the BARI result must be interpreted cautiously because in a retrospective subgroup analysis the observed difference in outcome between the two groups of diabetic patients may be due to chance. Further research is required before firm recommendations can be made about the choice of myocardial revascularization procedure for diabetic patients.

Myocardial Infarction

The reported rates of myocardial infarction differed between the trials, probably because of differences in methods of detection and classification, as well as real differences in the rates of myocardial infarction. For example, EAST reported comparatively high rates of myocardial infarction, possibly because the diagnosis was based on the appearance of new electrocardiographic abnormalities even in the absence of a clinical event. Nevertheless, the results of all nine trials suggest that in patients in whom either method of revascularization is feasible, PTCA and CABG are associated with a similar risk of death or nonfatal myocardial infarction. During a mean 3.6 years of follow-up, there were 306 deaths or nonfatal myocardial infarctions (11.9%) among patients assigned to an initial strategy of CABG, and 329 such events (12.5%) among patients assigned to an initial strategy of PTCA (fixed-effects estimate of RR 1.06, 95% CI 0.92–1.23; heterogeneity test χ^2 10.89, $P = 0.21$).

The use of myocardial infarction as a major component of a composite endpoint has several important limitations. The interpretation of electrocardiographic abnormalities and elevated cardiac enzyme levels in patients undergoing myocardial revascularization procedures may be difficult, and criteria for diagnosing myocardial infarction in these patients have not been clearly defined. In several of the trials the diagnosis of myocardial infarction was validated by an endpoint committee blinded to treatment assignment, but even with this precaution the possiblity of bias in open trials cannot be excluded completely. Moreover, the assumption that a diagnosis of myocardial infarction has the same long-term clinical significance in PTCA patients and in CABG patients, implicit in the use of myocardial infarction as an important trial endpoint, has not been validated prospectively. For example, in EAST the difference in the rate of perioperative myocardial infarction between the two treatment groups was not associated with any difference in clinical outcome or ejection fraction over 3 years of follow-up.[36]

Angina and Additional Revascularization Procedures

The trials confirm that PTCA and CABG are both effective treatments for angina, although most of the trials suggest that CABG is slightly more effective during the first 1–3 years after revascularization. This advantage of CABG over PTCA attenuated with time,[48] probably because of occlusion of saphenous vein grafts in the CABG patients[3,61] and treatment of incomplete revascularization and restenosis in the PTCA patients.

Angina is a subjective measure of health, and it is difficult to exclude the possibility of bias when such endpoints are evaluated in an open trial. In several trials the use of antianginal drugs was considered as a surrogate for angina: during follow-up antianginal drugs were used more widely among PTCA patients than among CABG patients, although in some patients these drugs may have been prescribed for reasons other than symptom relief.

In all the trials, the patients treated with PTCA had a greater requirement for additional revascularization procedures than did those treated with CABG. The risk of a nonrandomized CABG procedure in patients initially assigned to PTCA was about 20% over 2–3 years, compared with less than 5% in the CABG group.[48] Overall, about one-third of patients assigned to an initial strategy of PTCA required an additional revascularization procedure within 1 year, but thereafter the reintervention rate was much lower. In several of the trials the occurrence of additional revascularization procedures formed part of a composite trial endpoint, but in trials designed to compare two initial treatment strategies it may be more appropriate to consider these procedures as part of the overall treatment process.

Late Follow-up

As yet several of the trials have only reported medium term (1–3 year) follow-up, and it is possible that important differences between the two revascularization strategies will only emerge with longer term follow-up. After PTCA, restenosis usually occurs within 6 months of the procedure and late restenosis is rare, but late outcome may also be influenced by the effects of incomplete revascularization at the initial procedure. After CABG, 20% of saphenous vein grafts occlude within 1 year with an annual graft attrition of up to 5% thereafter,[3,61] and effects of saphenous vein graft occlusion may only become apparent after several years. Late clinical outcome may also be influenced by disease progression in both treatment groups, and the 5–10 year results of the trials will be of considerable importance to clinicians managing patients with angina.

New Technologies

The trials of PTCA and CABG recruited patients during the mid to late 1980s, since when there have been important advances in interventional cardiology and cardiac surgery. In particular, the STRESS and BENESTENTtrials demonstrated that in selected patients coronary stents reduce the risk of restenosis and the subsequent clinical event rate.[62–64] In these studies stents were associated with an increased risk of hemorrhage due to intensive anticoagulation, but it is now recognized that anticoagulation is unnecessary, provided that the stent is optimally deployed.[65–68]

New pharmacological interventions may also improve the acute and long-term results of coronary angioplasty. The EPIC trial suggested that the glycoprotein IIb/IIIa receptor blocker abciximab improves acute outcome after coronary angioplasty, and this benefit may be sustained in the long-term.[69,70] In addition, lipid-lowering drug therapy improves clinical outcome in patients with coronary artery disease,[71] but whether this beneficial effect is similar in patients treated with CABG and with PTCA is not known.

These important advances in cardiology limit the relevance of the trials of PTCA versus CABG to current clinical practice. In particular, the expanding role of coronary stenting in interventional cardiology may alter the balance of risks, benefits and costs between the two revascularization procedures, and further clinical trials comparing optimal interventional and surgical treatment strategies are now required.

Economic Considerations

The economic analyses of the trials are remarkably consistent, and indicate that CABG is initially twice the cost of PTCA, reflecting a greater requirement for specialized nursing and inpatient care during the initial surgical procedure. However, this cost difference attenuates during subsequent follow-up because of the greater requirement for additional procedures in the PTCA group, with little difference in cost between the two revascularization strategies over 3–5 years. As yet none of the trials have reported an analysis of cost-effectiveness.

Conclusions

The trials of coronary angioplasty versus CABG surgery are well designed, properly randomized studies, and provide important evidence about the comparative long-term effects of the two revascularization procedures. Although the trials are subject to limitations, the results provide clinicians with valuable information on which the choice of revascularization strategy for patients can be based.

Individually, the trials do not have sufficient statistical power to detect small but potentially important differences in mortality between the two treatment strategies. However, in the absence of evidence of a major difference in long-term mortality, risk of myocardial infarction or treatment cost, patients who are suitable for either procedure can be offered a choice. On the one hand, an initial strategy of PTCA usually involves a short admission to hospital, followed by a rapid return to normal activity. PTCA relieves angina but is somewhat less effective than CABG during the first 1–3 years, and is associated with a one in three risk of additional revascularization procedures during the first year of follow-up. On the other hand, the more invasive coronary bypass operation is usually followed by a 2–3 month convalescence. Thereafter, CABG is associated with a relatively stable clinical course, with relief of angina and a low requirement for additional procedures over several years.

In the light of this information some clinicians may prefer to individualize treatment. For instance, PTCA may be recommended in young patients in the hope of deferring CABG and of avoiding the risks of a second surgical procedure in the longer term. PTCA may also be preferred in the frail elderly, or patients with other pathologies that increase the risk of CABG. In other situations, patients who are suitable for either treatment method may choose between the short-term convenience of the simpler angioplasty procedure, and the more certain medium-term outcome of the more invasive bypass operation.

The late effects of graft occlusion in the CABG patients, restenosis, and incomplete revascularization in the PTCA patients, and disease progression in both treatment groups will be elucidated by further follow-up of the randomized patients. The relative merits of the two revascularization procedures may change as these longer term follow-up results become available.

Acknowledgment

I am grateful to Stephen Sharp for help with the meta-analyses in this chapter.

References

1. Favaloro RG. Saphenous vein autograft replacement of severe segmental coronary artery occlusion. Operative technique. *Ann Thorac Surg* 1968; **5**: 334–9.
2. Garrett HE, Dennis EW, DeBakey ME. Aortocoronary bypass with saphenous vein graft: seven-year follow-up. *JAMA* 1973; **223**: 792–4.
3. Loop FD, Lytle BW, Cosgrove DM, *et al*. Influence of the internal-mammary-artery graft on 10 year survival and other cardiac events. *N Engl J Med* 1986; **314**: 1–6.

63. Macaya C, Serruys P, Ruygrok P, *et al*. Continued benefit of coronary stenting versus balloon angioplasty: one-year clinical follow-up of Benestent trial. *J Am Coll Cardiol* 1996; **27**: 255–61.
64. Savage MP, Fischman DL, Schatz RA, *et al*. Long-term angiographic and clinical outcome after implantation of a balloon-expandable stent in the native coronary circulation. Palmaz–Schatz Stent Study Group. *J Am Coll Cardiol* 1994; **24**: 1207–12.
65. Colombo A, Hall P, Nakamura S, *et al*. Intracoronary stenting without anticoagulation accomplished with intravascular ultrasound guidance. *Circulation* 1995; **91**: 1676–88.
66. Hall P, Nakamura S, Mailello L, *et al*. A randomized comparison of combined ticlopidine and aspirin therapy versus aspirin therapy alone after successful intravascular ultrasound-guided stent implantation. *Circulation* 1996; **93**: 215–22.
67. Schömig A, Neumann FJ, Kastrati A, *et al*. A randomized comparison of antiplatelet and anticoagulant therapy after the placement of coronary-artery stents. *N Engl J Med* 1996: **334**: 1084–9.
68. Serruys PW, Emanuelsson H, van der Giessen W, *et al*. Heparin-coated Palmaz–Schatz stents in human coronary arteries. Early outcome of the Benestent-II pilot study. *Circulation* 1996; **93**: 412–22.
69. Topol EJ, Califf RM, Weisman HF, *et al*. Randomised trial of coronary intervention with antibody against platelet IIb/IIIa integrin for reduction of clinical restenosis: results at six months. *Lancet* 1994; **343**: 881–6.
70. The EPIC Investigators. Use of a monoclonal antibody directed against the platelet glycoprotein IIb/IIIa receptor in high risk coronary angioplasty. *N Engl J Med* 1994; **330**: 956–61.
71. Scandinavian Simvastatin Survival Study Group. Randomised trial of cholesterol lowering in 4444 patients with coronary heart disease: the Scandinavian simvastatin survival study (4S). *Lancet* 1994; **344**: 1383–9.

13

Thrombolysis

Harvey D. White

Introduction

Each year, between 1.5 and 2 million patients worldwide are admitted to hospital with acute myocardial infarction. Over 200 000 patients have been randomized in clinical trials evaluating the effects of thrombolytic therapy in patients with acute infarction. About 65 000 patients have been randomized to thrombolytic therapy versus placebo or control therapy, and about 140 000 patients to comparisons of different thrombolytic agents. In no other area of medicine has a treatment been so extensively investigated with such firm scientific evidence available on which to base recommendations for clinical practice.

Clinical trials of thrombolytic therapy have investigated a number of endpoints including infarct artery recanalization, patency, infarct size, left ventricular function, and mortality. Mechanistic trials evaluating pathophysiology have clearly shown that lysis of the infarct artery thrombus results in limitation of infarct size[1] and preservation of left ventricular function.[2] A number of mortality trials have shown that thrombolytic therapy reduces mortality. The Global Use of Streptokinase and Tissue Plasminogen Activator for Occluded Coronary Arteries (GUSTO) study combined a mechanistic angiographic substudy in 2431 patients within an overall mortality study of 41 041 patients to underpin infarct artery patency as the mechanism by which a greater mortality reduction was achieved with an accelerated tissue plasminogen activator (t-PA) compared with streptokinase.[3] The aim of thrombolytic therapy is to accelerate fibrinolysis. Endogenous fibrinolysis in the presence of antithrombin therapy slowly achieves infarct artery patency, but the earlier and more completely reperfusion is achieved, the greater the benefit.[3] In this chapter the only trials discussed in detail are those of sufficient size (>1000 patients) and with mortality as their endpoint.

Historical Aspects

The use of intravenous streptokinase in patients with acute myocardial infarction was first reported in 1958,[4] and 24 trials were performed in the early 1960s and 1970s.[5] By today's standards these trials had major design flaws, with randomization of patients up to 72 hours after the onset of infarction and the use of low doses of streptokinase, for example 250 000 iu over 30 minutes followed by 100 000 iu h^{-1}. The mortality rates were around 30%, and no trial showed a clear reduction in mortality. Furthermore, the theoretical basis for the use of thrombolytic therapy was insecure, based partly on the known vasodilatory

Table 13.2 Electrocardiographic, time, and age elibility for thrombolytic therapy in large mortality trials

| Trial | Time from symptom onset (h) | Age restriction (years) | ST elevation (mm) | | | ST depression (number of leads) | Other criteria |
			Limb leads (number)	Leads V_1 to V_3 (number)	Leads V_4 to V_6 (number)		
GISSI[13]	≤12	No	≥1 (1)	≥2 (1)	≥2 (1)	As for ST elevation	–
ISAM[20]	≤6	<76	≥1 (1)	≥2 (1)	≥2 (1)	Not eligible	–
AIMS[21]	≤6	<70	≥1 (2)	≥2 (2)	≥2 (2)	Not eligible	–
SIS-2[16]	≤24	No	–	–	–	–	Acute infarction clinically suspected
ASSET[18]	≤5	<75	–	–	–	–	Acute infarction clinically suspected
USIM[24]	≤4	No	≥1 (1)	≥2 (1)	≥2 (1)	As for ST elevation	–
GISSI-2[7]	≤6	No	≥1	≥2 (1)	≥2 (1)	Not eligible	–
ISIS-3[8]	>24	No	–	–	–	–	Acute infarction clinically suspected
EMERAS[14]	6-24	No	–	–	–	–	Acute infarction clinically suspected
LATE[26]	6-24	No	≥1 (2)	≥2 (2)	≥2 (2)	≥2 mm (2)	Abnormal Q- or T-waves (≥2 leads)
GUSTO[9]	≤6	No	≥1 (2)	≥2 (2)	≥2 (2)	Not eligible	–
EMIP[27]	<6	No	≥1 (2)	≥2 (2)	≥2 (2)	Eligible	QRS >0.12, tall T-waves
INJECT[37]	<12	No	≥1 (2)	≥2 (2)	≥2 (2)	Not eligible	Bundle branch block

Table 13.3 Early mortality and stroke rates in large mortality trials

Trial	Time from symptom onset (h)	Mortality (%)		Stroke (%)		Probable intracranial hemorrhage (%)	
		Thrombolytic	Control	Thrombolytic	Control	Thrombolytic	Control
GISSI[13]	<6	10.2	12.8	0.84	0.68	0.46	0.13
ISAM[20]	<6	5.9	7.0	–	–	0.47	0
AIMS[21]	<6	6.3	12.2	1.3	0.63	0.32	0.15
ISIS-2[16]	<6	8.8	12.1	0.71	0.78	0.31	0.15
ASSET[18]	<5	7.2	9.8	1.1	1.0	0.28	0.08
USIM[24]	<4	8.0	8.3	0.3	0.2	–	–
GISSI-2[27]	<6	Streptokinase, 9.2 t-PA, 9.6	– –	0.9 1.3	– –	0.3 0.4	– –
ISIS-3[8]	<6	Streptokinase, 10.6 t-PA, 10.3 Anistreplase, 10.5	– – –	Streptokinase, 1.0 t-PA, 1.4 Anistreplase, 1.26	– – –	0.2 0.7 0.5	– – –
EMERAS[14]	6–24	11.9	12.4	1.5	1.1	0.8	0.3
LATE[26]	6–24	8.8	10.3	2.3	1.2	0.8	0.2
GUSTO[9]	<6	Streptokinase s.c., 7.2 Streptokinase i.v., 7.4 t-PA, 6.3 t-PA + streptokinase, 7.0	– – – –	1.2 1.4 1.5 1.6	– – – –	0.5 0.5 0.7 0.9	– – – –
EMIP[27]	<6	Early anistreplase, 9.7 Hospital anistreplase, 11.1	– –	Early, 1.6 Hospital, 1.5	– –	Early, 0.8 Hospital, 0.8	– –
INJECT[37]	<12	Streptokinase, 9.5 Reteplase, 9.0	– –	Streptokinase, 1.0 Reteplase, 1.2	– –	Streptokinase, 0.4 Reteplase, 0.8	– –

i.v., Intravenous; s.c., subcutaneous; t-PA, tissue plasminogen activator.

Table 13.4   t-PA dosage (mg) by time in GUSTO[9] compared with the standard regimen in GISSI-2[7]

Time (min)	GUSTO		GISSI-2
	Accelerated t-PA	Combination[a] (t-PA + 1 000 000 iu streptokinase)	(standard t-PA)
30	65	40	35
60	82.5	80	60
90	100	80	70

t-PA, Tissue plasminogen activator.
[a]t-PA + 1 000 000 iu streptokinase.

7.4%; $P = 0.01$). Mortality in the combination-therapy group was 7.0%. The incidence of stroke was increased with t-PA, being 1.55%, versus 1.22% for streptokinase plus subcutaneous heparin, 1.4% for streptokinase plus intravenous heparin, and 1.64% for combination therapy. Infarct artery reocclusion rates were low and were similar in all four treatment groups in the angiographic substudy 5–7 days after thrombolysis (4.9–6.4%).[35]

Although adjunctive intravenous heparin was probably important for maintaining the high 90-minute TIMI-3 patency rate (54%) seen with the accelerated t-PA regimen, heparin in the doses used has not been shown to accelerate reperfusion,[36] and the major explanation for the benefit seen in the GUSTO study is the better 90-minute patency rates achieved by the accelerated t-PA regimen.[3,34]

Patients in the combination thrombolytic therapy group received a t-PA regimen similar to that administered in the GISSI-2/International study[7,28] and in ISIS-3[8] (Table 13.4). By 90 minutes, which is the time at which patency has been shown to be importantly related to mortality outcome,[3] the amount of t-PA administered was slightly greater than that administered in the standard regimen used in the GISSI-2/International study. Intravenous heparin was also given to patients in the combined-therapy group, and yet the mortality was similar to that in the streptokinase-treated patients. The GUSTO study therefore validates the previous left ventricular function trials[31] and the GISSI-2/International study[7,28] and ISIS-3[8] mortality trials, by again showing that the conventional regimen of t-PA, even when given with adjunctive intravenous heparin, is no better than streptokinase.

The GUSTO investigators used an innovative prespecified net clinical outcome endpoint to avoid double-counting of stroke events (i.e. in both the mortality and stroke statistics) and to allow interpretation of events going in opposite directions (mortality rates decreasing but stroke rates increasing).[9] Nonfatal disabling stroke was prospectively defined as an inability to carry out normal activities. This combined endpoint is very important for patients, as a stroke from which a patient recovers fully may not matter much. However, whether a patient has a disability or not depends on where in the brain the hemorrhage occurs, which may relate to a number of factors, including the presence of Bouchard aneurysms, or to chance. Also, functional outcome is highly dependent on the type of stroke, with primary intracerebral hemorrhage resulting in more severe deficits.[10] Other net clinical endpoints that have been used are mortality plus total stroke, or mortality plus hemorrhagic stroke. Both of these are important assessments for comparing thrombolytic agents, with the preferred agent being the one with a lower stroke rate, even if disability rates are similar.

In the GUSTO study the incidence of the combined endpoint of death plus nonfatal disabling stroke was 6.9% in the accelerated t-PA group, 7.7% in the streptokinase plus subcutaneous heparin group, and 7.9% in the streptokinase plus intravenous heparin group ($P = 0.006$), while for death plus nonfatal stroke the figures were 7.2% versus 7.9%

and 8.2%, respectively (P = 0.006 for accelerated t-PA versus both streptokinase groups).[9] Overall, accelerated t-PA was the best regimen in most subgroups, and its effect was greatest in those at the greatest risk of death.

The GUSTO study showed that there was a close association between patency rates, as judged by the TIMI infarct artery flow grading system[30] at 90 minutes, and mortality.[3] The mortality rates for the various TIMI flow rates were TIMI-0 (no reflow) 8.4%, TIMI-1 (penetration) 9.2%, TIMI-2 (slow flow) 7.9%, and TIMI-3 (normal flow) 4.0%. This provides a basis for mechanistic assessment of new thrombolytic regimens. However, assessment of TIMI-3 flow alone should not be seen as a basis for recommending widespread clinical use of new treatments, as simply assessing TIMI-3 flow ignores the possible adverse effects of therapy, such as intracranial hemorrhage or other major bleeding.

The INJECT (International Joint Efficacy Comparison of Thrombolytics) study randomized 6010 patients presenting within 12 hours to receive either streptokinase or double-bolus reteplase (two boluses of 10 000 000 iu 30 minutes apart).[37] The trial was double-blind and used a double-dummy technique. The primary endpoint was 35-day mortality, but the trialists aimed to show 'equivalence' of the treatments rather than superiority. This is a new concept for megatrials of thrombolytic therapy. The assumption was made that the treatments could be assumed to be 'equivalent' if the upper 90% confidence limit for reteplase was not more than 2.1% greater than that for streptokinase. This determination was based on a meta-analysis of 13 placebo-controlled trials, showing an overall benefit of thrombolysis over placebo of 2.7%, with the lower 90% confidence limit being 2.1%.[37]

At 35 days the mortality in the reteplase group was 9.02% versus 9.53% in the streptokinase group. The 90% confidence level for the lower mortality with reteplase was -1.74 to 0.73%. This confidence interval includes zero, and the study therefore does not show reteplase to be superior to streptokinase. The stroke rate was 1.23% in the reteplase-treated patients and 1.0% in the streptokinase-treated patients (90% CI -0.21 to 0.68). It can be concluded that reteplase is 'equivalent' to streptokinase in terms of mortality reduction. However, the confidence limits are such that it is possible that reteplase might produce seven extra strokes per 1000 patients treated.

Analysis of Subgroups

In recommending treatments for individual patients, it can usually be assumed that there will be a similar relative reduction in risk among different patient subgroups, but the size of the absolute risk reduction will vary according to the baseline risk. Thus larger benefits will be seen in patients at high absolute risk. However, subgroups need to be considered separately if there is evidence of heterogeneity of a treatment effect between subgroups, or if there is an *a priori* pathophysiological basis why a subgroup may be different. When the GISSI Study[13] was published, some commentators evaluated subgroups, looking for patients in whom thrombolytic therapy might not have been beneficial. These groups included patients with inferior infarction, the elderly, those with previous infarction, and those with cardiogenic shock. There are no reasons why thrombolytic therapy might not be beneficial in any of these subgroups, although the risks of therapy increase in the elderly. Misinterpretation of data derived from these subgroups has probably led to hundreds of thousands of patients worldwide being denied a very effective therapy. The ISIS Collaborative Group illustrated the unreliability of subgroup analysis by analyzing their results according to astrology.[16] Aspirin appeared not to be effective in Libra or Gemini patients, but was highly effective in patients born under other signs. Unfortunately, these sorts of misinterpretation are still being propagated.

In the GISSI study patients with inferior infarction treated with streptokinase had a mortality of 7.8%, while those treated with conventional treatment had a mortality of 7.2% (NS).[13] It has recently been advocated that patients with inferior infarction should not be treated with thrombolysis, but with conventional therapy,[38] despite the fact that the FTT overview showed a reduction in mortality from 8.1% to 7.1% (95% CI −24 to 0) for patients with inferior ST-segment elevation randomized within 12 hours of symptom onset to receive either thrombolysis or control therapy. Patients with inferior infarction are a heterogeneous group, and some will benefit more than others. Patients with inferior infarction and anterior ST-segment depression are at particularly high risk,[39] and those with associated right ventricular infarction, which occurs in 30% of patients with inferior infarction,[40] have a mortality of 30%.[41] Many patients with inferior infarction are at high risk of dying, and identification of high- and low-risk patients may be difficult at presentation, when the decision whether or not to give thrombolysis has to be made quickly. It is inappropriate to recommend that 40% of patients who are currently eligible to receive thrombolysis (presenting within 12 hours of symptom onset with ST-segment elevation or bundle branch block)[42] should be denied thrombolysis.[43]

The elderly are at high absolute risk of dying after myocardial infarction and, although the risk of stroke is higher in the elderly, the FTT overview showed that the reduction in mortality per 1000 patients treated is 10 lives, versus 11 lives for patients aged less than 55 years.[42] Thrombolysis is also very cost-effective in elderly patients.[11] Age should therefore not be considered an exclusion criterion for administration of thrombolytic therapy. Thrombolytic therapy still remains underutilized, and the elderly are often inappropriately denied treatment. In a recent US registry, 50% of patients under 60 years received thrombolysis, but only 28% of patients over 60 years were treated ($P < 0.001$).[44]

Patients with hypotension (blood pressure <100 mmHg) have a mortality in excess of 35%,[42] and those with cardiogenic shock have a mortality of >75%.[45] In the GISSI study there were only 280 patients with cardiogenic shock (Killip class IV), and streptokinase was not beneficial in this group, but the 95% confidence interval was consistent with a mortality reduction of 25–30%.[13] In the FTT overview mortality was significantly reduced in patients with a blood pressure of <100 mmHg, with a saving of approximately 60 lives per 1000 patients treated ($P < 0.01$).[42] Although these patients may not fulfil strict criteria for the diagnosis of cardiogenic shock, the only major strategy that is likely to have an impact on the mortality rate in these patients is to open the infarct-related artery. Thrombolysis is an appropriate treatment for these patients if angioplasty or bypass surgery are not available. It is to be noted that there have been no randomized trials of these revascularization procedures in patients with cardiogenic shock.

In the GISSI study patients with previous infarction who received streptokinase had a relative reduction in mortality of 1% (NS), while for those without previous infarction there was a reduction in mortality of 23%.[13] In the FTT overview, the relative reduction in mortality in patients with previous infarction was 13% ($P < 0.02$) versus 20% in those without previous infarction.[42] This represents 15 lives saved per 1000 patients treated with previous infarction versus 20 lives saved in those without previous infarction. Patients with impaired left ventricular function from previous infarction cannot afford to lose any more myocardium. They have a high mortality rate, and should be treated with thrombolytic therapy.

Patients with ST-segment Depression

The pathophysiology of patients with acute ischemic syndromes and electrocardiographic ST-segment depression is different from those with ST-segment elevation. In patients with ST-segment depression the coronary artery thrombus is usually nonocclu-sive rather than occlusive.[46] Therefore, the benefit of thrombolytic therapy is likely to be less than in patients with total coronary artery occlusion, but the risks of therapy are likely to be similar. Also, thrombolytic therapy is procoagulant,[47] and it is possible that treatment with a thrombolytic agent may convert a nonocclusive thrombus to an occlusive one. It is interesting that several small randomized trials of thrombolytic therapy in patients with ST-segment depression have shown an increased infarction rate in patients randomized to receive thrombolytic therapy.[48] In the FTT overview, 3563 patients with ST-segment depression were randomized, and the 35-day mortality was 15.2% with thrombolytic therapy and 13.8% with placebo or control (odds ratio 1.12, 99% CI 0.88–1.44).[42] The mortality for patients with ST-segment depression is high and is affected by the degree of ST-segment depression, previous infarction, left ventricular function, and coronary artery anatomy. It is possible that some patients within this group, for example those with total circumflex artery occlusions, could benefit from thrombolytic therapy. However, it is very unlikely, given the 99% confidence interval for the FTT data, that thrombolysis will be beneficial overall in patients with ST-segment depression, i.e. there is a <1% chance that thrombolytic therapy will reduce mortality by 15%. Thrombolytic therapy is therefore not recommended in patients with ST-segment depression.

Cost-effectiveness

Thrombolytic therapy with streptokinase has been shown, in various cost-effectiveness models using retrospective data and varying assumptions, to be very cost-effective.[49] A major resource issue is whether t-PA (US$2750 per standard dose) is cost-effective compared with streptokinase (US$300 per standard dose). For decision-making about the appropriate allocation of scarce health resources, clinical trials in the future must prospectively collect cost data. These data should be collected in different countries and across different health systems with different price structures and resource use; for example, lower rates of outpatient visits or angioplasty. Country-specific data can then be used to assess cost-effectiveness given the overall results of the trial. The GUSTO study is the only trial that prospectively collected details of all hospital and medical charges in a subgroup.[11] The incorporation of prospective collection of cost-effectiveness data as part of the GUSTO study was an important advance.

The GUSTO study showed that the extra cost of accelerated t-PA per extra life-year saved, compared with streptokinase therapy, was US$27 382 (1992).[11] The cost-effective-ness varied according to age and the site of infarction (*Table 13.5*).

Table 13.5 Cost-effectiveness of accelerated t-PA versus streptokinase (US$ per life-year added)

Age (years)	Anterior infarction	Inferior infarction
≤40	76 417	99 510
41–60	35 123	46 639
61–75	21 885	24 956
>76	17 893	18 967

ineffective when hypotension is present.[55] Although streptokinase may produce hypotension in 4–13% of patients,[9,13,16] the incidence is not related to the level of the initial blood pressure,[16] and the hypotension is usually rapidly resolved by stopping the infusion and recommencing 10–15 minutes later after fluid administration. Given some pathophysiologic basis and the subgroup findings in two trials,[56] it may be reasonable to choose streptokinase for these patients if angioplasty or bypass surgery are not appropriate alternatives. Note that these data are based on retrospective subgroup analysis.

Early Treatment

There are still unacceptable delays in administering thrombolytic therapy. Much of the delay from symptom onset is related to patients not seeking help early after symptom onset, but there are still important delays after patient presentation. For prehospital administration of thrombolysis, major organizational requirements and resources are needed, including double-manning of ambulances and provision of defibrillators. Also, it has been reported that as few as 4% of patients seen by ambulance services fulfil eligibility criteria for thrombolysis.[57] It would therefore seem appropriate to transfer patients rapidly by ambulance to hospital for administration of thrombolytic therapy if the transport delay is less than an hour, rather than developing services for prehospital administration of thrombolytic therapy. However, in some rural communities and cities with long transport delays, prehospital administration is likely to have an important impact on patient outcome after myocardial infarction.

Delay in hospital continues to be a major component of the delay in administering thrombolytic therapy. In the GUSTO study, which was undertaken in 15 countries, 59% of patients had a delay of more than 60 minutes from hospitalization to administration of thrombolytic therapy,[9] while in a recent US registry the hospital delay was 99 minutes.[44] Improving the 'door-to-needle' time in hospital is clearly very important, and this should be carefully monitored with corrective measures as appropriate. *Table 13.6* details reasonable goals of treatment.

Late Treatment

EMERAS[14] and the LATE study[26] increase the amount of information available about treatment of patients presenting between 6 and 12 hours after symptom onset. The 12-hour time window for administration of thrombolytic therapy is now widely accepted.[58] Although patients may have stuttering infarction, or the infarct-related artery may open and close,[59] it is unlikely that myocardial salvage is the mechanism of benefit for patients treated after 6 hours. Animal studies have shown that myocardial necrosis is almost complete 6 hours after coronary occlusion.[60] Patency of the infarct artery has been shown to be an independent long-term prognostic factor.[61] The major mechanism of late benefit is

Table 13.6 Goals of treatment

- All patients should receive aspirin immediately if there are no contraindications
- Patients should seek medical help within 1 hour of the onset of symptoms
- An electrocardiogram should be performed within 5 minutes of arrival at hospital
- Thrombolytic therapy should be administered within 30 minutes of arrival at hospital if there are no contraindications

probably infarct artery patency, which decreases left ventricular remodelling and dilatation.[62-64] Left ventricular dilatation is the most important modifiable adverse prognostic factor.[65] Patency of the infarct-related artery can also reduce the propensity for life-threatening ventricular arrhythmias[66,67] and potentially supply collateral blood flow to another infarct artery territory if another infarction occurs in the future. The benefits of late treatment are, therefore, not so critically time dependent as those of early treatment. Accelerated t-PA is more effective than streptokinase in achieving 90-minute patency, but streptokinase 'catches up' by 3 hours,[32,68] and the patency rates for the two thrombolytic agents are then equivalent.[9] The 'late' patency rates achieved by streptokinase and t-PA would, therefore, be expected to be similar. Streptokinase therapy is associated with lower stroke rates; there were an extra four strokes per 1000 patients treated with streptokinase in EMERAS,[14] and an extra 11 strokes per 1000 patients treated with t-PA in the LATE study.[26]

Conclusion

The randomized controlled trial remains the most scientifically rigorous method for comparing two therapies. Over the last decade investigators and patients throughout the world have made major contributions to our understanding of the role of thrombolytic therapy. The large mortality trials have shown clear-cut benefits in a large range of patients. Although much remains to be learned, it is incumbent upon practicing physicians that the results of these trials are translated into everyday clinical practice. As many patients as possible without contraindications should be treated as early as possible with thrombolytic therapy if they present within 12 hours of symptom onset with ST-segment elevation or new bundle branch block.

References

1. Simoons ML, Serruys PW, van den Brand M, *et al*. Early thrombolysis in acute myocardial infarction: limitation of infarct size and improved survival. *J Am Coll Cardiol* 1986; **7**: 717–28.
2. White HD, Norris RM, Brown MA, *et al*. Effect of intravenous streptokinase on left ventricular function and early survival after acute myocardial infarction. *N Engl J Med* 1987; **317**: 850–5.
3. Simes RJ, Topol EJ, Holmes DR, *et al*. Link between the angiographic substudy and mortality outcomes in a large randomized trial of myocardial reperfusion: importance of early and complete infarct artery reperfusion. *Circulation* 1995; **91**: 1923–8.
4. Fletcher AP, Alkjaersig N, Smyrniotis FE, *et al*. The treatment of patients suffering from early myocardial infarction with massive and prolonged streptokinase therapy. *Trans Assoc Am Physicians* 1958; **71**: 287–96.
5. Yusuf S, Collins R, Peto R, *et al*. Intravenous and intracoronary fibrinolytic therapy in acute myocardial infarction: overview of results on mortality, reinfarction and side-effects from 33 randomized controlled trials. *Eur Heart J* 1985; **6**: 556–85.
6. European Cooperative Study Group for Streptokinase Treatment in Acute Myocardial Infarction. Streptokinase in acute myocardial infarction. *N Engl J Med* 1979; **301**: 797–802.
7. Gruppo Italiano per lo Studio della Sopravvivenza nell'Infarto Miocardico. GISSI-2: a factorial randomized trial of alteplase versus streptokinase and heparin versus no heparin among 12 490 patients with acute myocardial infarction. *Lancet* 1990; **336**: 65–71.
8. ISIS-3 (Third International Study of Infarct Survival) Collaborative Group. ISIS-3: a randomised comparison of streptokinase vs tissue plasminogen activator vs anistreplase and of aspirin plus heparin vs aspirin along among 41 299 cases of suspected acute myocardial infarction. *Lancet* 1992; **339**; 753–70.
9. The GUSTO Investigators. An international randomized trial comparing four thrombolytic strategies for acute myocardial infarction. *N Engl J Med* 1993; **329**: 673–82.
10. Gore JM, Granger CB, Simoons ML, *et al*. Stroke after thrombolysis: mortality and functional outcomes in the GUSTO-I trial. *Circulation* 1995; **92**: 2811–18.

11. Mark DB, Hlatky MA, Califf RM, *et al*. Cost effectiveness of thrombolytic therapy with tissue plasminogen activator as compared with streptokinase for acute myocardial infarction. *N Engl J Med* 1995; **332**: 1418–24.
12. Kleiman NS, White HD, Ohman EM, *et al*. Mortality within 24 hours of thrombolysis for myocardial infarction: the importance of early reperfusion. *Circulation* 1994; **90**: 2658–65.
13. Gruppo Italiano per lo Studio della Streptochinasi nell'Infarto Miocardico (GISSI). Effectiveness of intravenous thrombolytic treatment in acute myocardial infarction. *Lancet* 1986; **i**: 397–402.
14. EMERAS (Estudio Multicéntrico Estreptoquinasa Repúblicas de América del Sur) Collaborative Group. Randomized trial of late thrombolysis in patients with suspected acute myocardial infarction. *Lancet* 1993; **342**: 767–72.
15. The TIMI IIIB Investigators. Effects of tissue plasminogen activator and a comparison of early invasive and conservative strategies in unstable angina and non-Q-wave myocardial infarction: results of the TIMI IIIB trial. *Circulation* 1994; **89**: 1545–56.
16. ISIS-2 (Second International Study of Infarct Survival) Collaborative Group. Randomised trial of intravenous streptokinase, oral aspirin, both, or neither among 17 187 cases of suspected acute myocardial infarction: ISIS-2. *Lancet* 1988; **ii**: 349–60.
17. Col NF, Gurwitz JH, Alpert JS, *et al*. Frequency of inclusion of patients with cardiogenic shock in trials of thrombolytic therapy. *Am J Cardiol* 1994; **73**: 149–57.
18. Wilcox RG, von der Lippe G, Ollson CG, *et al*. Trial of tissue plasminogen activation for mortality reduction in acute myocardial infarction: Anglo-Scandinavian Study of Early Thrombolysis (ASSET). *Lancet* 1988; **ii**: 525–30.
19. Gruppo Italiano per lo Studio della Streptochi-nasi nell'Infarto Miocardico (GISSI). Long-term effects of intravenous thrombolysis in acute myocardial infarction: final report of the GISSI Study. *Lancet* 1987; **ii**: 871–4.
20. The ISAM Study Group. A prospective trial of intravenous streptokinase in acute myocardial infarction (ISAM): mortality, morbidity, and infarct size at 21 days. *N Engl J Med* 1986; **314**: 1465–71.
21. AIMS Trial Study Group. Effect of intravenous APSAC on mortality after acute myocardial infarction: preliminary report of a placebo-controlled clinical trial. *Lancet* 1988; **i**: 545–9.
22. O'Brien PC, Fleming TR. A multiple testing procedure for clinical trials. *Biometrics* 1979; **35**: 549–56.
23. ISIS Steering Committee. Intravenous streptokinase given within 0–4 hours of onset of myocardial infarction reduced mortality in ISIS-2. *Lancet* 1987; **i**: 502 (letter).
24. Rossi P, Bolognese L, on behalf of Urochinasi per via Sistemica nell'Infarto Miocardico (USIM) Collaborative Group. Comparison of intravenous urokinase plus heparin versus heparin alone in acute myocardial infarction. *Am J Cardiol* 1991; **68**: 585–92.
25. Neuhaus K, Tebbe U, Gottwik M, *et al*. Intravenous recombinant tissue plasminogen activator (rt-PA) and urokinase in acute myocardial infarction: results of the German Activator Urokinase Study (GAUS). *J Am Coll Cardiol* 1988; **12**: 581–7.
26. LATE Study Group. Late Assessment of Thrombolytic Efficacy (LATE) study with alteplase 6–24 hours after onset of acute myocardial infarction. *Lancet* 1993; **342**: 759–66.
27. The European Myocardial Infarction Project Group. Prehospital thrombolytic therapy in patients with suspected acute myocardial infarction. *N Engl J Med* 1993; **329**: 385–9.
28. The International Study Group. In-hospital mortality and clinical course of 20 891 patients with suspected acute myocardial infarction randomised between alteplase and streptokinase with or without heparin. *Lancet* 1990; **336**: 71–5.
29. GISSI-2 and International Study Group. Six-month survival in 20 891 patients with acute myocardial infarction randomized between alteplase and streptokinase with or without heparin. *Eur Heart J* 1992; **13**: 1692–7.
30. Chesebro JH, Knatterud G, Roberts R, *et al*. Thrombolysis in Myocardial Infarction (TIMI) Trial, Phase I: a comparison between intravenous tissue plasminogen activator and intravenous streptokinase: clinical findings through hospital discharge. *Circulation* 1987; **76**: 142–54.
31. White HD, Rivers JT, Maslowski AH, *et al*. Effect of intravenous streptokinase as compared with that of tissue plasminogen activator on left ventricular function after first myocardial infarction. *N Engl J Med* 1989; **320**: 817–21.
32. White HD. GISSI-2 and the heparin controversy. *Lancet* 1990; **336**: 297–8.
33. Sobel BE, Collen D. Questions unresolved by the Third International Study of Infarct Survival. *Am J Cardiol* 1992; **70**: 385–9.
34. Neuhaus KL, Feuerer W, Jeep-Tebbe S, *et al*. Improved thrombolysis with a modified dose regimen of recombinant tissue-type plasminogen activator. *J Am Coll Cardiol* 1989; **14**: 1566–9.
35. Reiner JS, Lundergan CF, van den Brand M, *et al*. Early angiography cannot predict postthrombolytic coronary reocclusion: observations from the GUSTO Angiographic Study. *J Am Coll Cardiol* 1994; **24**: 1439–44.
36. Topol EJ, George BS, Kereiakes DJ, *et al*. A randomized controlled trial of intravenous tissue plasminogen activator and early intravenous heparin in acute myocardial infarction. *Circulation* 1989; **79**: 281–6.
37. International Joint Efficacy Comparison of Thrombolytics. Randomized, double-blind comparison of reteplase double-bolus administration with streptokinase in acute myocardial infarction (INJECT): trial to investigate equivalence. *Lancet* 1995; **346**: 329–36.
38. Tobé TJM. Is thrombolytic therapy in acute inferior myocardial infarction really better than conventional treatment? *Br Heart J* 1995; **73**: 108–9.
39. Bates ER, Clemmensen PM, Califf RM, *et al*. Precordial ST segment depression predicts a worse prognosis in inferior infarction despite reperfusion therapy. *J Am Coll Cardiol* 1990; **16**: 1538–44.
40. Berger PB, Ryan T. Inferior myocardial infarction: high-risk subgroups. *Circulation* 1990; **81**: 401–11.

41. Zehender M, Kasper W, Kauder E, *et al*. Right ventricular infarction as an independent predictor of prognosis after acute inferior myocardial infarction. *N Engl J Med* 1993; **328**: 981–8.
42. Fibrinolytic Therapy Trialists' (FTT) Collaborative Group. Indications for fibrinolytic therapy in suspected acute myocardial infarction: collaborative overview of early mortality and major morbidity results from all randomised trials of more than 1000 patients. *Lancet* 1994; **343**: 311–22.
43. Ellis CJ, French JK, White HD. Is thrombolytic therapy really better than conventional treatment in acute inferior myocardial infarction? *Br Heart J* 1995; **74**: 476–7 (letter).
44. Rogers WJ, Bowlby LJ, Chandra NC, *et al*. Treatment of myocardial infarction in the United States (1990 to 1993): observations from the National Registry of Myocardial Infarction. *Circulation* 1994; **90**: 2103–14.
45 O'Neill WW. Angioplasty therapy of cardiogenic shock: are randomized trials necessary? *J Am Coll Cardiol* 1992; **19**: 915–17.
46. DeWood MA, Spores J, Notske R, *et al*. Prevalence of total coronary occlusion during the early hours of transmural myocardial infarction. *N Engl J Med* 1980; **303**: 897–902.
47. Fitzgerald DJ, Catella F, Roy L, *et al*. Marked platelet activation in vivo after intravenous streptokinase in patients with acute myocardial infarction. *Circulation* 1988; **77**: 142–50.
48. Waters D, Lam JYT. Is thrombolytic therapy striking out in unstable angina? *Circulation* 1992; **86**: 1642–4.
49. Woo KS, White HD. Pharmacoeconomic aspects of treatment of acute myocardial infarction with thrombolytic agents. *PharmacoEconomics* 1993; **3(3)**: 192–204.
50. Lau J, Antman EM, Jimenez-Silva J, *et al*. Cumulative meta-analysis of therapeutic trials for myocardial infarction. *N Engl J Med* 1992; **327**: 248–54.
51. Ketley D, Woods KL. Impact of clinical trials on clinical practice: example of thrombolysis for acute myocardial infarction. *Lancet* 1993; **342**: 891–4.
52. White HD. Selecting a thrombolytic agent. *Cardiol Clin* 1995; **13**: 347–54.
53. Elliott JM, Cross DB, Cederholm-Williams SA, *et al*. Neutralizing antibodies to streptokinase four years after intravenous thrombolytic therapy. *Am J Cardiol* 1993; **71**: 640–5.
54. White HD. Thrombolytic treatment for recurrent myocardial infarction: avoid repeating streptokinase or anistreplase. *Br Med J* 1991; **302**: 429–30.
55. Prewitt RM, Gu S, Garber PJ, *et al*. Marked systemic hypotension depresses coronary thrombolysis induced by intracoronary administration of recombinant tissue-type plasminogen activator. *J Am Coll Cardiol* 1992; **20**: 1626–33.
56. Oxman AD, Guyatt GH. A consumer's guide to subgroup analyses. *Ann Intern Med* 1992; **116**: 78–84.
57. Weaver WD, Eisenberg MS, Martin JS, *et al*. Myocardial Infarction Triage and Intervention Project – Phase I: patient characteristics and feasibility of prehospital initiation of thrombolytic therapy. *J Am Coll Cardiol* 1990; **15**: 925–31.
58. White HD. Thrombolytic therapy for patients with myocardial infarction presenting after six hours. *Lancet* 1992; **340**: 221–2.
59. Hackett D, Davies G, Chierchia S, *et al*. Intermittent coronary occlusion in acute myocardial infarction: value of combined thrombolytic and vasodilator therapy. *N Engl J Med* 1987; **317**: 1055–9.
60. Reimer KA, Lowe JE, Rasmussen MM, *et al*. The wave-front phenomenon of ischemic cell death. I. Myocardial infarct size vs duration of coronary occlusion in dogs. *Circulation* 1977; **56**: 786–94.
61. White HD, Cross DB, Elliott JM, *et al*. Long-term prognostic importance of patency of the infarct-related coronary artery after thrombolytic therapy for acute myocardial infarction. *Circulation* 1994; **89**: 61–7.
62. White HD. Mechanism of late benefit in ISIS-2. *Lancet* 1988; **ii**: 914 (letter).
63. Hochman JS, Choo H. Limitation of myocardial infarct expansion by reperfusion independent of myocardial salvage. *Circulation* 1987; **75**: 299–306.
64. Bonaduce D, Petretta M, Villari B, *et al*. Effects of late administration of tissue-type plasminogen activator on left ventricular remodeling and function after myocardial infarction. *J Am Coll Cardiol* 1990; **16**: 1561–8.
65. White HD, Norris RM, Brown MA, *et al*. Left ventricular end-systolic volume as the major determinant of survival after recovery from myocardial infarction. *Circulation* 1987; **76**: 44–51.
66. Gang ES, Lew AS, Hong M, *et al*. Decreased incidence of ventricular late potentials after successful thrombolytic therapy for acute myocardial infarction. *N Engl J Med* 1989; **321**: 712.
67. Sager PT, Perlmutter RA, Rosenfeld LE, *et al*. Electrophysiologic effects of thrombolytic therapy in patients with a transmural anterior myocardial infarction complicated by left ventricular aneurysm formation. *J Am Coll Cardiol* 1988; **12**: 19–24.
68. Sherry S, Marder VJ. Streptokinase and recombinant tissue plasminogen activator (rt-PA) are equally effective in treating acute myocardial infarction. *Ann Intern Med* 1991; **114**: 417–23.

14

Antiplatelet and Anticoagulant Therapy

Freek W. A. Verheugt

Introduction

Thrombosis plays a major role in the pathogenesis of cardiovascular disease. Thromboses in both coronary and cerebral arteries are complications of atherosclerosis, the most important single cause of mortality in the Western world. Both myocardial and cerebral infarction cause impressive mortality and morbidity in millions of patients each year. Not only arterial thrombosis, but also thrombosis in the heart cavities, is responsible for major morbidity and mortality of cardiovascular disease. Intracardiac thrombosis can be seen in atrial fibrillation, in patients with artificial valves and in those with left ventricular aneurysm. Since the 1950s, antithrombotic therapy has been applied with large success to prevent these frequently fatal thrombotic complications.

Pharmacology of Antiplatelet and Anticoagulant Therapy

Pharmacology of Antiplatelet Agents

The most regularly used antiplatelet agents in cardiovascular disease are aspirin (acetyl-salicylic acid) and dipyridamole.[1] Aspirin irreversibly blocks cyclo-oxygenase in the blood platelet, and therefore prevents the formation of the proaggregatory and vasoconstrictive thromboxane A_2. Because endothelial cells are nucleated, the blockage of cyclo-oxygenase in these cells is almost immediately reversible. The antiaggregatory and vasodilating endothelial prostaglandin (PGI_2 or prostacyclin) is not blocked by low-dose aspirin and a favorable imbalance in the interaction between platelet and vessel wall is achieved with aspirin. The most widely used and effective dosage of aspirin in cardiovascular disease is 75–325 mg daily. Usually, life-long administration of aspirin is recommended in cardiac patients. Since the 1980s low-dose aspirin has been introduced and found to be as effective as high-dose aspirin,[1] the latter being associated with gastrointestinal ulceration and subsequent bleeding.

Dipyridamole inhibits phosphodiesterase in the platelet, and therefore diminishes platelet adhesion and possibly subsequent aggregation. Its clinical efficacy as a single agent is questionable.[1] It is almost uniformly used in combination with aspirin, but the benefit of its addition to aspirin is debatable.[1] The usual dosage of dipyridamole is 75–100 mg three times daily.

Ticlopidine and clopidogrel inhibit platelet aggregation independently from the cyclo-oxygenase and thromboxane pathway, the phosphodiesterase metabolism or intracellular cyclic AMP. It inhibits mainly ADP-induced platelet aggregation, probably by interfering with fibrinogen and von Willebrand factor interaction with platelets. Bleeding time is prolonged. The usual dose of ticlopidine is 250 mg twice daily. Neutropenia is seen in 2% of patients, most cases occurring during the first weeks of treatment. Clopidogrel lacks this side effect and is given in a dose of 250 mg daily.

The platelet glycoprotein IIb/IIIa receptor binds fibrinogen during the aggregation process. Inhibition of this binding prevents platelet aggregation independently of the stimulus (ADP, thrombin, arachidonic acid, adrenalin). Therefore, glycoprotein IIb/IIIa receptor blocking agents inhibit the final pathway of platelet aggregation and prolong bleeding time profoundly. Monoclonal antibodies (7E3) to this receptor are available for clinical use. In the future nonpeptide blockers will be developed.

Pharmacology of Anticoagulant Agents

Heparin consists of a mix of compounds that inhibit the fluid phase of antithrombin III, and therefore both the extrinsic and intrinsic coagulation cascades are inhibited by heparin. Given intravenously, heparin acts immediately and can be antagonized by intravenous protamine. Subcutaneous application is more slow acting, needs twice-daily administration, and is suitable for ambulatory use. Heparinization usually is monitored by the activated partial thromboplastin time (APTT). Heparin is notoriously difficult to monitor. Recently, direct and specific antithrombins have been developed, which do not need plasma cofactors. Recombinant hirudin and hirulog are complex molecules, but smaller molecules such as argatroban have been developed and tested. They are more easily titratable than heparin using APTT.

Oral anticoagulants are derivatives of coumarin. They inhibit vitamin K dependent carboxylation of factors II, VII, IX, and X in the liver. Both the extrinsic and intrinsic coagulation cascades are inhibited by these agents. As the vitamin K dependent factors have a half-life of 12 hours to several days, the action of oral anticoagulant therapy starts after a few days. On the other hand, discontinuation of therapy results in a delayed termination of action. Usually, these drugs are used with target ranges of the inhibition of the prothrombin time, the latter now being expressed as the international normalized ratio (INR). These drugs are usually given on a life-long basis in cardiovascular disease. Since frequent INR checks by thrombosis laboratories are necessary, patients should be mobile and cooperative.

Trials with Antiplatelet Therapy in Cardiology

Antiplatelet agents are proven to be effective in the primary and secondary prevention of myocardial infarction, in unstable angina, in coronary artery bypass grafting, in percutaneous transluminal coronary angioplasty (PTCA), in atrial fibrillation, and in patients with prosthetic heart valves. These data have recently been summarized in the overview published by the Antiplatelet Trialists Collaboration.[1] This overview consists of a meta-analysis of nearly 300 randomized controlled trials in over 100 000 patients with vascular disease. In the present chapter, trials on antiplatelet therapy in cardiology will be addressed. It should be realized that meta-analytic documentation necessarily includes publication bias and might overestimate drug efficacy and safety.

The first part of this section covers trials with antiplatelet drugs in the primary prevention of myocardial infarction, in the treatment of acute myocardial infarction, in the secondary prevention of myocardial infarction, and in the treatment of unstable angina pectoris. The second part will deal with the use of antiplatelet drugs in unstable angina, PTCA, and coronary artery bypass surgery. The third part will address the role of antiplatelet therapy in patients with atrial fibrillation and those with artificial heart valves.

Antiplatelet Drugs in the Prevention and Treatment of Myocardial Infarction

Acute myocardial infarction is generally associated with partial or complete occlusion of coronary arteries. In addition to coronary artery spasm, platelet embolization, and plaque hemorrhage and/or rupture, thrombosis is assumed to contribute to the development of coronary artery occlusion. Platelets are known to be involved in the formation of thrombi. As recently formed thrombi are mainly composed of aggregated platelets, vasoactive mediators such as thromboxane A_2 released from platelets may further occlude the coronary vessels. It has therefore been suggested that antiplatelet drugs may be active in the secondary, and possibly also in the primary, prevention of myocardial infarction. Indeed, in a retrospective study involving 473 patients treated with aspirin for rheumatoid arthritis the drug seemed to reduce the incidence of myocardial infarction, angina pectoris, sudden death, and cerebral infarction.[2] Statistical significance, however, was not reached. Several large-scale, randomized, placebo-controlled trials of aspirin in doses of 75–1500 mg daily in the secondary prevention of myocardial infarction have been completed (see below).

The efficacy of antiplatelet drugs in the prevention and treatment of myocardial infarction is illustrated in *Figure 14.1*, which is based on data from the Antiplatelet Trialists Collaboration.[1] In the indications with a high event rate in the control groups, acute and chronic treatment with antiplatelet agents is very effective in preventing vascular events. In trials where the event rate in the control groups is very low (e.g. primary prevention), antiplatelet agents do not seem to be efficacious.

Antiplatelet Agents in the Primary Prevention of Acute Myocardial Infarction

The efficacy of aspirin in the primary prevention of myocardial infarction has been studied in two large-scale trials: The American Physicians' Health Study[3] and The British Doctors' Study.[4]

In the American randomized, double-blind, placebo-controlled study, 22 071 male physicians received either 325 mg of aspirin every other day or placebo. The average follow-up period was 60 months. A reduction in the risk of myocardial infarction of 44% was found ($P < 0.00001$). The effect was only apparent in those who were 50 years or older. The risk of stroke was slightly, but not significantly ($P = 0.06$), enhanced.

In the British study, which was randomized but not blinded, 5139 male physicians received aspirin 500 mg daily or no treatment for 6 years. Treatment with aspirin did not influence the incidence of myocardial infarction or stroke. However, total mortality was 14% lower in the aspirin group. This difference was not statistically significant.

Ridker *et al.*[5] evaluated the efficacy of low-dose aspirin in the primary prevention of myocardial infarction in 333 patients with chronic stable angina in a randomized, double-blind trial. Patients were treated with aspirin 325 mg on alternate days or given placebo,

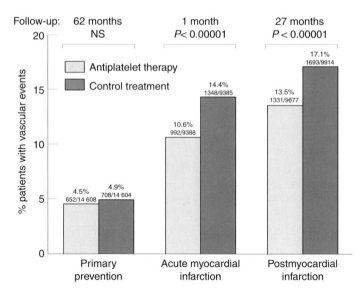

Figure 14.1   Prevention of vascular events with antiplatelet therapy compared to control treatment in healthy individuals, in patients with acute myocardial infarction, and in patients with prior myocardial infarction. The time of follow-up is also given. (Adapted from Ref. 1.)

and were followed for an average of 60 months for the occurrence of myocardial infarction, stroke, or cardiovascular death. During follow-up, 27 patients had confirmed myocardial infarction: 7 were in the aspirin-treated group and 20 in the placebo-treated group, a risk reduction of 70% (*P* = 0.003). The incidence of stroke, however, seemed to be increased in the aspirin group.

Juul-Möller *et al.*[6] studied over 2000 patients with stable angina pectoris with a follow-up of over 4 years. The study shows a risk reduction of 39% in nonfatal myocardial infarction (*P* < 0.01) and 38% in sudden death (*P* < 0.10). Any vascular event was reduced by 32% (*P* < 0.001) and total mortality by 22% (*P* = 0.10).

Earlier data were given by Chesebro *et al.*,[7] who randomized 370 patients with stable angina pectoris and coronary angiography to high-dose aspirin 975 mg daily with dipyridamole 225 mg daily or placebo. At 5 years, angiographic and clinical follow-up was available in 283 (76%) patients. The outcome shows 5% of myocardial infarction with aspirin/dipyridamole and 12% with placebo (risk reduction 56%; *P* = 0.05). At follow up, neither the degree of coronary stenosis nor mortality was changed by aspirin/dipyridamole. However, new coronary lesions were observed in 23% of aspirin/dipyridamole patients and in 35% of placebo patients (risk reduction 34%; *P* = 0.04).

In view of the opposing results of the large American and British trials, the value of aspirin in the primary prevention of myocardial infarction remains controversial (*Figure 14.2*). In making the decision of whether to use aspirin for the primary prevention of myocardial infarction, the cardiovascular risk profile of the patient and the risks and benefits of therapy with aspirin should be taken into account.

Miller[8] reported the results of a pilot study on a low dose of warfarin in middle-aged men at high risk but without clinical coronary heart disease. The average dose of warfarin needed to meet the target level of anticoagulation appeared to be 4–6 mg daily. At this dose side-effects were minimal. A thrombosis trial has been launched to demonstrate a 30% reduction in the incidence of myocardial infarction in 6000 men at high risk. In this respect

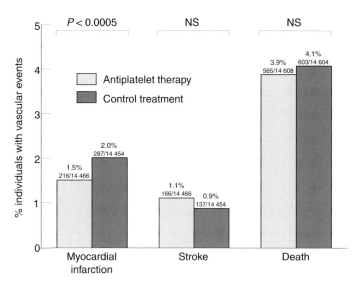

Figure 14.2 Primary prevention of vascular events with antiplatelet therapy compared to control treatment in healthy individuals. (Adapted from Ref. 1.)

the effects of low-dose warfarin in combination with low-dose aspirin (75 mg daily) as a film-coated, sustained-release preparation will be studied in middle-aged men at high risk. The recruitment ended in 1992 and results are due in 1997.[8] In 1992 the first safety data were published. Minor bleeding was reported in 15% of placebo patients, in 20% of the aspirin alone and warfarin alone arm groups, and in nearly 30% of the combination group.[9]

The Women's Health Study has recruited over 40 000 healthy women over 50 years old, and randomized them to aspirin 50 mg daily or placebo, vitamin E or placebo, and β-carotene or placebo in a 2 × 2 × 2 design. Cardiovascular mortality and morbidity will be the endpoint and results are expected after 2000.[10]

In the HOT study, nearly 20 000 patients with hypertension have been randomized to several doses of felodipine, to aspirin 75 mg daily, or to placebo with the aim of looking at prevention of cardiovascular mortality and morbidity. Results will be available in 1997.[10]

Antiplatelet Agents in the Treatment of Acute Myocardial Infarction

In the Medical Research Council (MRC) trial, a randomized, controlled, double-blind trial by Elwood and Sweetnam,[11] 1682 patients who had had a myocardial infarction were treated with aspirin 300 mg 3 times daily, for 1 year. Twenty-five percent of the patients were admitted to the trial within 3 days following the infarction, and 50% within 7 days. Total mortality was 12.3% in patients given aspirin and 14.8% in those given placebo. The reduction in total mortality (17%) was not statistically significant. The reduction of specific ischemic heart disease was 22%. Aspirin appeared less effective in women than in men.

In the Second International Study on Infarct Survival (ISIS-2),[12] a randomized, double-blind, placebo-controlled multicenter trial, the value of low-dose aspirin in the treatment of myocardial infarction was evaluated. In this study, 17 187 patients were randomized at 417 hospitals to receive early, after the onset of myocardial infarction: (1) a 1-hour intravenous infusion of 1.5 million iu of streptokinase; (2) 1 month of 160 mg daily enteric coated aspirin; (3) both treatments, or (4) neither treatment.

Streptokinase alone and aspirin alone significantly reduced 5-week vascular mortality: 9.2% of patients allocated to streptokinase infusion and 12.0% of those treated with placebo, a risk reduction of 25% ($P < 0.00001$); and 94% vascular deaths among patients allocated to aspirin versus 11.8% among those treated with placebo, a risk reduction of 25% ($P < 0.00001$). The effect of the drugs appeared additive: 8.0% vascular deaths among patients allocated to both streptokinase and aspirin versus 13.2% among those allocated to placebo, a reduction in vascular mortality of 42% ($P < 0.0001$). Subgroup analysis indicated that patients treated late after myocardial infarction (13–24 hours) also benefited from treatment with each of the agents. The authors suggested that a daily aspirin dose of 40 mg or higher might be sufficient to reduce the incidence of myocardial infarction if inhibition of cyclo-oxygenase dependent platelet aggregation is the main mechanism of action. As higher doses of aspirin are associated with more severe gastrotoxic effects than lower doses, it has been concluded that, following myocardial infarction, unstable angina, transient cerebral ischemia, or stroke, a dose of about 160 mg daily is preferred. The combination of streptokinase and aspirin reduced the risk of disabling, fatal stroke, and mortality more substantially than either of the drugs alone. The serious side-effects related to the combination were not more frequent than those resulting from streptokinase alone. Platelet activity is known to be increased in patients with myocardial infarction. Fibrinolytic therapy may further increase platelet activity, resulting in an increased risk of myocardial reinfarction. The streptokinase-induced increase in platelet activity can be counteracted by aspirin. In ISIS-2 the increased risk of reinfarction produced by strepto-kinase was avoided by giving streptokinase in combination with aspirin. Since ISIS-2, aspirin has been given after thrombolytic therapy for acute myocardial infarction.

Verheugt et al.[13] studied the effect of low-dose aspirin in a prospective, randomized, double-blind, placebo-controlled trial after early thrombolysis in 50 patients with first anterior wall acute myocardial infarction. After treatment with 1 500 000 iu of strepto-kinase, patients received 100 mg of aspirin daily. Heparin 5000 iu twice daily subcuta-neously was also given. The results of this study with respect to myocardial reinfarction within 3 months were in agreement with those of the ISIS-2 trial described above: in the placebo and the aspirin-treated groups, the incidence of reinfarction was 6 and 1, respectively. In this study aspirin was ineffective in reducing the rate of left ventricular thrombus development, the primary endpoint of the study.

The effects of antiplatelet therapy in the treatment of acute myocardial infarction are summarized in *Figure 14.3*.

Antiplatelet Agents in the Secondary Prevention of Acute Myocardial Infarction

In the trials on antiplatelet agents in the secondary prevention of acute myocardial infarction, the moment of inclusion after the index myocardial infarction is crucial. Some trials included patients in the coronary care unit,[12] some included patients up to 5 years after infarction.[14] In addition, some studies had a short follow-up of only a few weeks,[12] while some had a follow-up of several years.[14]

In the German–Austrian Multicenter Prospective Clinical Trial (GAMIS) involving 946 patients who had survived at least one myocardial infarction for 30–42 days,[15] aspirin 1500 mg daily was compared with treatment with an anticoagulant (phenprocoumon in a dose leading to prothrombin time values between 15% and 25%) or placebo. Patients were followed for up to 2 years. Compared to placebo and phenprocoumon, aspirin reduced the incidence of coronary death ($P = 0.05$) and all coronary events ($P = 0.07$). Interruptions

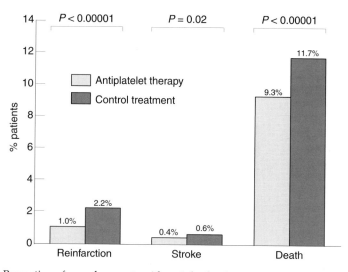

Figure 14.3 Prevention of vascular events with antiplatelet therapy compared to control treatment in patients with acute myocardial infarction. (Adapted from Ref. 1.)

because of side-effects occurred more frequently with aspirin treatment than with phenprocoumon.

Elwood and Williams[16] reported the results of a randomized controlled trial of a single dose of aspirin 300 mg in 1705 patients who might have suffered a myocardial infarction. A single dose of aspirin appeared not to be effective in preventing early mortality at 28 days.

In the controlled, randomized, double-blind Persantine–Aspirin Reinfarction Study (PARIS) I trial[14] involving 2026 patients, three subgroups of patients were treated with aspirin 324 mg three times daily, dipyridamole 75 mg plus aspirin 324 mg daily, or placebo. Patients were entered in the study 2–60 months after myocardial infarction. Treatment with aspirin or with aspirin plus dipyridamole tended to decrease the incidence of total mortality, coronary mortality, and nonfatal myocardial infarction. In a subgroup of patients who entered the study within 6 months after myocardial infarction the reduction of total and coronary mortality was proportionally greater. This result prompted the PARIS II trial.

In the PARIS II trial, a randomized, controlled, double-blind study,[17] the effectiveness of aspirin 330 mg in combination with dipyridamole 75 mg three times daily was studied in 3128 patients. The average length of follow-up was 23 months. Coronary incidence was significantly lower in the aspirin plus dipyridamole group than in the placebo group, both at 1 year (30% reduction) and at the end of the study (24% reduction). Coronary mortality was 20% lower in the aspirin plus dipyridamole treated patients than in placebo treated patients. The difference, however, was not statistically significant. Side-effects in the aspirin plus dipyridamole treated group included stomach pain, heartburn, nausea, gastrointestinal irritation, and gastrointestinal bleeding.

The Enquete de Prevention Secondaire de l'Infarctus de Myocarde (EPSIM)[18] research group compared the effects of aspirin 1500 mg daily with those of anticoagulants on mortality after myocardial infarction in 1307 patients in a multicenter, randomized, prospective trial. The mean time to entry in the study following myocardial infarction was 11 months. No significant differences in mortality or coronary incidence were found between the groups treated with the different regimens. In the oral anticoagulant treated

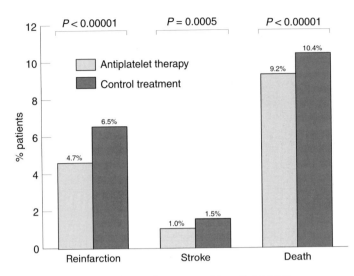

Figure 14.4 Secondary prevention of vascular events with antiplatelet therapy compared to control treatment in patients who had sustained a myocardial infarction. (Adapted from Ref. 1.)

group, 16% of patients had at least one episode of bleeding, as compared with 5% in the aspirin treated group. Of those taking anticoagulants, 3% had severe bleeding, of whom 8 patients died, and 1% taking aspirin had severe bleeding, of whom 4 patients died. Gastritis and peptic ulcer were more frequent among those taking aspirin; 3% reported gastritis and 3% had confirmed peptic ulcer.

Although the ISIS-2 trial (described above) was an intervention trial, the results apply also to secondary prevention. Aspirin 160 mg daily for 5 weeks reduced recurrent infarction, stroke, and death by about 25%.[12]

Küpper *et al.*[19] described a prospective, randomized, placebo-controlled study on the influence of low-dose aspirin 100 mg on the incidence of left ventricular thrombosis in 100 patients with a first anterior wall acute myocardial infarction. In this study aspirin was ineffective in reducing the rate of thrombus development.

The Aspirin Myocardial Infarction Study (AMIS) randomized over 4500 patients to 1000 mg aspirin daily or placebo at a mean time of over 2 years after myocardial infarction.[20] After 3 years, total mortality was similar in aspirin-treated patients (10.8%) versus 9.7% in the placebo group. Reinfarction tended to be less with aspirin (9.5% versus 11.6%).

The effects of antiplatelet therapy in the secondary prevention of vascular events after myocardial infarction are summarized in *Figure 14.4.*

Antiplatelet Agents in the Treatment of Unstable Angina Pectoris, in PTCA and in Coronary Bypass Surgery

Antiplatelet Agents in the Treatment of Unstable Angina Pectoris

It is well recognized that unstable angina pectoris is associated with a high risk of myocardial infarction and sudden death. The occurrence of thrombosis followed by atherosclerotic plaque rupture is an important factor in these conditions.[21] The presence of platelet thrombi in the coronary vessel distal to the site of active coronary disease and the presence of layers of platelet thrombi at the site of coronary occlusion indicate that platelets play a major role in the pathogenesis of unstable angina.[22,23] In addition, FitzGerald *et al.*[24] showed that about 80% of episodes of chest pain in patients with angina are associated with increased platelet activity, resulting in an increased thromboxane and prostacyclin synthesis. Platelets are known to release vasoactive substances such as thromboxane A_2, serotonin, and platelet-derived growth factors, which induce vasoconstriction and thereby reduce the coronary flow further.[25] It has therefore been anticipated that antiplatelet agents may reduce the risk of myocardial infarction and sudden death in patients with unstable angina. The effectiveness of aspirin in unstable angina has been investigated in four large-scale randomized, double-blind, placebo-controlled trials.

The Veterans Administration Cooperative Study investigated the effects of aspirin 324 mg once daily for a period of 12 weeks in 1266 male patients with unstable angina in a multicenter, double-blind, placebo-controlled, randomized trial.[26] The principal endpoints were death and myocardial infarction. The combined incidence of death and acute myocardial infarction in patients treated with aspirin and placebo was 5.0% and 10.1%, respectively. The difference was highly significant ($P = 0.0005$). Similarly, the frequency of nonfatal acute myocardial infarction was reduced by 51% in the aspirin group: (21 (3.4%) versus 44 (6.9%), respectively; $P = 0.005$). The overall mortality in the aspirin group was also reduced (1.6% versus 3.3% in the placebo group). This difference was not statistically significant ($P = 0.054$). All deaths were thought to be cardiac in origin. No formal follow-up visits were carried out after the initial 12-week treatment period; however, survival data 1 year after entry into the study were available on 86% of the patients, and showed a significant ($P = 0.008$) reduction in the mortality rate in the aspirin-treated group (5.5%) compared to the placebo group (9.6%). No difference with respect to gastrointestinal symptoms or evidence of blood loss between the treatment and control groups was observed.

The beneficial effects of aspirin in patients with unstable angina have been confirmed in a multicenter, randomized, double-blind, placebo-controlled study in 555 patients.[27] In contrast to the Veterans Administration Study, women (20–30%) were included. The patients were randomized to aspirin 1300 mg daily, sulfinpyrazone 800 mg daily, a combination of aspirin and sulfinpyrazone in the same doses, or matching placebo tablets. The patients were followed for up to 2 years (mean 18 months). The primary endpoints were cardiac death and nonfatal myocardial infarction. In the groups treated with aspirin and aspirin plus sulfinpyrazone, the incidence of cardiac death and nonfatal myocardial infarction considered together was 8.6%; in the other groups the incidence was 17%, representing a risk reduction of 51% ($P = 0.008$). If only those patients in the aspirin alone and placebo groups are compared, the incidence of death or acute myocardial infarction was 5.8% in the aspirin group and 12.9% in the placebo group, a risk reduction of 55%. The corresponding figures for cardiac death were 2.2% in the patients given aspirin alone and 8.6% in the placebo group, a risk reduction of 74%. If all patients receiving aspirin are compared with those not receiving aspirin, the reduction in cardiac death was almost identical (71%; $P = 0.004$). As in the Veterans Administration Study, all deaths were thought to be cardiac in origin. Although the number of women in each group was rather small, the observed benefit of aspirin was similar in men and women. Analysis of the results on an intention-to-treat basis yielded smaller risk reductions in the aspirin-treated patients: 30% ($P = 0.072$) and 56% ($P = 0.009$) for the incidence of cardiac death and nonfatal acute myocardial infarction and for cardiac death alone, respectively. Gastrointestinal side-effects were 29% more common in patients given aspirin than in the other groups. Suspected gastrointestinal hemorrhage and peptic ulcers were considered to be potentially dangerous gastrointestinal side-effects.

Théroux et al.[28] studied the effects of aspirin and heparin in a randomized, double-blind, placebo-controlled trial involving 479 patients. Patients received 325 mg of aspirin twice daily, 1000 units of heparin per hour by intravenous infusion, a combination of both agents, or placebo. Refractory angina, myocardial infarction, and death were the major endpoints. Heparin and the combination of heparin and aspirin decreased the occurrence of refractory angina ($P = 0.002$). The incidence of myocardial infarction was significantly reduced in the groups receiving aspirin (3%; $P = 0.01$), heparin (0.8%; $P < 0.001$), and aspirin plus heparin (1.6%; $P = 0.003$). No deaths occurred in these groups. Overall, there were too few deaths to permit evaluation of the effect of treatment on this endpoint. It has been shown that in the acute phase of unstable angina, either aspirin or heparin treatment is associated with a reduced incidence of myocardial infarction. Complications and side-effects were relatively infrequent in this study. Bleeding occurred in 20 patients receiving heparin, which was twice as frequently as in patients not receiving the drug. Serious bleeding, defined as the need for transfusion, was more frequent in the group treated with aspirin plus heparin. Patients cannot be weaned from heparin unless aspirin is given. Heparin shows rebound after cessation in patients with unstable angina.[29]

In the randomized, double-blind, placebo-controlled RISC trial involving 796 men with unstable coronary artery disease, the effect of aspirin 75 mg daily and/or 5 days of intermittent heparin was investigated.[30] After 5 days the risk was 0.43, at 1 month it was 0.31 and at 3 months it was 0.36. Aspirin significantly ($P < 0.05$) reduced the incidence of myocardial infarction and death. Heparin did not influence these parameters. Hematological side-effects due to aspirin were rare and minor. Gastrointestinal symptoms were more frequent in the aspirin (5.2–6.5%) than the placebo (0.7–1.9%) group after 3 months.

Ticlopidine, in comparison to placebo, also protects patients with unstable angina against myocardial infarction and death, with a risk reduction of about 50%, as was shown in an Italian study in 665 patients.[31]

The first trial in unstable angina with antiplatelet therapy combined with heparin followed by oral anticoagulant therapy has been published recently, and a positive result was found. A total of 214 patients with unstable angina or non-Q-wave myocardial infarction were randomized to aspirin alone (daily dose 162.5 mg), or to aspirin plus intravenous heparin followed by oral warfarin (target INR 2.0–3.0). It was found that the event rate was significantly lower than with the combination therapy, both at 14 days (62% reduction) and at 3 months (48% reduction). Bleeding, however, was insignificantly increased by the combination therapy, leading to more withdrawals.

In conclusion, the results of four randomized controlled trials have shown the beneficial effect of aspirin in the prevention of myocardial infarction and death in patients with unstable angina. The same may be true for ticlopidine, but more studies on this drug are needed. The addition of heparin followed by oral anticoagulation in patients with unstable angina may be another improvement in medical treatment, and is now being tested in large randomized trials.

Antiplatelet Agents in PTCA

After successful PTCA, the incidence of restenosis is approximately 40%. Whether or not aspirin prevents the incidence of restenosis remains uncertain. Schwartz et al.[33] studied the influence of 330 mg aspirin, three times daily, in combination with dipyridamole or placebo in 376 patients undergoing PTCA. With respect to restenosis observed by angiography no difference between antiplatelet therapy and placebo was seen. However, the incidence of transmural myocardial infarction was significantly reduced in aspirin plus dipyridamole treated patients. In order to reduce the incidence of myocardial infarction it has been recommended to apply short-term treatment with antiplatelet agents during PTCA.[33] In fact this is the only large randomized trial on conventional antiplatelet therapy in PTCA, but such therapy is uniformly initiated before and continued after PTCA.

In high-risk PTCA (lesions with thrombus, unstable angina, acute myocardial infarction) monoclonal antibodies against platelet glycoprotein IIb/IIIa receptor together with 325 mg aspirin daily are superior to aspirin alone in the prevention of major ischemic events by 35% in the short term[34] and by 23% in the longer term.[35] This was found in the Evaluation of 7E3 for the Prevention of Ischemic Complications (EPIC) trial in 2098 patients undergoing high-risk PTCA randomized to bolus antibody, to bolus followed by 24-hour infusion, and to placebo. Bolus and infusion provided the best protection. The same effects were observed in a smaller trial with 60 patients with unstable angina undergoing PTCA.[36]

When coronary stents are implanted as a bail-out procedure, ticlopidine 250 mg twice daily should be given in addition to aspirin.[37]

Antiplatelet Agents in Coronary Bypass Surgery

Vein graft occlusion is one of the main causes of morbidity following coronary artery bypass surgery. The pathogenesis of vein graft occlusion has been divided into four stages.[38] During the early phase, endothelial damage as the cause of the high pressure arterial system results in platelet disposition. This and the subsequent release of platelet factors initiate mural and occlusive thrombus formation. During the late phase, occlusion appears to be related to the rapid progression of initial hyperplasia and chronic smooth muscle cell and connective tissue proliferation. Finally, beyond the first year after operation there is further connective tissue synthesis from smooth muscle cells and fibroblasts, which may be followed by incorporation of lipids into the lesions closely resembling arterial atherosclerotic disease.[38] The results from a number of trials on aspirin, either alone or in combination with dipyridamole, in the prevention of occlusion of coronary artery vein grafts have been reviewed in the literature.[39]

McEnany *et al.*[40] compared the influence of aspirin 600 mg twice daily with warfarin treatment in a randomized, double-blind, placebo-controlled trial involving 216 patients. Aspirin and warfarin tended to improve graft patency. The difference, however, was not statistically significant ($P > 0.05$).

Lorenz *et al.*[41] reported on a small randomized, double-blind, placebo-controlled study (60 patients) comparing aspirin 100 mg daily with placebo given within 24 hours of operation. Aspirin significantly reduced the number of occluded grafts 4 months after surgery (10% aspirin versus 32% placebo; $P = 0.012$). Ventricular arrhythmias after surgery were more frequently observed in patients on placebo (12/18) than in patients on aspirin (5/17). No side-effects were reported.

Brown *et al.*[42] compared the effect of aspirin alone (975 mg) with aspirin plus dipyridamole, and placebo in a randomized, double-blind, placebo-controlled study involving 174 coronary bypass patients. Repeated coronary angiography 12 months after bypass surgery was performed in 86% of the patients. The percentage of occluded grafts was smaller in the two treatment groups when compared with placebo (13% versus 21%; $P < 0.05$), but there was no significant difference between aspirin alone and the aspirin plus dipyridamole combination.

In a randomized, double-blind, placebo-controlled study by Goldman *et al.*,[43] 555 patients were treated with aspirin 325 mg once daily, aspirin 325 mg three times daily, aspirin 325 mg three times daily with dipyridamole 75 mg three times daily, sulfinpyrazone 267 mg three times daily, or placebo. Treatment with aspirin was started 12 hours before operation. Angiography was carried out within 2 months postoperatively. Analysis of early graft patency revealed the following graft patency percentages: aspirin once daily 93.5; aspirin three times daily 92.3; aspirin and dipyridamole 91.9; sulfinpyrazone 90.2; and placebo 85.2. The aspirin-containing regimens significantly ($P < 0.05$) improved graft patency. In the three treatment groups chest-tube blood loss was increased.

The influence of aspirin 330 mg three times daily plus dipyridamole 75 mg three times daily for 6 months postoperatively was studied by Rajay et al.[44] in 125 patients who underwent aortocoronary bypass grafting. Anticoagulants were administered as additional treatment for the first 3 months after operation. Therapy was started preoperatively, the first dose being administered on the evening prior to surgery. Angiography was repeated 6 months later on 82% of the patients: 8% of the grafts were occluded in the treated group compared with 25% in the placebo group ($P < 0.01$). In the treatment groups blood loss was slightly but not significantly less severe than in the untreated group. Side-effects were generally not serious, except in two patients who were withdrawn from the study because of gastric upset and headache.

Brooks et al.[45] described a randomized, double-blind, placebo-controlled study on the effect of combination therapy with aspirin 330 mg and dipyridamole 225 mg three times daily for 12 months in 320 bypass graft patients. Warfarin was given for 3 months. Repeated coronary angiography was performed on 266 patients. Treatment with this regimen slightly increased coronary patency. The difference, however, was not statistically significant ($P > 0.05$). Active treatment was associated with a significantly higher incidence of gastrointestinal side-effects.

In a randomized, double-blind, placebo-controlled study of 407 patients, Chesebro et al.[46,47] examined the effect of aspirin 325 mg plus dipyridamole 75 mg three times daily on the frequency of both early (median time of assessment 8 days postoperatively) and late (6–18 months) graft occlusion. Although treatment with dipyridamole was initiated prior to surgery, the first dose of aspirin was not given until 7 hours postoperatively. Within 1 month of operation, 10 to 351 (3%) distal anastomoses were occluded in the treatment group compared with 38 of 362 (10%) in the placebo group. Similarly, 8% of the treated patients had at least one occluded graft compared with 21% of those on placebo ($P = 0.003$). The benefit of aspirin plus dipyridamole on prevention of late occlusion was much less striking, with 16% of treated patients having occluded grafts when re-examined 6–18 months after surgery versus 27% of patients in the placebo group ($P = 0.038$).

Pfisterer et al.[48] described a randomized trial comparing the effectiveness of aspirin plus dipyridamole with standard anticoagulant therapy in 285 patients. Patients were treated with either anticoagulants or aspirin 25 mg and dipyridamole 200 mg twice daily. Antiplatelet therapy was started 2 days preoperatively with dipyridamole 200 mg twice daily, followed by the combination of aspirin 25 mg and dipyridamole 200 mg twice daily on the morning of surgery. After 3 months of treatment, in half of the patients active treatment was replaced by placebo. Dipyridamole plus low-dose aspirin appeared similarly effective in preventing early and late aortocoronary vein bypass graft occlusion. Replacement of active treatment by placebo after 3 months long-term treatment decreased graft patency. Treatment with the drugs was well tolerated and did not influence perioperative blood loss.

In a multicenter, randomized, double-blind, placebo-controlled trial, Sanz et al.[49] have studied the effect of aspirin alone and in combination with dipyridamole in 1112 patients who were undergoing saphenous vein aortocoronary bypass surgery. Patients received aspirin 50 mg three times daily, aspirin 50 mg three times daily plus dipyridamole 75 mg three times daily, or placebo. All patients were given dipyridamole 100 mg four times daily, beginning 2 days before surgery. The vein graft occlusion rate was 18% for the placebo group compared with 14.2% ($P = 0.058$) and 12.9% ($P = 0.017$) for the aspirin and aspirin plus dipyridamole groups. The proportion of patients with at least one occluded graft was significantly lower in the group of patients receiving aspirin plus dipyridamole than in the placebo group (24.3% versus 33%; $P < 0.01$). There were no statistically significant differences between the aspirin and placebo groups nor between the different aspirin dosage groups. Thus, low-dose aspirin plus dipyridamole improved early aorto-coronary bypass surgery, the effect being additive to preoperative treatment with dipyridamole. Chest-tube blood loss was slightly increased in both the aspirin alone and in the aspirin plus dipyridamole treated groups. Total blood loss in the aspirin and aspirin plus dipyridamole groups was 629 and 713 ml over 24 hours, respectively, the quantities being lower than observed in studies using higher doses of aspirin.[49]

In conclusion, either alone or in combination with dipyridamole, aspirin has been shown to be effective in the prevention of early graft occlusion. The benefit was most apparent in those studies in which treatment was started prior to or within 24 hours of surgery. Treatment should be continued for at least 1 year.[46,48]

Antiplatelet Agents in the Treatment of Atrial Fibrillation and in Patients with Artificial Heart Valves

Antiplatelet Agents in the Treatment of Atrial Fibrillation

Atrial fibrillation is associated with an increased risk of thromboembolism. Antiplatelet agents may be effective in preventing this complication. The Danish AFASAK Study and the American Stroke Prevention in Atrial Fibrillation Study studied the influence of aspirin or warfarin versus placebo on the risk of thrombotic embolism in patients with atrial fibrillation.

In the Danish study, 1007 patients with chronic nonrheumatic atrial fibrillation were followed for 2 years.[50] The effects of aspirin 75 mg daily, warfarin, and placebo treatment were compared.

The American study compared the effects of aspirin 325 mg given once daily, warfarin, and placebo in 1244 patients.[51] In this setting both aspirin and warfarin decreased the incidence of thrombotic embolism. It should be noted that, in contrast to the Danish study, the American study investigated whether or not patients were eligible for treatment with warfarin.

Aspirin reduced the rate of thromboembolism in the two studies (2264 patient-years) by 30% compared to placebo.

Antiplatelet Agents in the Treatment of Patients with Artificial Heart Valves

Anticoagulants are the most important component of drug therapy for the prevention of thromboembolism in patients with prosthetic heart valves. The combination of anti-coagulants and high-dose aspirin may be dangerous, but the combination with low-dose aspirin may be beneficial (see later).

Trials of Anticoagulant Therapy in Cardiology

After antiplatelet therapy, anticoagulant therapy offers the second most important protection against thrombotic and thromboembolic complications of cardiovascular disease. Intravenous and subcutaneous anticoagulant therapy usually consist of heparin or, more recently, specific antithrombin agents such as hirudin, hirulog, and argatroban. Oral anticoagulants can be used in-hospital, in which case their use is often preceded by heparin therapy. Oral anticoagulants are ideal for ambulatory use, but need laboratory control.

In this section, the role of anticoagulants in the treatment of ischemic heart disease, valvular heart disease, atrial fibrillation, and coronary bypass surgery is reviewed.

Heparin and Thrombin Inhibitors in Ischemic Heart Disease

Heparin is valuable in the treatment and protection of patients with unstable angina. Théroux et al.[28] studied the effects of aspirin and heparin in a randomized, double-blind, placebo-controlled trial involving 479 patients. Patients received aspirin 325 mg given twice daily, heparin 1000 iu h^{-1} by intravenous infusion, a combination of both agents, or placebo. Refractory angina, myocardial infarction, and death were the major endpoints. Heparin and the combination of heparin and aspirin decreased the occurrence of refractory angina ($P = 0.002$). The incidence of myocardial infarction was significantly reduced in the groups receiving aspirin (3%; $P = 0.01$), heparin (0.8%; $P < 0.001$), and aspirin plus heparin (1.6%; $P = 0.003$). No deaths occurred in these groups. Overall, there were too few deaths to permit evaluation of the effect of treatment on this endpoint. It has been shown that, in the acute phase of unstable angina, either aspirin or heparin treatment is associated with a reduced incidence of myocardial infarction. Complications and side-effects were relatively infrequent in this study. Bleeding occurred in 20 patients receiving heparin, which was twice as frequent as in patients not receiving the drug. Serious bleeding, defined as the need for transfusion, was more frequent in the group treated with aspirin plus heparin. Patients cannot be weaned from heparin unless aspirin is given. Heparin shows rebound after cessation in patients with unstable angina.[29] Subcutaneous low-molecular-weight heparin (dalteparin) 120 iu kg^{-1} twice daily is an effective alternative.[52]

Hirudin bolus followed by infusion was superior to heparin in a relatively small angiographic dose-finding study[53] in 75 patients with unstable angina. Also, argatroban bolus and infusion tested in 43 patients with unstable angina seems to be effective and superior to heparin.[54]

The role of intravenous heparin in acute myocardial infarction has been controversial, because in the prethrombolytic era proper clinical trials on early treatment with heparin were lacking. Subcutaneous heparin 12 500 iu twice daily may reduce the incidence of left ventricular thrombosis and subsequent stroke in patients with anterior myocardial infarction.[55]

Since the introduction of thrombolytic therapy, intravenous heparin has been increasingly used in patients with acute myocardial infarction. In two thrombolytic agent megatrials GISSI-2[56] and ISIS-3,[57] subcutaneous heparin 12 500 iu twice daily did not improve survival, but increased bleeding risk. Intravenous heparin as an adjunct to alteplase improves early patency of the infarct-related artery[58–60] and was associated with the lowest 30-day mortality in the GUSTO trial.[61] The scheme used was a 5000 iu bolus injection prior to alteplase and subsequent infusion with an APTT between 60 and 85 seconds. Intravenous heparin as adjuncts to streptokinase or anistreplase is not associated with better outcome compared to subcutaneous or no heparin.[61,62]

Relatively small angiographic studies with hirudin[63] and hirulog[64] as adjuncts to thrombolysis showed benefit in early patency and reocclusion over heparin. Hirudin with or without thrombolysis in a bolus of 6 mg kg^{-1} followed by an infusion of 0.2 mg

$kg^{-1} h^{-1}$ was associated with more than 50% higher cerebral bleeding risk compared to the standard heparin regimens in three prematurely discontinued trials.[65–67] Two of these trials are being continued with a lower hirudin dosing scheme, consisting of a 1 mg kg^{-1} bolus followed by an infusion of 0.1 mg $kg^{-1} h^{-1}$.

Oral Anticoagulants in Ischemic Heart Disease

Secondary prevention of myocardial infarction with oral anticoagulants has been thoroughly investigated. However, many trials were done in the 1960s and 1970s and lacked a proper prospective, placebo control and a randomized design. The first breakthrough for oral anticoagulants in ischemic heart disease was the Sixty Plus Reinfarction trial,[68] which showed that discontinuation of oral anticoagulation after myocardial infarction can lead to reinfarction and death. These data initiated two large prospective, placebo-controlled, randomized trials on the efficacy of oral anticoagulation in secondary prevention after acute myocardial infarction.

The first of these studies was the WARIS study[69] conducted in Norway, which consisted of 1214 patients who were randomized to warfarin or placebo. It was shown that a 25% reduction in death, 35% in reinfarction, and 55% in stroke can be achieved by proper anticoagulation. The risk of oral anticoagulation in this study was highly acceptable. Interestingly, the prevention of ischemic stroke was even more pronounced than death or reinfarction. A second similar study, ASPECT, was conducted in The Netherlands in 3034 patients.[70] This study showed a 10% (not significant) reduction in death, 50% in reinfarction, and 40% in stroke in comparison to placebo. In both trials the bleeding risk was acceptable and the risk reduction for ischemic stroke largely outweighed the small increased risk of cerebral bleeding. The optimum INR range was found to be 2.0–4.0.[71]

Both WARIS and ASPECT were placebo-controlled trials. Nowadays, antiplatelet therapy is the common secondary preventive measure after myocardial infarction. The efficacy of oral anticoagulation relative to antiplatelet therapy was studied in the prethrombolytic era. No specific benefit of oral anticoagulation over aspirin was established in the EPSIM or GAMIS studies (see above). However, this issue is under investigation in currently running trials (see below).

Combination oral anticoagulation therapy with low-dose aspirin has recently been studied in a small trial and was found to be beneficial (see above).

Oral Anticoagulants in Coronary Artery Bypass Surgery

McEnany *et al.*[40] compared the influence of aspirin 600 mg twice daily with warfarin treatment in a randomized, double-blind, placebo-controlled trial involving 216 patients. Aspirin and warfarin tended to improve graft patency. The difference, however, was not statistically significant ($P > 0.05$).

Pfisterer *et al.*[48] described a randomized trial comparing the effectiveness of aspirin plus dipyridamole with standard anticoagulant therapy in 285 patients. Patients were treated with either anticoagulants or aspirin 25 mg and dipyridamole 200 mg twice daily. Antiplatelet therapy was started 2 days preoperatively with dipyridamole 200 mg twice daily followed by the combination of aspirin 25 mg and dipyridamole 200 mg twice daily started on the morning of surgery. After 3 months of treatment, in half the patients active treatment was replaced by placebo. Dipyridamole plus low-dose aspirin appeared similarly effective in preventing early and late aortocoronary vein bypass graft occlusion. Replacement of active treatment by placebo after 3 months of long-term treatment decreased graft patency. Treatment with the drugs was well tolerated and did not influence perioperative blood loss.

In another direct comparison in nearly 1000 patients, the CABADAS trial found no differences in 1-year patency of vein grafts between aspirin 50 mg daily combined with dipyridamole 75 mg three times daily, aspirin 50 mg daily alone, and oral anticoagulation. All treatments were started preoperatively and were equally safe.[72]

Oral Anticoagulants in Atrial Fibrillation

Atrial fibrillation is associated with an increased risk of thromboembolism. Both oral anticoagulant therapy and antiplatelet agents are effective in preventing this complication.

In five randomized controlled trials with a total of 3692 patient-years warfarin reduced the rate of thromboembolism by 70% compared to placebo.[50,51,73–75] Interestingly, in two studies[73,75] warfarin was given in low intensity (INR around 2.0). As shown above, aspirin reduces thromboembolism by only 30%. However, in a direct comparison in 1165 patients with atrial fibrillation, warfarin reduced thromboembolism better than aspirin, but at the cost of more intracerebral breeding in patients over the age of 75 years, thus resulting in overall equivalence in stroke prevention.[76]

Electric cardioversion of atrial fibrillation seems to increase the risk of postprocedural thromboembolism, which can be prevented with oral anticoagulation,[77] although more studies are necessary.

Once thromboembolism has occurred in patients with atrial fibrillation, oral anticoagulation is more effective than aspirin in preventing recurrent thromboembolism.[78] However, aspirin is more effective than placebo in these patients.

Oral Anticoagulants in Heart Valve Disease

Artificial heart valves can thrombose with subsequent malfunction and/or thromboembolism. Oral anticoagulation therapy is always indicated in patients with artificial heart valves. The optimum intensity of oral anticoagulation in patients with artificial heart valves is still under debate.[79–81] Full intensity oral anticoagulation (target INR 3.0–4.0) is the most usual treatment of patients with artificial heart valves. Although many feel that antiplatelet drugs should not be combined with full oral anticoagulation, the results of combined oral anticoagulant and antiplatelet therapy in patients with artificial heart valves are promising and show acceptable safety. Three trials[82–84] of the combined therapy using full intensity oral anticoagulation and high-dose aspirin were published in the early 1980s. The trials showed a significant reduction in thromboembolism by the combination therapy of 60% in a total of 1366 patient-years. Major bleeding, however, was doubled by the combination therapy. Therefore, lower doses of aspirin in combination with full intensity oral anticoagulation was tested. In over 600 patient-years, low-dose aspirin (100 mg aspirin, slow release, once daily) combined with full intensity oral anticoagulation (mean INR 2.8) diminished thromboembolism and death significantly by 65% in 370 patients with artificial heart valves, compared to placebo,[85] but bleeding was increased by 27% (not significant).

Conclusions and Perspectives

Both antiplatelet and anticoagulant therapy are effective in preventing thrombotic and thromboembolic complications of cardiovascular disease when compared to placebo. Ischemic heart disease, atrial fibrillation, and valvular heart disease are the classic indications for these forms of prophylactic treatment. Antiplatelet therapy is preferred in most indications in ischemic heart disease, and anticoagulants are preferred in many cases of atrial fibrillation and all patients with artificial heart valves.

As both strategies have completely different modes of action, it might well be possible that they could be synergistic. However, bleeding complications are common to both therapies, and therefore synergism might also lead to increased bleeding. The first trials with combined antiplatelet and anticoagulant therapy provided promising results. WARIS-2 is running in Norway in patients who have survived myocardial infarction, and is comparing aspirin alone with either full intensity oral anticoagulation (target INR 2.8–4.2) alone or a combination of low-dose aspirin and low intensity oral anticoagulation (target INR 2.0–3.0). In the USA, the Coumadin Aspirin Reinfarction Study (CARS) is comparing low-dose aspirin alone (160 mg daily) versus low-dose aspirin (80 mg daily) combined with low intensity fixed dose oral anticoagulation. Other postmyocardial infarction studies in progress, where combined oral anticoagulation and antiplatelet therapy is compared with aspirin alone or with full oral anticoagulation alone, are APRICOT-2, ASPECT-2, CHAMP, and LOWASA.

Studies of combined therapy are also in progress in patients with atrial fibrillation (AFASAK-2 and SPAF-3). These studies compare combined oral anticoagulant and antiplatelet therapy with anticoagulant therapy alone in the primary prevention of thromboembolism in patients with atrial fibrillation.

Finally, the glycoprotein IIb/IIIa receptor antagonists are promising new antiplatelet agents, of which many trials are underway.

References

1. Antiplatelet Trialists' Collaboration. Collaborative overview of randomised trials of antiplatelet therapy I: prevention of death, myocardial infarction, and stroke by prolonged antiplatelet therapy in various categories of patients. *Br Med J* 1994; **308**: 81–106.
2. Linos A, Worthington JW, O'Fallon W, Fuster V, Whisnant JP, Kurland LT. Effect of aspirin on prevention of coronary and cerebrovascular disease in patients with rheumatoid arthritis. *Mayo Clin Proc* 1978; **53**: 581–6.
3. The Steering Committee of The Physicians' Health Study. Final report on the aspirin component of the ongoing Physicians' Health Study. *N Engl J Med* 1989; **321**: 129–35.
4. Peto R, Gray R, Collins C, *et al*. Randomised trial of prophylactic daily aspirin in British male doctors. *Br Med J* 1988; **296**: 313–16.
5. Ridker PM, Manson JE, Gaziano JM, Buring JE, Hennekens CH. Low-dose aspirin therapy for chronic stable angina. A randomized, placebo-controlled clinical trial. *Ann Intern Med* 1991; **114**: 835–9.
6. Juul-Möller S, Edvardsson N, Jahnmatz B, Rosén A, Sorensen S, Omblus R. Double-blind trial of aspirin in primary prevention of myocardial infarction in patients with stable chronic angina pectoris. *Lancet* 1992; **340**: 1421–5.
7. Chesebro JH, Webster MWI, Smith HC, *et al*. Antiplatelet therapy in coronary disease progression reduced infarct and new lesion formation. *Circulation* 1989; **80**(Suppl II): II–266 (abstract).
8. Miller GJ. Antithrombotic therapy in the primary prevention of acute myocardial infarction. *Am J Cardiol* 1989; **64**: 29B–32B.
9. Meade TW, Roderick PJ, Brennan PJ, Wilkes HC, Kelleher CC. Extra-cranial bleeding and other symptoms due to low dose aspirin and low intensity oral anticoagulation. *Thromb Haemostas* 1992; **68**: 1–6.
10. Patrono C. Aspirin as an antiplatelet drug. *N Engl J Med* 1994; **330**: 1287–94.
11. Elwood PC, Sweetnam PM. Aspirin and secondary mortality after myocardial infarction. *Lancet* 1979; **ii**: 1313–15.
12. ISIS-2 (Second International Study of Infarct Survival) Collaborative Group. Randomised trial of intravenous streptokinase, oral aspirin, both, or neither among 17 187 cases of suspected acute myocardial infarction: ISIS-2. *Lancet* 1988; **ii**: 349–60.

13. Verheugt FWA, Funke Kupper AJ, Galema TW, Roos JP. Low dose aspirin after early thrombolysis in anterior wall acute myocardial infarction. *Am J Cardiol* 1988; **61**: 904–6.

14. The Persantine–Aspirin Reinfarction Study Research Group. Persantine and aspirin in coronary heart disease. *Circulation* 1980; **62**: 449–61.

15. Breddin K, Loew D, Lechner K, Oberla K, Walter E. The German Aspirin Trial: A comparison of acetylsalicylic acid, placebo and phenprocoumon in secondary prevention of myocardial infarction. *Circulation* 1980; **62**(Suppl V): V63–72.

16. Elwood PC, Williams WO. A randomized controlled trial of aspirin in the prevention of early mortality in myocardial infarction. *J R Coll Gen Pract* 1979; **29**: 413–16.

17. Klimt CR, Knatterud GL, Stamler J, Meier P. Persantine–Aspirin Reinfarction Study. Part II. Secondary coronary prevention with persantine and aspirin. *J Am Coll Cardiol* 1986; **7**: 251–69.

18. The EPSIM Research Group. A controlled comparison of aspirin and oral anticoagulants in prevention of death after myocardial infarction. *N Engl J Med* 1982; **307**: 701–8.

19. Küpper AJF, Verheugt FWA, Peels CH, Galema TW, Den Hollander W, Roos JP. Effect of low dose aspirin on the frequency and hematologic activity of left ventricular thrombus in anterior wall acute myocardial infarction. *Am J Cardiol* 1989; **63**: 917–20.

20. Aspirin Myocardial Infarction Study Research Group. A randomized, controlled trial of aspirin in persons recovered from myocardial infarction. *JAMA* 1980; **243**: 661–9.

21. Sherman CT, Litvack F, Grundfest W, *et al*. Coronary angioscopy in patients with unstable angina pectoris. *N Engl J Med* 1986; **315**: 913–19.

22. Davies MJ, Path FRC, Thomas AC, *et al*. Intramyocardial platelet aggregation in patients with unstable angina suffering sudden ischemic cardiac death. *Circulation* 1986; **73**: 418–27.

23. Falk E. Unstable angina with fatal outcome: dynamic coronary thrombosis leading to infarction and/or sudden death. *Circulation* 1985; **71**: 699–708.

24. Fitzgerald DJ, Catella F, Roy L, FitzGerald GA. Marked platelet activation after streptokinase in patients with acute myocardial infarction. *Circulation* 1988; **77**: 142–50.

25. Lam JYT, Chesebro JH, Steele PM, *et al*. Antithrombotic therapy for deep arterial injury by angioplasty. Efficacy of common platelet inhibition compared with thrombin inhibition in pigs. *Circulation* 1991; **84**: 814–20.

26. Lewis HD, Davis JW, Archibald DG, *et al*. Protective effects of aspirin against acute myocardial infarction and death in men with unstable angina. *N Engl J Med* 1983; **309**: 396–403.

27. Cairns JA, Gent M, Singer J, *et al*. Aspirin, sulfinpyrazone, or both in unstable angina. *N Engl J Med* 1985; **313**: 1369–75.

28. Théroux P, Ouimet H, McCans J, *et al*. Aspirin, heparin, or both to treat acute unstable angina. *N Engl J Med* 1988; **319**: 1105–11.

29. Théroux P, Waters D, Lam J, Juneau M, Cairns J. Reactivation of unstable angina after the discontinuation of heparin. *N Engl J Med* 1992; **327**: 192–4.

30. The RISC Group. Risk of myocardial infarction and death during treatment with low dose aspirin and intravenous heparin in men with unstable coronary artery disease. *Lancet* 1990; **336**: 827–30.

31. Balsano F, Rizzon P, Violi F, *et al*. Antiplatelet treatment with ticlopidine in unstable angina. A controlled multicenter clinical trial. *Circulation* 1990; **82**: 17–26.

32. Cohen M, Adams PC, Parry G, *et al*. Combination antithrombotic therapy in unstable rest angina and non-Q-wave infarction in nonprior aspirin users. Primary endpoints analysis from the ATACS trial. *Circulation* 1994; **89**: 81–8.

33. Schwartz L, Bourassa MG, Lespérance J, *et al*. Aspirin and dipyridamole in the prevention of restenosis after percutaneous transluminal coronary angioplasty. *N Engl J Med* 1988; **318**: 1714–19.

34. The EPIC Investigation. Use of a monoclonal antibody directed against the platelet glycoprotein IIb/IIIa receptor in high-risk coronary angioplasty. *N Engl J Med* 1994; **330**: 956–61.

35. Topol EJ, Califf RM, Weisman HF, *et al*. Randomised trial of coronary intervention with antibody against platelet IIb/IIIa integrin for reduction of clinical restenosis: results at six months. *Lancet* 1994; **343**: 881–6.

36. Simoons ML, De Boer MJ, Van den Brand MJ, *et al*. Randomised trial of a GP IIb/IIIa platelet receptor blocker in refractory unstable angina. *Circulation* 1994; **89**: 596–603.

37. Schömig A, Neumann FJ, Kastrati A, *et al*. A randomized comparison of antiplatelet and anticoagulant therapy after the placement of coronary-artery stents. *N Engl J Med* 1996; **334**: 1084–9.

38. Fuster V, Adams PC, Badimon JJ, Chesebro JH. Platelet-inhibitor drugs' role in coronary artery disease. *Prog Cardiovasc Dis* 1987; **29**: 325–46.

39. Verstraete M, Brown BG, Chesebro JH, *et al*. Evaluation of antiplatelet agents in the prevention of aorto-coronary bypass occlusion. *Eur Heart J* 1986; **7**: 4–13.

40. McEnany MT, Salzman EW, Mundt ED, *et al*. The effect of antithrombotic therapy on patency rates of saphenous vein coronary artery bypass grafts. *J Thorac Cardiovasc Surg* 1983; **83**: 81–9.

41. Lorenz RL, Weber M, Kotzur J, *et al*. Improved aortocoronary bypass patency by low-dose aspirin (100 mg daily). *Lancet* 1984; **i**: 1261–4.

42. Brown BG, Cukingnan RA, DeRouen T, *et al*. Improved graft patency in patients treated with platelet-inhibiting therapy after coronary bypass surgery. *Circulation* 1985; **72**: 138–46.

43. Goldman S, Copeland J, Moritz T. Improvement in early saphenous vein graft patency after coronary artery bypass surgery with antiplatelet therapy: results of a Veterans Administration Cooperative Study. *Circulation* 1988; **77**: 1324–32.

44. Rajay SM, Salter MCP, Donaldson DR, *et al*. Aspirin and dipyridamole improve the early patency of aorta-coronary bypass grafts. *J Thorac Cardiovasc Surg* 1985; **90**: 373–7.

45. Brooks N, Wright J, Sturridge M, *et al.* Randomised placebo controlled trial of aspirin and dipyridamole in the prevention of coronary vein graft occlusion. *Br Heart J* 1985; **53**: 201–7.
46. Chesebro JH, Fuster V, Elveback LR. Effect of dipyridamole and aspirin on late vein-graft patency after coronary bypass operations. *N Engl J Med* 1984; **310**: 209–14.
47. Chesebro JH, Clements IP, Fuster V, *et al.* A platelet-inhibitor-drug trial in coronary-artery bypass operations. *N Engl J Med* 1982; **307**: 73–8.
48. Pfisterer M, Jockers G, Regenass S, *et al.* Trial of low-dose aspirin plus dipyridamole versus anticoagulants for prevention of aortocoronary vein graft occlusion. *Lancet* 1989; **ii**: 1–6.
49. Sanz G, Pajarón A, Alegría E, *et al.* Prevention of early aortocoronary bypass occlusion by low-dose aspirin and dipyridamole. *Circulation* 1990; **82**: 765–73.
50. Petersen P, Boysen G, Godtfredsen J, Andersen ED, Andersen B. Placebo-controlled, randomized trial of warfarin and aspirin for prevention of thromboembolic complications in chronic atrial fibrillation: the Copenhagen AFASAK study. *Lancet* 1989; **i**: 175–9.
51. Stroke Prevention in Atrial Fibrillation Study Group Investigators. Final results. *Circulation* 1991; **84**: 527–39.
52. FRISC Study Group. Low-molecular-weight heparin during instability in coronary artery disease. *Lancet* 1996; **347**: 561–8.
53. Topol EJ, Fuster V, Harrington RA, *et al.* Recombinant hirudin for unstable angina pectoris. A multicenter, randomized angiographic trial. *Circulation* 1994; **89**: 1557–66.
54. Gold HK, Torres FW, Garabedian HD, *et al.* Evidence for a rebound coagulation phenomenon after cessation of a 4-hour infusion of a specific thrombin inhibitor in patients with unstable angina pectoris. *J Am Coll Cardiol* 1993; **21**: 1039–47.
55. Turpie AGG, Robinson JG, Doyle DJ, *et al.* Comparison of high-dose with low-dose subcutaneous heparin to prevent left ventricular mural thrombosis in patients with acute transmural anterior myocardial infarction. *N Engl J Med* 1989; **320**: 352–7.
56. The International Study Group. In-hospital mortality and clinical course of 20 891 patients with suspected acute myocardial infarction randomised between alteplase and streptokinase with or without heparin. *Lancet* 1990; **336**: 71–5.
57. ISIS-3 (Third International Study of Infarct Survival) Collaborative Group. A randomised comparison of streptokinase vs tissue plasminogen activator vs anistreplase and of aspirin plus heparin vs aspirin alone among 41 299 cases of suspected acute myocardial infarction: ISIS-3. *Lancet* 1992; **339**: 753–70.
58. Bono D de, Simoons ML, Tijssen J, *et al.* Effect of early intravenous heparin on coronary patency, infarct size, and bleeding complications after alteplase thrombolysis: results of a randomized double blind European Cooperative Study Group trial. *Br Heart J* 1992; **67**: 122–8.
59. Hsia J, Hamilton WP, Kleiman N, *et al.* A comparison between heparin and low-dose aspirin as adjunctive therapy with tissue plasminogen activator for acute myocardial infarction. *N Engl J Med* 1990; **323**: 1433–7.
60. Bleich SD, Nichols T, Schumacher RR, Cooke DH, Tate DA, Teichman SL. Effect of heparin on coronary arterial patency after thrombolysis with tissue plasminogen activator in acute myocardial infarction. *Am J Cardiol* 1990; **66**: 1412–17.
61. GUSTO Investigators. An International randomized trial comparing four thrombolytic strategies for acute myocardial infarction. *N Engl J Med* 1993; **329**: 673–82.
62. O'Connor CM, Meese R, Carney R, *et al.* A randomized trial of intravenous heparin in conjunction with anistreplase (anisoylated plasminogen streptokinase activator complex) in acute myocardial infarction: the Duke University Clinical Cardiology Study (DUCCS)-1. *J Am Coll Cardiol* 1994; **23**: 11–18.
63. Cannon CP, McCabe CH, Henry TD, *et al.* A pilot trial of recombinant desulfatohirudin compared with heparin in conjunction with tissue plasminogen activator and aspirin in acute myocardial infarction: results of the Thrombolysis in Myocardial Infarction (TIMI) 5 trial. *J Am Coll Cardiol* 1994; **23**: 993–1003.
64. Théroux P, Perez-Villa F, Waters D, Lesperance J, Shabani F, Bonan R. Randomized double-blind comparison of two doses of hirulog with heparin as adjunctive therapy to streptokinase to promote early patency of the infarct-related artery in acute myocardial infarction. *Circulation* 1995; **91**: 2132–9.
65. GUSTO-IIa Investigators. Randomized trial of intravenous heparin versus recombinant hirudin for acute coronary syndromes. *Circulation* 1994; **90**: 1631–7.
66. Neuhaus KL, Von Essen R, Tebbe U, *et al.* Safety observations from the pilot phase of the randomized r-Hirudin for Improvement of Thrombolysis (HIT-III) Study. *Circulation* 1994; **90**: 1638–42.
67. Antman ER. Hirudin in acute myocardial infarction. Safety report from the Thrombolysis and Thrombin Inhibition in Myocardial Infarction (TIMI) 9A trial. *Circulation* 1994; **90**: 1624–30.
68. Sixty Plus Reinfarction Study Research Group. A double-blind trial to assess long-term oral anticoagulant therapy in elderly patients after myocardial infarction. *Lancet* 1980; **ii**: 989–4.
69. Smith P, Arnesen H, Holme I. The effect of warfarin on mortality and reinfarction after myocardial infarctions. *N Engl J Med* 1990; **323**: 147–52.
70. Anticoagulants in the Secondary Prevention of Events in Coronary Thrombosis (ASPECT) Research Group. Effect of long-term oral anticoagulant treatment on mortality and cardiovascular morbidity after myocardial infarction. *Lancet* 1994; **343**: 499–503.
71. Azar JA, Cannegieter SC, Deckers JW, *et al.* Optimal intensity of oral anticoagulant therapy after myocardial infarction. *J Am Coll Cardiol* 1996; **27**: 1349–55.
72. Van der Meer J, Hillige HL, Kootstra GJ, *et al.* Prevention of one-year vein-graft occlusion after aortocoronary bypass

surgery: a comparison of low-dose aspirin, low-dose aspirin plus dipyridamole, and oral anticoagulants. *Lancet* 1993; **342**: 257–64.

73. Ezekowitz ME, Bridgers SL, James KE, *et al.*, and the VA SPINAF Investigators. Warfarin in the prevention of stroke associated with nonrheumatic atrial fibrillation. *N Engl J Med* 1992; **327**: 1406–12.

74. Connolly SJ, Laupaucis A, Gent M, *et al.*, and the CAFA Study Co-investigators. Canadian Atrial Fibrillation Anticoagulation (CAFA) Study. *J Am Coll Cardiol* 1991; **18**: 349–55.

75. Boston Area Anticoagulation Trial for Atrial Fibrillation (BAATAF) Investigators. The effect of low-dose warfarin on the risk of stroke in patients with nonrheumatic atrial fibrillation. *N Engl J Med* 1990; **323**: 1505–11.

76. Stroke Prevention in Atrial Fibrillation Investigators. Warfarin versus aspirin for prevention of thromboembolism in atrial fibrillation: Stroke Prevention in Atrial Fibrillation II Study. *Lancet* 1994; **343**: 687–91.

77. Arnold AZ, Mick MJ, Mazurek RP, Loop FD, Trohman RG. Role of prophylactic anticoagulation for direct current cardioversion in patients with atrial fibrillation. *J Am Coll Cardiol* 1992; **15**: 851–5.

78. EAFT (European Atrial Fibrillation Trial) Study Group. Secondary prevention of non-rheumatic atrial fibrillation after transient ischaemic attack or minor stroke. *Lancet* 1993; **342**: 1255–62.

79. Saour JN, Sieck JO, Mamo LAR, Gallus AS. Trial of different intensities of anticoagulation in patients with prosthetic heart valves. *N Engl J Med* 1990; **322**: 428–32.

80. Cannegieter SC, Rosendaal FR, Briët E. Thromboembolic and bleeding complications in patients with mechanical heart valve prostheses. *Circulation* 1994; **89**: 635–41.

81. Cannegieter SC, Rosendaal FR, Wintzen AR, Van der Meer FJ, Vandenbroucke JP, Briët E. Optimal oral anticoagulant therapy in patients with mechanical heart valves. *N Engl J Med* 1995; **333**: 11–17.

82. Dale J, Myhre E, Rootwelt K. Effects of dipyridamole and acetylsalicylic acid on platelet functions in patients with aortic ball-valve prostheses. *Am Heart J* 1975; **89**: 613–18.

83. Altman R, Boullon F, Rouvier J, Raca R, de la Fuente L, Favaloro R. Aspirin and prophylaxis of thromboembolic complications in patients with substitute heart valves. *J Thorac Cardiovasc Surg* 1976; **72**: 127–9.

84. Chesebro JH, Fuster V, Elveback LR. Trial of combined warfarin plus dipyridamole or aspirin therapy in prosthetic heart valve replacement: danger of aspirin compared with dipyridamole. *Am J Cardiol* 1983; **51**: 1537–41.

85. Turpie AGG, Gent M, Laupacis A, *et al.* A comparison of aspirin with placebo in patients treated with warfarin after heart-valve replacement. *N Engl J Med* 1993; **329**: 524–9.

15

ACE Inhibitors in and after Myocardial Infarction

Alistair S. Hall, Gordon D. Murray and
Stephen G. Ball

Introduction

The randomized controlled trials of angiotensin converting enzyme (ACE) inhibitor therapy following acute myocardial infarction collectively represent a fascinating case study of modern trial design. Eight investigations were of an adequate size to comment on the effect of treatment on all-cause mortality, while many more smaller investigations have addressed surrogate clinical endpoints such as left ventricular dilatation.[1] We will focus our comments only on the larger mortality studies, the details of which are summarized in *Table 15.1*. These can be considered in a number of different ways, based on design features such as method for selecting patients, timing of treatment initiation, duration of maintenance therapy, number of patients recruited, and the type of ACE inhibitor studied.

Although each analytical approach provides important information for the 'frontline' clinician, it should be remembered that, owing to the intrinsic heterogeneity of these investigations, any one perspective or trial in isolation is an inadequate means of understanding the whole picture. Here we consider a number of key methodological issues, which are relevant to all eight trials both in isolation and when combined. In particular, we hope to draw attention to the concept that large patient numbers, while reducing random errors, may unmask systematic biases. Consequently, increasing size should not automatically be equated to greater reliability when considering the results of the individual trials in this series. By critical appraisal we aim to help the practicing clinician appreciate the strengths and weaknesses of the various trials, with the emphasis on appropriate patient care, while encouraging a rigorous approach to the design, conduct, and interpretation of future trials.

Trial Protocols and Primary Reports

The findings of each of the trials discussed in this chapter have now been published,[2-8] although with varying levels of completeness.[9] Furthermore, the protocols and design considerations on which some of these investigations were based have also been reported

Table 15.1 Summary of the design and findings of major mortality trials with ACE inhibitors after acute myocardial infarction

	AIRE[8,13,14]	TRACE[6,16]	SAVE[4,12]	SMILE[7,15]	CONSENSUS-II[5]	ISIS-4[2,11]	GISSI-3[3,10]	CCS-1[9]
Sample size	2006	1749	2231	1556	6090	58 050	19 394	13 634
Inclusion criteria	LVF	WMI < 1.2	EF < 40%	Anterior >6 h, no lysis	'All'	'All'	'All'	'All'
ACE inhibitor	Ramipril	Trandolapril	Captopril	Zofenopril	Enalapril	Captopril	Lisinopril	Captopril
Start day (hours from symptom onset)	2–9 (>24 h)	2–6 (>24 h)	2–15 (>24 h)	0 (<24 h)	0 (<24 h)	0 (<24 h)	0 (<24 h)	0–1 (<36 h)
Consent	Yes	Yes	Yes	Yes	Yes	No[a]	No[a]	?
Confirmed MI	Yes	Yes	Yes	No[a]	No[a]	No[a]	No[a]	No[a]
Placebo	Yes	Yes	Yes	Yes	No[a]	Yes	No[a]	Yes
Double-blind	Yes	Yes	Yes	Yes	Yes	Yes	No[a]	?
Duration	15 months	24 months	42 months	42 days (12 months)[b]	6 months	35 days	42 days	28 days
RRR (%)	11	9	3	Negative	Negative	<1	<1	Negative
95% CL[c]				(6)[b]				
No. patients lost to analysis	1	0	6	0	0	1742	499	?
Sensitivity analysis	Yes	–	Yes	–	–	No	No	?

CL, confidence limit; EF, ejection fraction; LVF, left ventricular failure; MI, myocardial infarction; RRR, relative risk reduction; WMI, wall motion index.
[a] Indicates no stated protocol requirement for prospective consent.
[b] The SMILE study primary endpoint was 42 days, although data are shown for a secondary analysis performed at 1 year.
[c] The lower 95% confidence limit provides the best summary statistic, reflecting both the magnitude and robustness of the result.

prior to the end of the study.[10-16] This permits an appraisal of the statistical analyses utilized in the primary report. Were these planned and stated prospectively or did they evolve during the course of the trial? When addressing this question to the published literature, it becomes apparent that two prominent trials in this area changed their primary statistical endpoints between publishing their protocols and results. The GISSI-3 trialists made the decision to drop 6-month all-cause mortality from their primary analysis.[3,10] Also, the ISIS-4 investigators opted to change from an intended primary analysis of vascular deaths, as stated in the opening sentence of their published protocol,[11] to a primary analysis of all-cause mortality.[2] However, the reasons for and the consequences of such changes in the most central aspect of each trial's design were either not mentioned[3] or inadequately dealt with[2] in the primary publications.

Secondary Analyses and Reports

Many additional reports, based almost entirely on retrospective 'exploratory analyses' have also been published.[17] Often it is stated that both the statistical endpoint measured and the details of the analyses were determined prospectively, i.e. prior to any knowledge of the trial results. Indeed, this can be readily supported by publishing a long list of all possible secondary analyses prior to the close of the trial. However, unless rigorously controlled (e.g. by techniques for adjusting P values each time an additional statistical test is performed), such data are well recognized to have the potential to seriously mislead.[18]

Practical Objectives in Clinical Trial Design

Although often employing high technology and based on established sciences, the actual practice of medicine is often not amenable to detailed scientific investigation using strict methodologies. Most clinicians will agree that to care for an individual patient involves complex judgments that are difficult to make without sufficient personal experience. Years of predominantly theoretical education culminate in an apprenticeship on the wards where diagnostic and therapeutic skills are developed. However, ultimately, the competent practice of medicine requires both theoretical knowledge and practical experience. A good clinical trial or series of trials should supply new knowledge in a form that can be readily understood and applied by individual doctors to individual patients.

In order to establish that an observed relationship between a therapeutic intervention and a subsequent effect on mortality is one of cause and effect, certain methodological criteria should, ideally, be applied (*Table 15.2*). However, in clinical practice these methodologies can be restrictive to the extent that relevant questions cannot be answered easily. Consequently, there has been a move towards more pragmatic trial design.[19] Ultimately this approach has led to a compromise of many conventional methodological criteria, with the exception of the absolute need for randomization and a definitive endpoint such as all-cause mortality. However, the extent to which conventional trial methodologies can or should be dispensed with remains a matter of current concern.[20,21]

The Pragmatic Trial

The randomized controlled trial (RCT) represents a singular tool for clinical research and for the evaluation of new clinical treatment strategies. At the core of this methodological

Table 15.2   Standard methodological/scientific criteria for a survival study

- The patient population under investigation should be readily identifiable (achieved by applying defined inclusion and exclusion criteria)
- Patients taking part in the investigation should be aware of any possible risks or benefits (achieved by obtaining informed consent)
- The effect of the intervention in one group of patients should be compared to a reference or control group of patients who did not receive the intervention (achieved by parallel-group design)
- The two groups should be matched in all respects apart from the intervention under investigation (achieved by randomization)
- The possibility of introducing bias or confounding effects during the course of the trial should be avoided (achieved by double-blinding and placebo control)
- The possibility of introducing bias or confounding effects when analyzing the effect of the intervention on outcome should be avoided (achieved by analyzing a prestated primary endpoint of all-cause mortality at a prestated time using the intention-to-treat methodology)
- When the survival status of some patients is not known, a sensitivity analysis should be performed to assess the robustness of the observed outcome

approach is the philosophy that *a fact can only be considered to be true if it cannot be proven to be false*. Consequently, RCTs aim to disprove the null hypothesis, which states that a treatment strategy is ineffectual. However, the medical literature is full of trials that claim to have disproven the null hypothesis based on a quoted low P value (conventionally $P <$ 0.05). Because such a finding may still occur purely as a result of chance, particularly when multiple analysis are performed, trials should specify a single endpoint (e.g. death from all causes up to a prestated time point) to be evaluated in a primary intention-to-treat statistical analysis.

A pragmatic trial assesses the effect of an entire treatment strategy rather than the direct effect of the treatment itself. Consequently, the GISSI-3 trial was designed to assess the effect on survival of the ACE inhibitor lisinopril when given rapidly (<24 hours) after the onset of symptoms of suspected acute myocardial infarction and continued for 42 days. This approach was compared with a second treatment strategy in which the use of all ACE inhibitors was avoided unless overt signs of congestive heart failure developed. A total of 19 394 patients was randomly allocated to one or other strategy and then followed-up in order to assess survival status at 42 and 180 days. At the first time point there was a small reduction in the mortality observed for patients randomized to the lisinopril strategy ($P =$ 0.03), but when the effects of the overall strategy were assessed (at 180 days) the null hypothesis could not be disproved.[22] Furthermore, the initial analysis compared lisinopril alone, nitrates alone, and the two combined against patients randomized to receive neither. The lack of any correction to the P value for such multiple comparisons deserves critical comment, as this would have raised the initial (42 day) P value above the level of conventional significance.

The Mega-trial

In order to reduce the possibility of a random error occurring in the GISSI-3 study, approximately 20 000 patients were recruited. Combined with the randomization procedure, this ensured that each group of patients was comparable in all respects other than the treatment strategy being tested. However, such equity is likely to have been short lived owing to the complete absence of treatment blinding. Consequently, both the patients and their physicians may have been influenced by knowledge of treatment allocation, this possibly resulting in a systematic error or bias.[23] Major differences in adjunctive drug therapy, for example, is a potent mechanism for introducing error (the relevant data were not published by the GISSI investigators). Most importantly, such a bias, even if small, would be unmasked by the large number of patients entered into the trial. By analogy, the even outcome of tossing a coin (heads versus tails) would be emphasized by repetition only if the coin were balanced. A very slight bias towards tails, although not apparent after a small number of tosses, would become manifest by repetition. Similarly, while minimizing random errors, mega-trials accentuate any systematic errors, such as those resulting from lack of treatment blinding.

Trials in Context

The GISSI-3 trial assumes a slightly different significance in the light of other similarly designed trials. The CONSENSUS-II trial randomized patients with suspected AMI to receive intravenous enalapril or placebo within the first 24 hours of onset of symptoms.[5] When the trial was stopped prematurely owing to concerns regarding safety,[24] a nonsignificant trend towards harm was observed. This was provisionally reported by the CONSENSUS-II investigators prior to the initiation of the GISSI-3 trial.[25] Such knowledge will necessarily have influenced the GISSI-3 trial, which cannot therefore be considered to be entirely independent of CONSENSUS-II. Nevertheless, in conjunction with the long-term results of GISSI-3, the negative findings of the CONSENSUS-II trial do not lend support to the rapid, nonselective use of ACE-inhibitor drugs in patients with suspected acute myocardial infarction.

The ISIS-4 trial recruited 58 050 patients into a placebo-controlled study of captopril therapy, administered within the first 24 hours, continued for 28 days and then withdrawn.[2] ACE inhibitor therapy was subsequently permitted in both groups of patients if considered necessary based on clinical examination or diagnostic investigation. In contrast with GISSI-3, the ISIS-4 trial was conducted double-blind, thereby reducing one possible source of systematic error. However, a second potential source of error was clearly apparent; the 35-day survival status of 1742 of the patients recruited into the study was not known. Given that the mortality rates first reported for this study in 1993 (captopril 6.87%, placebo 7.33%)[26] were approximately 0.3% lower than those finally reported in 1995 (captopril 7.19%, placebo 7.69%),[2] it would appear that delayed reporting of survival status was more commonly associated with the occurrence of death.

From this one might surmise that a major reason for patients being missing from the final analysis is that they had died. The relative proportions of patients missing from the placebo and captopril groups at time of hospital discharge (placebo 1.6%, captopril 1.8%) further suggest the possibility of a systematic bias that may have influenced the study outcome. Certainly, the application of a strict sensitivity analysis (in which all missing patients randomized to captopril are assumed to be dead and all missing patients randomized to placebo are assumed to be alive) would have erased any suggestion of benefit from active therapy, as would adjustment of P values to allow for the multiple comparisons of a $2 \times 2 \times 2$ factorial design. The fact that no such analyses were reported is unfortunate, as these would have left clinicians in no doubt as to the ineffectiveness of the early/nonselective treatment strategy. Furthermore, the fact that the marginal treatment benefit initially observed was no longer statistically significant at 1 year should have been emphasized, and ought not to be excused by the fact that still more patients (18 576) were lost to the intention-to-treat analysis.[2]

The Chinese Captopril Study[9] provided an 'interim' report on the effect of captopril therapy in 13 634 patients for whom follow-up data were available. There is no statement in the paper regarding the number of patients lost to follow-up, nor is it clear whether the investigation was double-blind or whether patient consent was obtained prospectively. Other aspects of the trial's design and its investigators' intent remain similarly obscure. However, to date the trial shows early, nonselective administration of captopril to be ineffective ($2P = 0.3$). Given that the prestated objective of the trial was to recruit 10 000 patients, one must wonder at what stage this trial will be considered to be complete and whether an appropriately detailed publication (with suitably adjusted P values) will follow.

Meta-analysis of the Mega-trials

By definition, a mega-trial is a trial designed to be large enough to be definitive. On the other hand, a meta-analysis is usually used to combine the results of trials that on their own are less than definitive. Consequently, the notion that the primary outcome of the mega-trials of early nonselective ACE inhibition after acute myocardial infarction should require meta-analysis in order to assume any practical relevance is a major indicator of the treatment strategy's scientific destitution.

Independently, the negative long-term findings of the CONSENSUS-II, GISSI-3, Chinese Captopril and ISIS-4[2,3,5,9] trials do little to disprove the null hypothesis concerning early nonselective use of ACE inhibitors after acute myocardial infarction. However, a meta-analysis of the short-term results of these trials[2] suggests a marginal, but statistically significant ($P = 0.006$), benefit from this treatment strategy (4.6 lives saved per 1000 patients treated; SD 1.7). Importantly, such an analysis will have compounded systematic errors present within the individual trials, yet assumes spurious authority from the combined large number of patients. Consequently, it is to be hoped that the superficial message from such data is not being transposed into directive clinical guidelines. Furthermore, the summary statistic derived from a meta-analysis of the short-term outcome of the mega-trials fails to alert the physician to the high rate of associated adverse effects, nor does it inform him or her of the absence of long-term benefit.

Balancing Risks and Benefits

The adverse events reported by each of the mega-trials are consistent, although they have not yet featured in any published meta-analysis. The ISIS-4 investigators[2] report a major excess of the following in-hospital adverse events: profound hypotension (99 extra events per 1000 patients given captopril; $2P < 0.0001$), confirmation of infarction (5 extra events per 1000 patients given captopril; $2P < 0.01$), cardiogenic shock (5 extra events per 1000 patients given captopril; $2P < 0.01$), and renal dysfunction (5 extra events per 1000 patients given captopril; $2P < 0.0001$). Importantly, the adverse event rates up to the 35-day primary endpoint of the trial are not reported, but, it would appear that the marginal mortality benefit of five fewer deaths observed at this time is only part of the complete picture.

'Creating' a Consensus

A meeting of 'all' the key investigators of ACE inhibitor use after acute myocardial infarction took place at the European Congress in Berlin in 1994, being announced in a letter to *The Lancet*.[27] Subsequently, a paper was drafted to summarize 'expert opinion' in this area, and this was published in *Circulation* in 1995.[25] To this paper was appended an acknowledgement, although not a clarification, of some dissent concerning the presentation and interpretation of secondary analyses from the GISSI-3 and ISIS-4 trials. Importantly the first histogram (day 0 and 1) depicted in figure 2 of this publication[25] relates to deaths occurring up to 48 hours after randomization, without giving the profile for benefit or harm within the first 24 hours after acute myocardial infarction. Much is made of the consistency of findings between GISSI-3 and ISIS-4 in the first 48 hours, but not the lack of consistency in the subsequent week and beyond between the trials. Furthermore, the reasons for selecting both this and the other time periods, while neglecting the excess of deaths that occurred in GISSI-3 between days 42 and 180, is not stated.

In our view, the contents of this important 'expert statement' had a clear bias, which was apparent also in the erroneous suggestion that the early nonselective strategy produced a greater survival benefit over the first month of treatment than was observed in the more selective trials (see table 2 in Ref. 25). Such analyses are in stark contrast to the intended authoritative nature of this 'expert' statement, the stature of which is consequently diminished.

Patient Selection – an Alternative Approach

Four trials prospectively selected patients in whom the benefits from ACE inhibition might be maximized and any unwanted adverse effects minimized.[28] The results of these investigations have been published and debated fully.[4,6,7,8] They remain without serious criticism of methods or findings. This probably results from the fact that similar trials performed in patients with chronic congestive cardiac failure provide important supportive data.[29,30] Sensible interpretation of the early nonselective trials relies heavily on the results of selective studies such as SAVE, AIRE, SMILE, and TRACE. Consequently, criticisms may have been, understandably, restrained. Perhaps the best evaluation of the potential weaknesses of the selective studies comes from the investigators themselves.

The SAVE investigators studied patients selected on the basis of a low ejection fraction, although later they commented that the benefit seen with captopril would probably have been greater had they also included patients with overt left ventricular dysfunction.[31] Such patients were included in the AIRE study, while those without overt left ventricular dysfunction would have been excluded. Consequently, SAVE and AIRE are complementary, but not independently comprehensive, studies.

Further examples of restrictive entry criteria can be found with the TRACE and SMILE studies. The TRACE trialists reported excluding many high-risk subjects, despite vigorous attempts to include them in the study.[6] Among these were some patients with overt heart failure with a measured wall motion index of >1.2 and a few excluded owing to problems with obtaining a suitable echocardiographic image. TRACE undoubtedly also excluded some patients with clinical heart failure of a severity which would have excluded them from AIRE. The SMILE study selected only patients with anterior acute myocardial infarction who were not eligible for thrombolysis owing to late presentation (>6 hours from onset of symptoms to admission), thereby excluding many other important categories of patient.[7]

Finally, and with particular relevance to the discussion of the issue of patient selection, is the fact that large numbers of patients will also have been excluded from the mega-trials. Although patients were largely 'unselected' according to the trial protocols, physician discretion was encouraged and will certainly have been exercised. The findings of other completed trials such as CONSENSUS-II as well as the perceived needs for other treatments factored into the design (e.g. nitrates) must have influenced clinicians, causing them to exclude many types of patient. Consequently, it is likely that the eventual study populations are a poor representation of the population of unselected patients with suspected myocardial infarction that clinicians face daily. In-hospital mortality after myocardial infarction in 'all patients' is three times the 35-day mortality reported in ISIS-4. Once again, large numbers will have exaggerated rather than diminished any selection bias.

No Meta-analysis Required for the Micro-trials

The SAVE, AIRE, TRACE, and SMILE studies were each double-blind, placebo-controlled studies. In two cases the primary publication reported the outcome of a sensitivity analysis performed to assess the effect of covert deaths occurring in any patients in whom survival status was not known at the end of the study.[4,8] In the other two trials no such analysis was required owing to complete follow-up data.[6,7] Consequently, this potential source of systematic bias, which was discussed previously in relation to mega-trials, was not present. Each trial reported a major reduction in the long-term relative risk of all-cause mortality, although in the case of the SMILE trial this occurred only at a *post hoc* secondary endpoint time of 1 year. Consequently, this result should be interpreted with caution.

In each case the null hypothesis was convincingly rejected, with treatment benefit of the order of 40 lives saved per 1000 patients treated for 1 year.[32] Each study demonstrated an increasing benefit with time, although AIRE, TRACE, and SMILE, but not SAVE, observed benefit within the first month. No meta-analysis of the primary endpoint of these trials has yet been performed, and clearly one is not needed owing to the conclusive nature of the independent data. However, analysis of the effect of treatment in subgroups enlarged by combination may provide further guidance to clinicians caring for patients with specific subgroup characteristics, such as a prior history of diabetes or hypertension.

Concluding Remarks

The key lesson for trial design which may be drawn from the studies reviewed here is that big is not always better. While random errors associated with confounding baseline differences can be minimized by using the large/pragmatic approach, systematic errors such as those associated with lack of blinding and incomplete patient follow-up, may be revealed. Ultimately, there must be a point at which a trial is pragmatic to a fault. Obtaining a suitable balance between pragmatism (short-term practical expediency) and conventional scientific principles must be a very major priority for future clinical trials.

The critical appraisal of the methodologies utilized by trials of ACE inhibitors after acute myocardial infarction reveals a number of other salutary scientific points. However, whether an understanding of such issues will enhance or diminish the appropriate use of this highly beneficial mode of therapy is a necessary cause for concern. Busy clinicians seek authoritative and unambiguous guidance from clinical trials and their investigators. We have not sought to provide such advice up to this point, though would like to do so here.

Perhaps the strongest clinical argument in favor of applying clinical judgment when targeting ACE-inhibitor therapy is the fact that, because individual patients are different, so also are the potential risks and benefits that they may accrue.[33] In our opinion, ACE inhibitor therapy should be strongly considered in all patients who have confirmed evidence of acute myocardial infarction in association with: (a) clinical evidence of heart failure, and/or (b) a reduced left ventricular ejection fraction, and/or (c) a left ventricular wall motion index of less than 1.2, and/or (d) anterior location plus a contraindication to thrombolysis. Furthermore, given the overall logic of these indications, other surrogates of ventricular damage (e.g. electrocardiographic or enzyme criteria) might also be usefully considered. However, for all patients selected, we would advise indefinite continuation of appropriately dosed maintenance therapy, and that due caution (taking particular account of on-going ischemic and hemodynamic compromise) be exercised if opting to initiate treatment within the first 24 hours after the onset of symptoms.

References

1. Pfeffer MA, Lamas GA, Vaughan DE, Parisi AF, Braunwald E. Effect of captopril on progressive dilatation after anterior myocardial infarction. *N Engl J Med* 1988; **319**: 80–6.
2. ISIS-4 Collaborative Group. Fourth International Study of Infarct Survival: a randomised factorial trial assessing early oral captopril, oral mononitrate, and intravenous magnesium sulphate in 58 050 patients with suspected acute myocardial infarction. *Lancet* 1995; **345**: 669–85.
3. Gruppo Italiano per lo Studio della Suprawivenza nell'Infarto Miocardico. GISSI-3: effects of lisinopril and transdermal glyceryl trinitrate singly and together on 6 week mortality and ventricular function after acute myocardial infarction. *Lancet* 1994; **343**: 1115–22.
4. Pfeffer MA, Braunwald E, Moye LA, *et al.*, on behalf of the SAVE Investigators. Effect of captopril on mortality and morbidity in patients with left ventricular dysfunction after myocardial infarction. *N Engl J Med* 1992; **327**: 669–77.
5. Swedberg K, Held P, Kjekshus J, *et al.* Effects of early administration of enalapril on mortality in patients with acute myocardial infarction: results of the Cooperative New Scandanavian Enalapril Survival Study II (CONSENSUS II). *N Engl J Med* 1992; **327**: 678–84.
6. Kober L, Torp-Pedersen C, Carlsen JE, *et al.*, for the TRAndolapril Cardiac Evaluation (TRACE) Study Group. A clinical trial of the angiotensin-converting enzyme inhibitor trandolapril in patients with left ventricular dysfunction after myocardial infarction. *N Engl J Med* 1995; **333**: 1670–6.
7. Ambrosioni E, Borghi C, Magnani, for the Survival of Myocardial Infarction Long-term Evaluation (SMILE) Study Investigators. The effect of the angiotensin converting-enzyme inhibitor zofenopril on mortality and morbidity after anterior myocardial infarction. *N Engl J Med* 1995; **332**: 80–5.
8. The AIRE Study Investigators. Effect of ramipril on mortality and morbidity of survivors of acute myocardial infarction with clinical evidence of heart failure. *Lancet* 1993; **342**: 821–8.
9. Chinese Cardiac Study Collaborative Group. Oral captopril versus placebo among 13 634 patients with suspected acute myocardial infarction: interim report from the Chinese Cardiac Study (CCS-1). *Lancet* 1995; **345**: 686–7.
10. GISSI-3 Gruppo Italiano per lo Studio della Sopravvivenza nell'Infarto Miocardico. GISSI-3 study protocol on the effects of lisinopril, of nitrates, and of their association in patients with acute myocardial infarction. *Am J Cardiol* 1992; **70**: 62C–9C.
11. ISIS-4 Collaborative Group. Fourth international Study of Infarct Survival: Protocol for a large simple study of the effects of oral mononitrate, of oral captopril, and of intravenous magnesium. *Am J Cardiol* 1991; **68**: 87D–100D.
12. Moye LA, Pfeffer MA. Rationale, design and baseline characteristics of the survival and left ventricular enlargement trial. *Am J Cardiol* 1991; **68**: 70D–9D.
13. Hall AS, Winter C, Bogle SM, Mackintosh AF, Murray GD, Ball SG. The Acute Infarction Ramipril Efficacy (AIRE) Study: rationale, design, organization and outcome definitions. *J Cardiovasc Pharmacol* 1991; **18**(Suppl 2): S105–9.
14. Cleland JGF, Erhardt L, Hall AS, Winter C, Ball SG. Validation of primary and secondary outcomes and classification of mode of death among patients with clinical evidence of heart failure after myocardial infarction. A report from the AIRE Study investigators. *J Cardiovasc Pharmacol* 1993; **22**(Suppl 10): S22–7.
15. Ambrosioni E, Borghi C, Magnani B, on behalf of the SMILE Study Investigators. Survival of myocardial infarction long-term evaluation (SMILE) study: rationale, design, organization and outcome definitions. *Controlled Clin Trials* 1994; **15**: 201–10.
16. The TRACE Study Group. The TRAndolopril Cardiac Evaluation (TRACE) Study: rationale, design and baseline characteristics of the screened population. *Am J Cardiol* 1994, **73**: 44C–50C.
17. Gangley CJ, Hung HMJ, Temple R. More on the survival and ventricular enlargement trial. *N Engl J Med* 1993; **329**: 1204–6.
18. Mills JL. Data torturing. *New Engl J Med* 1993; **329**: 1196–9.
19. Yusuf S, Collins R, Peto R. Why do we need some large, simple randomized trials? *Stat Med* 1994; **3**: 409–20.
20. Lubsen J, Tijssen JGP. Large trials with simple protocols: indications and contraindications. *Controlled Clin Trials* 1989; **10**: 151S–60S.
21. Hall AS. The context of consent. *Lancet* 1994; **344**: 618.
22. GISSI-3 Investigators. Presentation at the World Congress of Cardiology, Berlin, 1994.

23. Schultz KF, Chalmers I, Hayes RJ, Altman DG. Empirical evidence of bias – dimensions of methodological quality associated with estimates of treatment effect in controlled trials. *JAMA* 1995; **273**(5): 408–12.

24. Furberg CD, Campbell RWF, Pitt B. ACE inhibitors after myocardial infarction. *N Engl J Med* 1993; **328**: 967–68.

25. Latini R, Maggioni AP, Flather M, Sleight P, Tognoni G. ACE Inhibitors use in patients with myocardial infarction. Summary of evidence from clinical trials. *Circulation* 1995; **92**: 3132–7.

26. ISIS Collaborative Group, Oxford UK. ISIS-4: randomised study of oral isosorbide mononitrate in over 50,000 patients with suspected acute myocardial infarction. *Circulation* 1993; **88**: I–394.

27. Tognoni G. Role of angiotensin-converting enzyme inhibitors in myocardial infarction. *Lancet* 1994; **344**(8924): 758 (letter; comment).

28. Hall AS, Tan LB, Ball SG. Inhibition of ACE/kininase-II, acute myocardial infarction, and survival. *Cardiovasc Res* 1994; **28**: 190–8.

29. The CONSENSUS Trial Study Group. Effects of enalapril on mortality in severe congestive heart failure. Results of the Cooperative North Scandanavian Enalapril Survival Study (CONSENSUS). *N Engl J Med* 1987; **316**: 1429–35.

30. The SOLVD Investigators. Effect of enalapril on survival in patients with reduced left ventricular ejection fractions and congestive heart failure. *N Engl J Med* 1991; **325**: 293–302.

31. Rouleau JL, Packer M, Moye L, *et al.* Prognostic value of neurohumoral activation in patients with an acute myocardial infarction: effect of captopril. *J Am Coll Cardiol* 1994; **24**(3): 583–91.

32. Hall AS, Ball SG. ACE-inhibitor therapy after myocardial infarction – a new treatment strategy. *Z Kardiol* 1994; **83**(4): 57–62.

33. CAST Investigators. Preliminary report: effect of ecainide and flecainide on mortality in a randomized trial of arrhythmia suppression after myocardial infarction. *N Engl J Med* 1989; **321**: 406–12.

16

Beta-blockers, Calcium Blockers, Nitrates, and Magnesium in and after Myocardial Infarction

Steven Borzak and Sidney Goldstein

Introduction

Be prepared for the advice of today to be discarded or derided dogma of tomorrow. Remember that every treatment is really an experiment, so try to make it valuable for the future by recording it and, preferably, by making it part of a properly documented clinical trial so that my successor in the 1990's can offer some real advice.[1]

In the middle of the twentieth century, the realization that acute myocardial infarction represented a major clinical issue facing physicians led to a variety of treatments directed at the modification of its morbidity and mortality. They included hormones,[2] lipid-lowering,[2] antiplatelet,[3] and antiarrhythmic agents,[4,5] to name but a few. The results of these studies, with the exception of those exploring the use of aspirin, were 'underwhelming'. In spite of this lack of success, clinical trials provided major advances in our understanding of coronary heart disease and its natural history. The randomized clinical trial (RCT) has been used to its greatest extent in the solution of the issue of the postinfarction patient. An RCT, by its nature, is built on the premise that an obvious proof of benefit is not at hand. Its outcome is, by necessity, uncertain. It is, therefore, not surprising that treatment failures have emerged, the most noteworthy being in the Cardiac Arrhythmia Suppression Trial.[5]

RCTs have usually been initiated after pilot or laboratory studies have suggested that a theoretic basis exists upon which it is reasonable to test the benefit of an intervention. In some instances, pilot studies have strongly indicated that a particular therapy could be beneficial, as in the case of the use of nitrates and beta-adrenergic blocking agents after acute myocardial infarction. Even so, widespread skepticism existed in regard to their potential benefit. In some RCTs, pilot studies were few and the outcome failed to demonstrate a benefit, as in the case of calcium entry blockers. Still other issues have not been totally resolved by large RCTs, such as the use of high-dose magnesium or nitroglycerin for infarction patients.

Other issues still remain regarding the timing of administration and dose of these various drugs. Proof of benefit has also become more complex as we measure the drug

271

efficacy in diseases with low event rates. Perhaps a paradox of evaluating treatment in an age of effective therapies is that in disease states like myocardial infarction, still a very prevalent problem, issues of morbidity and mortality are of great clinical and public health importance, yet morbid events occur with relative low frequency. RCTs may, therefore, not achieve statistical significance owing to small sample size. Such was the case in the use of beta-blockers in acute myocardial infarction in the Metoprolol in Acute Myocardial Infarction (MIAMI) trial,[6] which examined early metoprolol therapy in approximately 5000 patients. The 13% decrease in mortality did not reach significance. Its beneficial effect was demonstrated when a larger sample of 16 000 patients tested the use of atenolol in the First International Study of Infarct Survival (ISIS-1)[7] and showed decreased mortality by 15% ($P < 0.001$). In this chapter we will describe these trials, highlighting their important features, and offer an interpretation in order for the results to be useful for the clinician.

Beta-adrenergic Blocking Agents

In 1945, Ahlquist[8] demonstrated the presence of beta-adrenergic receptors in the cardio-vascular system. Some years later, Black and Stephenson[9] described the effect of pharmacologic agents which were able to block these receptors, and proposed that this class of drugs could have an important role in the treatment of angina pectoris and hypertension. This led to a number of small clinical trials to test their effect in patients following acute myocardial infarction. These studies provided the foundation upon which two large RCTs were initiated, the Norwegian Timolol Trial (NTT)[10] and the Beta Blocker Heart Attack Trial (BHAT),[11] which separately examined the effect of timolol and propranolol in patients following an acute myocardial infarction (*Figures 16.1* and *16.2* and *Table 16.1*). These two contemporaneous RCTs were initiated and carried out within a 3-year period between 1978 and 1980 using a standard multicenter, double-blind, randomized study format with the intervention tested using the intention-to-treat methodology. NTT randomized 1884 patients and BHAT randomized 3837 patients. The

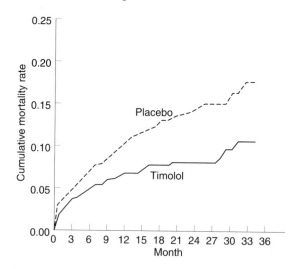

Figure 16.1 Mortality reduction due to timolol in the Norwegian timolol study. (Reproduced with permission from Ref. 10.)

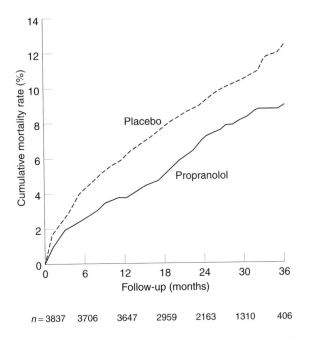

n = 3837   3706   3647   2959   2163   1310   406

Figure 16.2 Mortality reduction due to propranolol in the BHAT study. (Reproduced with permission from Ref. 11.)

patients in NTT were somewhat older, including patients up to the age of 75 years compared to maximum age of 69 years in BHAT. The patients were randomized after 5 days and as late as 21 days in NTT and 27 days in BHAT. The inclusion and exclusion criteria were similar in both studies. Confirmation of acute myocardial infarction depended upon the development of pathologic Q-waves or ST- and T-wave elevation followed by T-wave inversion, associated with either an elevation of the serum aspartate aminotransferase or lactate dehydrogenase in NTT and serum glutamic oxaloacetic transaminase in BHAT. As at that time the enzyme criteria for diagnosis of myocardial infarction were insensitive compared to current standards, patients randomized in these trials had relatively large myocardial infarctions and, therefore, are vastly different from patients diagnosed with acute myocardial infarction today using more sensitive laboratory measurements. Patients in NTT were followed for a minimum of 12 months and a

Table 16.1 Selected results of long-term beta-blocker trials for secondary prevention after acute myocardial infarction

Trial	No. of patients	Beta-blocker	Entry time from MI (days)	Mean follow-up (months)	Mortality (%) Drug	Mortality (%) Placebo	Reinfarction (%) Drug	Reinfarction (%) Placebo
NTT[10]	1884	Timolol	11.5	17	10.4	16.2[a]	10	14[a]
BHAT[11]	3738	Propranolol	13.8	25	7.2	9.8[a]	4	5[a]
APSI[22]	607	Acebutolol	2–22	10	5.7	11.0[a]	2	1.3

MI, Myocardial infarction.
[a]Statistically significant difference.

maximum of 36 months. BHAT had a similar period of follow-up of approximately 25 months.

Recruitment in both trials was difficult, owing to problems in identifying patients with acute myocardial infarction and to exclusion of individuals who might have contra-indications to beta-blockers. Of the 158 000 patients screened for the BHAT, 68% had myocardial infarction that met BHAT entry criteria.[12] Of these, 16 400 patients met the criteria, were age eligible, survived 5 days, and had no contraindications. The major exclusion criteria were the judgement that a contraindication to beta-blocker therapy existed; other patients were likely to receive a beta-blocker because of significant angina pectoris or they were unwilling to participate in the study. Of the 16 400 eligible patients, 23% were ultimately randomized. Similarly, in the NTT, 11 125 patients initially screened resulted in 1184 patients randomized. It is, therefore, clear that only a small percentage of patients screened were entered into the study. Whether or not they represented a typical or a unique population of myocardial infarction patients is uncertain, since there was no active follow-up of those patients who met the entry criteria but who were not randomized. Subsequent clinical trials, like the Coronary Artery Surgical Study (CASS),[13] did carry out this type of analysis and provided important information comparing the randomized patients to those who were excluded.

The treatment regimens were different in the two studies. Patients in NTT were given a fixed dose of timolol, starting with 5 mg twice daily initially for 2 days, increasing to 10 mg twice daily. BHAT used a dosage-adjustment methodology based on serum propranolol level. After an initial test of 20 mg of propranolol followed by six consecutive doses of 40 mg propranolol every 8 hours, a propranolol blood level was obtained. In those patients with a propranolol level <20 ng ml^{-1}, propranolol was increased to 80 mg three times daily and those with a blood level over 20 ng ml^{-1} were assigned to 60 mg three times daily. Of the 3837 enrolled, 82% were assigned to 180 mg, and 18% to a 240 mg daily dose.

The placebo mortality rates in the BHAT and NTT trials were 16.2% and 19.8%, respectively, probably reflecting a 5-year increased age range in NTT patients. The average age of the placebo population was 54.8 years in BHAT and 60.8 years in NTT. In NTT, a total mortality reduction of 39.4% was observed, compared to a 26% decrease in BHAT. A significant decrease in sudden death of 44.6% was observed in NTT using a criterion of death within 24 hours of the onset of symptoms. In BHAT, using a definition of death within 1 hour of onset of symptoms, sudden death was decreased by 28%. BHAT was terminated approximately 6 months prior to its planned ending, owing to a statistically significant benefit demonstrated in the propranolol-treated patients. The positive results of NTT also probably influenced the early termination of the trial.

In addition to the overall mortality, one of the objectives of NTT was to examine whether or not timolol had an effect on reinfarction or other cardiac events. Timolol demonstrated a statistically significant decrease of 28.4% in reinfarction. In BHAT, a secondary goal was to test the effect of propranolol on the occurrence of coronary heart disease mortality and nonfatal myocardial infarction.[14] Coronary heart disease mortality decreased by 27%, from 8.5% to 6.2%. Coronary incidence, defined as recurrent nonfatal reinfarction plus fatal myocardial infarction, was reduced by 23%. Although there was a decrease in definite nonfatal myocardial infarction by 15.6%, this did not reach statistical significance.

A question has been raised regarding the benefit of beta-blockers in patients with non-Q-wave myocardial infarction. Most of the patients included in the BHAT study, by nature of the enzyme requirements and clinical setting, had suffered a transmural myocardial infarction. A subgroup analysis of 601 patients in BHAT was carried out examining the benefit of propranolol in non-Q-wave acute myocardial infarction. These patients met the relatively insensitive enzyme criteria of that period and represented 17% of the BHAT population.[15] Propranolol had no effect on mortality or reinfarction rate. In the NTT study, however, there was a 46% reduction in mortality in non-Q-wave acute myocardial infarction, although the identification of this subset in NTT was less rigorous than that carried out in BHAT.

Subsequent analysis of both NTT and BHAT examined a variety of subgroups, including the duration of therapy,[16] the effect of the drugs on patients with ventricular ectopy,[17] and congestive heart failure.[18] In addition, BHAT was also examined in regard to the effect of propranolol on lipid metabolism and mortality in patients with abnormal blood lipid levels.[19] Although propranolol-treated patients had a slight decrease in HDL cholesterol and an increase in triglycerides, patients with elevated lipids experienced the same benefit as those with normal lipid levels. Adverse effects during the trial were examined extensively with regard to patients' complaints. In general, propranolol was well tolerated, although a statistically significant increase existed for withdrawal in patients owing to hypotension, reduced sexual activity, and minor gastrointestinal problems. In contrast, placebo was withdrawn more often due to the presence of serious ventricular arrhythmias. Interpretation of the side-effects of beta-blockers is clouded by frequent occurrence of a variety of physical and emotional events following an acute myocardial infarction. In NTT, patients took 90% of the prescribed dosage. In BHAT, a similar low percentage of patients were withdrawn from therapy in the propranolol-treated patients. At the last visit, 76% of the patients were taking the prescribed drug; 57% were taking a full protocol dose, and 19% were taking a reduced dose of the drug.

Both propranolol and timolol were nonselective beta-adrenergic blocking agents without any significant sympathomimetic activity. Studies with two drugs, pindolol[20] and oxprenolol,[21] both of which expressed increased sympathomimetic activity, raised questions about beta-blockers with these physiologic effects, since they failed to show benefit in RCTs. However, the Acebutolol et Prevention Secondaire de l'Infarctus (APSI) trial,[22] was a double-blind, placebo-controlled trial designed to evaluate acebutolol, a beta-blocker with intrinsic sympathomimetic activity, in high-risk patients with myocardial infarction (see *Table 16.1*). APSI demonstrated that acebutolol, in this population, resulted in a 48% decrease in total mortality. The study was prematurely terminated because the placebo group did not reach the predetermined mortality rate. Therefore, it appears that, at least at present, beta-blockers seem to have a generic benefit in patients who have suffered acute myocardial infarction, despite the fact that only five drugs (propranolol, metoprolol, timolol, atenolol, and acebutolol) have fully shown benefit in RCTs for long-term therapy.

Beta-blockers in the Acute Phase

The effect of beta-blockers in the acute phase of myocardial infarction was examined in three major trials, metoprolol in two, and atenolol in one. The initial study was the Göteborg Metoprolol Trial (GMT),[23] in which 1395 patients were randomized in either metoprolol or placebo. After initial intravenous therapy, patients continued on oral metoprolol or placebo for 3 months. At the end of 3 months, the overall mortality decreased by 35% in metoprolol-treated patients. Following this study, the Metoprolol in Acute Myocardial Infarction (MIAMI) trial[24] was initiated, in which 5778 patients were treated with intravenous metoprolol followed by 100 mg twice daily of oral metoprolol for 15 days. This study resulted in a 13% decrease in mortality, which did not reach significance. A subgroup analysis, however, suggested that metoprolol did have a significant impact on mortality in patients who were at high risk, i.e. those with prior myocardial infarction, congestive heart failure, diabetes, hypertension, angina, or receiving therapy with digoxin. The largest study to examine the effect of early beta-blocker therapy in AMI was ISIS-1,[7] in which 16 027 patients were randomized either to intravenous atenolol or to standard medical therapy. The study was not blinded and placebo control was not part of the design. Patients randomized to atenolol were treated for 7 days and then followed for 1 year, at the end of which time the initial 15% decrease in mortality at 14 days persisted. Although a somewhat impure methodology because of lack of blinding and a placebo control, it involved the largest population studied to date and the determination of the study endpoint (vascular mortality) was probably unbiased. The GMT study demonstrated a decrease in mortality,[23] beginning at approximately 5 days after the event. The patients in the MIAMI[24] and ISIS-1[7] trials expressed a decrease in mortality within 24 hours of initiation of therapy which persisted throughout the remaining follow-up of the study.

Patients enrolled in these studies were those suspected of having suffered an acute myocardial infarction, and, in general, included those patients with chest pain lasting at least 30 minutes, with electrocardiographic signs of acute myocardial infarction within the previous 48 hours. ISIS-1 randomized patients with onset of symptoms within 12 hours and who had not already been receiving a beta-blocker or verapamil. In each study the drug was administered in intravenous form, 5–10 mg of atenolol followed by an oral dose of 100 mg of atenolol in ISIS-1. In the GMT, 15 mg was given in one bolus, and in MIAMI, 5 mg of metoprolol was given every 5 minutes over a 15-minute period followed by oral metoprolol, initially 50 mg and then 100 mg daily.

The applicability of intravenous beta-blocker therapy in the thrombolytic era was examined in the Thrombolysis in Myocardial Infarction IIB (TIMI-IIB) study.[25] This study compared an early catheterization and angioplasty strategy with a conservative noninterventional therapy in patients who received thrombolytic therapy. A subgroup of 1390 patients who were eligible for short-term early beta-blocker therapy were randomly assigned to acute intravenous and then oral metoprolol and compared to a control group in whom the drug was administered orally on day 6. There was a significant decrease in the rate of reinfarction and recurrent ischemia in the intravenous metoprolol group, although there was no significant difference in the overall mortality or 6-week ejection fraction, the primary endpoints.

Impact of the Beta-blocker Trials on Treatment Strategies

Beta-blockers were the first drugs to be demonstrated by RCTs to have a beneficial effect on mortality after myocardial infarction. Initial estimates by investigators suggested that approximately three-quarters of patients with acute myocardial infarction could be acceptable candidates for therapy and did not have contraindications. Despite this, until recently, the use of beta-blockers in the USA was <50%. In a registry of patients kept between 1990 and 1993 receiving thrombolytic therapy, 17% of patients received intravenous beta-blockers and 36% received long-term oral beta-blocker therapy.[26] Use of beta-blockers in North America was in the range 29–38%, in comparison to 46–71% in Scandinavian countries.[27] Differences in drug usage were also observed between internists, family practitioners, cardiologists and even geographical areas of the USA.[28] Not only were beta-blockers used infrequently in patients after myocardial infarction, they were also often used at doses that were inappropriately low. In one international study, only 58% of infarct survivors with no contraindication to beta-blockers received the drug at the time of hospitalization.[29] Of these patients, only 11% received a dose equivalent to 50% of the effective dose used in the RCTs. The remaining patients received an even smaller dose. A variety of reasons were identified for this underprescription of beta-blockers. The presence of diabetes was often the reason stated by clinicians for failure-to-treat, in spite of the fact that a subgroup analysis of beta-blocker trials[30] indicated that diabetic patients actually achieve a relatively greater therapeutic benefit. In addition, there is little evidence to suggest that peripheral vascular disease is made worse by beta-blockers, yet this was an additional reason for failure to treat.[31] The presence of left ventricular dysfunction was also a frequent reason, yet the use of beta-blockers in the BHAT[18] and in other RCTs indicates that those individuals with decreased left ventricular dysfunction achieved, again, a relatively greater mortality benefit in both total mortality and sudden death. Physicians were also reluctant to administer beta-blockers to elderly patients for reasons that are not entirely clear. Again, the trials had shown that elderly patients tended to achieve a greater benefit.[32,33]

The precise mechanism by which beta-blockers expressed their effect is not clear. A simplistic approach suggests that the decrease in mortality can be explained by its modest decrease in blood pressure and pulse rate. It has been suggested that the decrease in mortality is directly related to the relative decrease in resting heart rate in the RCTs (*Figure 16.3*).[34] Other possibilities relate to the drugs' ability to suppress both supraventricular and ventricular arrhythmias. Although these are all possible explanations, there is no definitive answer to explain the benefit of the drugs.

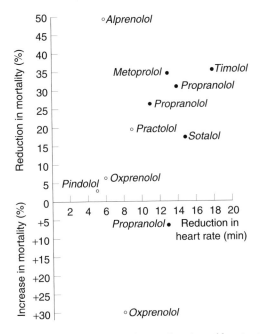

Figure 16.3 Mortality reduction after beta-blockade as a function of heart-rate reduction. The average heart-rate reduction by active treatment (*x* axis) is plotted for each trial against the effect on mortality (*y* axis). The figure illustrates the tendency for drugs with greater heart-rate reduction to have the most beneficial effect. (Reproduced with permission from Ref. 34.)

Calcium Channel Blockers

In the late 1970s calcium channel blockers were identified as drugs that could modify angina pectoris and myocardial ischemia in postinfarction patients. Based on preliminary observations, indicating a benefit in angina pectoris,[35,36] a number of RCTs were initiated to examine their effect on acute myocardial infarction. The Trial of Early Nifedipine and Acute Myocardial Infarction (TRENT),[37] the Secondary Prevention Reinfarction Israeli Nifedipine Trial (SPRINT-I),[38] and subsequently SPRINT-II[39] examined the use of nifedipine. Two studies, the Danish Verapamil Infarction Trial-I (DAVIT-I)[40] and DAVIT-II,[41] tested the use of verapamil. One study, the Multicenter Diltiazem Postinfarction Trial (MDPIT),[42] examined the use of diltiazem. These studies were similar in their design and were classic RCTs. A summary is given in *Table 16.2*.

Nifedipine

TRENT[35] randomized 4491 patients within 24 hours of the onset of symptoms, initially starting with sublingual nifedipine followed by 10 mg orally four times daily for 30 days. At 1-month follow-up, the mortality rate in the nifedipine group was 10.2% and that in the placebo group 9.3%. The SPRINT-I[38] trial randomized 2276 patients on days 7–21 to nifedipine 10 mg three times daily. The subsequent SPRINT-II[39] trial enrolled a somewhat smaller group of patients with high risk of acute myocardial infarction, those with prior myocardial infarction, and anterior location of myocardial infarction. SPRINT-I failed to demonstrate a beneficial effect and SPRINT-II was terminated early due to an excess mortality in the nifedipine group.

Verapamil

The DAVIT-I[40] trial examined the use of verapamil within the first 48 hours after myocardial infarction. The initial intravenous dose of 0.1 mg kg^{-1} was followed by 120

Table 16.2 Results of selected long-term randomized trials of calcium channel blockers in patients with suspected or confirmed myocardial infarction

Trial (Year)	No. of patients	Entry after symptoms	Minimum follow-up	Mortality (%) Drug[a]	Placebo	Reinfarction (%) Drug[a]	Placebo
Nifedipine							
TRENT (1986)	4491	24 h	30 days	10.2	9.3	2.2	1.5
SPRINT-I (1986)	2276	7–21 days	13 months	5.8	5.7	4.4	4.8
SPRINT-II (1988)	1373	48 h	6 months	15.4	13.2	?	?
Verapamil							
DAVIT-I (1984)	1436	48 h	6 months	12.8	13.9	7.0	8.3
DAVIT-II (1990)	1775	7–15 days	16 months	11.1	13.8	11.0	13.2
Diltiazem							
DRS (1986)	576	24–72 h	2 weeks	3.8	3.1	5.2	9.3
MDPIT (1988)	2466	3–5 days	25 months	10.3	10.0	8.0	9.4

[a]Intervention with a calcium channel blocker.

mg orally three times daily. At the end of 16 months there was no significant benefit, with a 12.8% mortality in the verapamil-treated patients and 13.9% in the placebo group. In contrast to DAVIT-I, DAVIT-II[41] examined the role of a delayed verapamil oral adminis-tration of 120 mg three times daily, 1–2 weeks after myocardial infarction. Again, no overall benefit was demonstrated, but a subgroup analysis indicated that pre-existing heart failure was related to an increased event rate in the treated group. In the patients without heart failure, the total mortality rate was 11.8% in the placebo group and 7.7% in the verapamil-treated patients. In those with heart failure there was no difference between the verapamil- and placebo-treated patients. When patients with heart failure were excluded from the analysis at 18 months, verapamil therapy resulted in a 28% reduction in mortality at 18 months.

Diltiazem

MDPIT[42] examined the use of diltiazem 60 mg every 6 hours over a 24-month period in patients randomized 3–4 days after myocardial infarction. The combined incidence of cardiac events, mortality, and reinfarction was 11.0% lower in the diltiazem-treated group, which was not significant. There was no effect on overall mortality, which was 10.3% in the diltiazem-treated patients and 10.0% in the placebo group. In a subgroup analysis of patients, representing 80% of the study population without pulmonary congestion on chest X-ray and ejection fractions of $>40\%$, there was a 30% reduction in cardiac events in the diltiazem-treated patients. In contrast, patients with pulmonary congestion and a lower ejection fraction experienced a 25% increase in cardiac events in the treatment group (*Figure 16.4*).

These studies were technically similar to the previously described beta-blocker studies. SPRINT-I and DAVIT-I initiated therapy within 24 and 48 hours, respectively, whereas the remaining trials randomized patients in the late postinfarction period. They were universally unsuccessful. Both the verapamil and diltiazem studies suggested an adverse effect in the presence of left ventricular dysfunction, although such subjects represented a minority of patients entering the studies. This phenomenon was not examined by subgroup analysis in the SPRINT-I and SPRINT-II trials.

Two special calcium blocker trials are also worth mentioning: the multicenter Diltiazem Reinfarction Study (DRS)[43] and the Holland Interuniversity Nifedipine/Metoprolol Trial (HINT).[44] The DRS randomized patients to 90 mg of diltiazem four times daily within the first 24–72 hours after the onset of symptoms in patients with non-Q-wave myocardial infarction, in order to test the effect of diltiazem in patients with active ischemia. Patients were followed with serial enzymes and electrocardiograms over the next 14 days. Approximately 60% of patients were receiving beta-blocker therapy and 80% were taking nitrates. There was a significant decrease in reinfarction from 9.3% to 5.2%, but no difference in mortality. A unique characteristic of this analysis was the achievement of statistical significance using a one-sided t-test, which presumed that there was no adverse effect of diltiazem in this population. Subsequently, based on the MDPIT, it was recognized that an adverse effect of diltiazem could exist in patients with acute myocardial infarction, particularly in those individuals with left ventricular dysfunction. This may explain the dissociation between the decrease in reinfarction rate observed in the DRS and any benefit in terms of mortality. In retrospect, a two-sided analysis would have been more appropriate, in which case statistical significance would not have been achieved.

HINT was a placebo-controlled trial which studied the effect of nifedipine, metoprolol, and a combination of both in 515 patients with preinfarction angina. Patients were

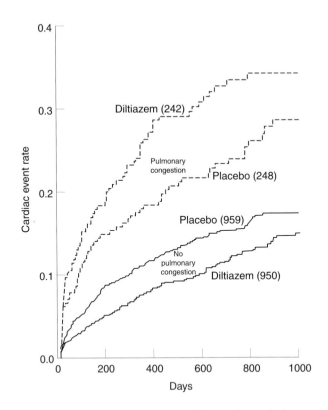

Figure 16.4   Effect of diltiazem on cardiac event rate (death or reinfarction) after myocardial infarction in the MDPIT study. While the overall effect was negligible, diltiazem appeared to increase events in patients with pulmonary congestion (– – – –) while it was favorable or neutral in patients without pulmonary congestion (———). (Reproduced with permission from Ref. 41.)

randomized to nifedipine 10 mg every 4 hours and metoprolol 100 mg twice daily, in combination or separately. The patients entering the study were those with persistent chest pain, which was thought to represent preinfarction angina. The occurrence of reinfarction or recurrent ischemia at 48 hours was the study endpoint. The trial was terminated early because the interim analysis indicated that patients receiving nifedipine alone had an increase in mortality events and infarction. Patients receiving a beta-blocker at the time of randomization to the combination of metoprolol and nifedipine did better than placebo. The combination of metoprolol and nifedipine did not appear to have any benefit over metoprolol alone.[44]

Impact of Calcium Blockers

Although there was general lack of benefit shown in all RCTs, calcium entry blockers continued to be widely prescribed. In early 1987, almost 60% of patients were receiving calcium blockers after myocardial infarction.[45] Shortly after the publication of SPRINT and MDPIT, the use of these drugs decreased to approximately 50%. As late as 1990, well after the last of these studies, 50% of patients were receiving calcium entry blockers as routine treatment following myocardial infarction. A registry of patients in 1993,[26] examining the use of thrombolytic agents in myocardial infarction patients, indicated 9.5% of patients received calcium blockers with thrombolytic therapy and 41.9% received calcium blockers without thrombolytic therapy. This is in contrast to oral beta-blockers, which were used in 36.3% and 29.5%, respectively. A recent survey of cardiologists, internists, and family practitioners regarding the use of calcium blockers indicated that, in patients with left ventricular dysfunction, diltiazem is thought to have a benefit by 2.4% of cardiologists, 5.8% of internists, and 16.5% of family practitioners in the USA.[28] Part of the general acceptance of calcium blockers by practitioners was the presumption that they had a relatively low side-effect profile compared to beta-blockers.

The RCTs proposed that intermittent ischemia was a major cause of mortality in ischemic heart disease and that calcium blockers could affect this phenomenon in acute transmural infarction and in patients with non-Q-wave myocardial infarctions. The trials were carried out at a time when coronary spasm was thought to be the dominant phenomenon in myocardial infarction and prior to the appreciation that recurrent coronary thrombosis was the likely pathogenesis of recurrent ischemia. However, all the calcium blockers studied express negative inotropic effects and can adversely affect patients with left ventricular dysfunction. It is possible that any positive effect they had was overwhelmed by their adverse effect in this subgroup. The atrioventricular block observed in some patients treated with diltiazem and verapamil could also explain some adverse effect. Nifedipine has been observed to sensitize the sympathetic nervous system, leading to reflex tachycardia and possible hypotension, both of which could lead to further ischemia and reinfarction.[46] Regardless of the mechanism, it is clear from these studies there does not appear to be any role for calcium blockers in the treatment of acute myocardial infarction patients.

Magnesium

The issues surrounding magnesium administration for acute myocardial infarction are numerous and complex. In particular, when the data from early clinical trials, a meta-analysis,[47] and a larger, contemporary trial[48] conflicted with the allegedly definitive 'mega-trial',[49] an aftermath of debate has led to introspective reviews and editorials[50–54] about the very nature of clinical trials and their implications, as well as a proposal for a subsequent large-scale trial on magnesium.[55] In no other area of the management of acute myocardial infarction have the methodologies of clinical trial design and analysis been more scrutinized.

Magnesium has been recognized as a mediator of cardiac function for many years. Several excellent reviews have discussed the many potential mechanisms of benefit of magnesium therapy in acute myocardial infarction.[56,57] Many of the putative properties of magnesium are ascribed to its actions as an inorganic calcium channel blocker and as a cofactor in enzymatic reactions, particularly those involving ATP. Magnesium has been described as a coronary vasodilatory, antiarrhythmic, and cytoprotective, which, when combined with a possible antiplatelet effect, forms a highly desirable set of functions for treating patients with acute myocardial infarction.[47]

Investigation of magnesium found a particular niche in the 1980s, also due to the evolving context of acute myocardial infarction management. Prophylactic lidocaine was largely abandoned owing to its ineffectiveness documented by pooled analysis,[58] and suppressing premature ventricular contractions after acute myocardial infarction was shown to be harmful in the Cardiac Arrhythmia Suppression Trial.[5] With the emergence of magnesium as an effective treatment for torsades de pointes,[59] perhaps by suppressing early afterdepolarizations and triggered activity,[60] came increased enthusiasm for a safe antiarrhythmic agent to be employed in the setting of acute ischemia.[56]

Early Clinical Trials

A series of seven small trials with a randomized and placebo-controlled design were published between 1981 and 1990.[47] These trials enrolled between 48 and 400 patients each, for a total of 1301 patients. In most cases, follow-up for mortality and morbidity events continued through hospitalization. Two of the studies showed significant reductions in mortality, while the other five were statistically neutral. However, publication of formal meta-analyses in 1991 and 1992 showed that, when individual trial results were analyzed together, magnesium appeared to reduce mortality by more than half.[47,61] One mechanism appeared to be a reduction in ventricular arrhythmias, although the definition of arrhythmia varied between the trials. In the pooled analysis, ventricular arrhythmias were significantly reduced by 50% overall. One trial found a reduction in the development of congestive heart failure, although this finding was not consistently seen.[47]

A much larger, single-center study, the Second Leicester Intravenous Magnesium Intervention (LIMIT-2) trial,[48] randomized 2316 patients within 24 hours of onset of suspected acute myocardial infarction to 73 mmol of magnesium sulfate or placebo given over 24 hours.[48] The dose was calculated rapidly to double and maintain the serum magnesium level throughout the infusion. Two-thirds of patients had confirmed infarctions; most of the remainder were thought to have angina. Thrombolysis and aspirin administration were routinely deployed during the course of the trial and, unlike earlier trials, were given to 35% and 65%, respectively, of the study population. Mortality at 28 days, the primary endpoint, was significantly reduced from 10.3% in the placebo patients to 7.8% in magnesium-treated patients, a reduction of 24% (95% confidence interval (CI) 1–43). No effect on progression to infarction was seen. Magnesium treatment was felt to be safe and well tolerated, except for transient flushing which was ascribed to the rapid bolus administration at initiation of the infusion.

Unlike the earlier meta-analysis, serious arrhythmias were not reduced overall or in a subset of 70 patients subjected to 24-hour Holter recording.[48] However, again, unlike the earlier trials, the incidence of heart failure was significantly reduced by 25%, whether measured clinically, radiologically, or by the need for loop diuretic or nitroprusside administration while in the coronary care unit. Aside from this surprising finding, benefit was independent of the effects of other treatments, and was not enhanced in any subgroup. The investigators thus postulated that magnesium may have a direct protective effect on myocardium, possibly by limiting injury caused by calcium overload during ischemia or during reperfusion.[48] The hypothesis that magnesium prevents reperfusion injury was fortified by the investigators when the long-term follow-up results were presented and benefit shown to persist.[62] In addition to being a plausible explanation for the treatment effect observed, this hypothesis also served to reconcile the absence of an effect of magnesium in ISIS-4, since the design of ISIS-4 and LIMIT-2 differed only in the proximity of magnesium infusion to randomization and/or thrombolytic administration (early in LIMIT-2 and later in ISIS-4).[55]

The ISIS-4 study initially intended to enroll 40 000 patients,[63] but was extended to 58 000 after an interim review.[49] Magnesium was given in a dose similar to that in the LIMIT-2 trial, but the loading bolus was given over 15 rather than 5 minutes, and the protocol advised to administer magnesium after initial stabilization and following thrombolytic

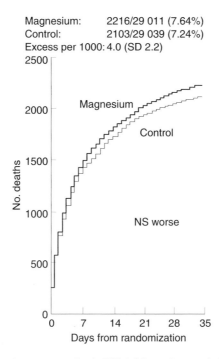

Magnesium: 2216/29 011 (7.64%)
Control: 2103/29 039 (7.24%)
Excess per 1000: 4.0 (SD 2.2)

Figure 16.5 Effect of magnesium on mortality in ISIS-4. Magnesium tended to increase mortality, but the results were not statistically significant. (Reproduced with permission from Ref. 49.)

administration.[63] The study randomized patients to magnesium or open control, since the occurrence of flushing with magnesium administration was felt to negate the blinding of placebo administration (*Figure 16.5*). The findings that magnesium had no effect on 35-day mortality (6% increase in mortality, 95% CI 0–12% increase) were a widespread disappointment. Magnesium failed to show benefit in any subgroup or to interact significantly with the other study drugs (captopril and mononitrate) or nonrandomized treatments prescribed by patients' physicians.[49]

That the negative ISIS-4 results differed so substantially from the promising results of the meta-analysis and the LIMIT-2 trial led to much discussion and analysis of the particular study designs, the more general nature of meta-analysis and its application to decision-making, and the impact of large, nonmechanistic trials on practice.

Mega-trials and the Role of Meta-analysis

When the LIMIT-2 results 'verified' the meta-analysis suggesting worthwhile benefit from magnesium, many coronary care units adopted the routine use of magnesium after endorsement by editorials.[64,65] This position was bolstered by the observation that evidence of treatment benefit may be available by meta-analysis long before a large trial had been conducted or the treatment widely embraced.[66] Similarly, when the ISIS-4 results 'invalidated' the meta-analysis, the method itself and its application to the clinical arena were both attacked[52,53] and defended.[51,54] Other authors suggested that, while the value of

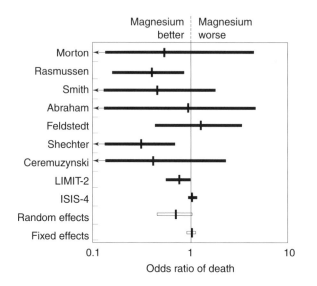

Figure 16.6   Magnesium trials and mortality reduction. Odds ratios for death in treatment versus control patients are shown for the seven early, small trials, and for the longer LIMIT-2 and ISIS-4 trials (closed bars). The results of two different techniques of meta-analysis (open bars) illustrate the discordance between the two techniques. (Reproduced with permission from Ref. 67.)

meta-analysis may not be at stake, important biological differences between the two large studies existed, and that a tenable role for magnesium in preventing reperfusion injury may not have been properly tested in ISIS-4.[62] A large, government-sponsored trial to resolve this issue is in the planning stages.[55]

We suggest that important philosophical and methodological differences exist between meta-analyses, which are inherently hypothesis-generating, and clinical trials, which are inherently hypothesis-testing.[67] As such, meta-analysis can never carry the weight of a properly conducted randomized trial, and even a meta-analysis of 10 studies of 100 patients each cannot favorably compare to a single trial of 1000 patients each.[68] The divergence between the large trial and the earlier meta-analysis is also less troublesome when the overall improvement in the management of acute myocardial infarction is considered,[69] an improvement which resulted in almost different populations studied in the 1970s and early 1980s (the studies forming the meta-analysis) and the late 1980s and early 1990s (the LIMIT-2 and ISIS-4 populations). Since meta-analysis assumes the absence of heterogeneity (fixed-effects method), or attempts to account for it statistically (random-effects method),[67] analysis of populations known to be different is problematic. The magnesium example, in fact, is an extreme and probably rare case where the two different methods of meta-analysis differed significantly[67] (*Figure 16.6*). As for the differences between the LIMIT-2 and ISIS-4 results, which appeared to include patients receiving similar treatments, the play of chance may be involved, with the larger trial potentially representing the 'true' result, or very early magnesium infusion may, in fact, prevent reperfusion injury, as suggested by the LIMIT-2 group.[50] This effect may or may not have been obscured by the design of ISIS-4, since the exact time of magnesium administration after enrollment and relative to other treatments was not collected as part of the trial data.[55]

Nitrates

Nitrates have been used to treat coronary artery disease for more than a century,[70] and are well established as safe and effective for the relief of angina. Until the 1970s, nitrates were considered to be dangerous and contraindicated for use in acute myocardial infarction. Investigation of nitroglycerin (TNG) for use in myocardial infarction began in earnest with the development of an intravenous preparation that could be easily titrated against physiologic parameters. Therapeutic goals examined in early trials included symptom relief, limitation of infarct size, preservation of left ventricular function, and, in the coronary care unit environment with the newly developed pulmonary artery catheter,[71] a reduction in filling pressures and improvement in other hemodynamic parameters. Only recently have clinical trials been large enough to address the issue of mortality reduction.

Early Clinical Trials

Seven small randomized trials that examined intravenous TNG were largely conducted and published by the 1980s. Together they encompassed fewer than 1000 patients.[72] The most compelling was also the largest study, conducted in a single center between 1981 and 1983 at the University of Alberta.[73] In this trial, intravenous TNG or placebo was administered in single-blind fashion to consecutive patients presenting within 12 hours of symptom onset, in a dose titrated to reduce mean arterial pressure by 10%, or 30% in initially hypertensive patients. The goals of the study were to assess the impact of therapy on infarct size and expansion, the latter being determined by echocardiography prior to discharge. In placebo patients, the ejection fraction declined from admission to predischarge, accompanied by an increase in left ventricular volume, but in TNG patients ejection fraction was preserved. Other favorable effects included smaller infarct size, as determined by creatine kinase MB release, and a reduced hospital mortality of 14% compared to 26% in controls.[73]

These results were considered together with other smaller studies in an early meta-analysis, and were also combined with a series of trials evaluating nitroprusside in nearly 1200 patients studied in a similar context. The benefit ascribed to early nitrates was a striking 24% mortality reduction for nitroprusside, a 49% reduction for TNG, and a 35% reduction for the two drugs taken together.[72] These findings, combined perhaps with the compelling theoretical and physiologic rationale for nitrate use, led to a nearly universal deployment of intravenous TNG in many North American centers.[26,69]

Nitrates have generally been perceived as safe, but reports have suggested that episodic hypotension and bradycardia may occur,[74] as well as possible interference with the actions of heparin[75] and perhaps thrombolytic agents.[76,77] Clinical effects on platelet function *in vivo* may be inhibitory, but are not fully understood. In addition, tolerance to the hemodynamic and presumably other favorable effects of continuous nitrates may develop soon after 24 hours.[80]

Large, Contemporary Trials

As with magnesium, strongly positive results from a meta-analysis were followed by large, randomized trials showing limited to no benefit. In the ISIS-4 trial, patients were randomized to oral isosorbide mononitrate or placebo, given initially as 30 mg and subsequently 60 mg daily for 30 days[49] (*Figure 16.7*). In the GISSI-3 study, patients were

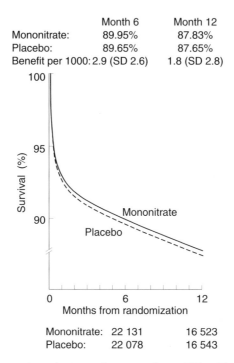

	Month 6	Month 12
Mononitrate:	89.95%	87.83%
Placebo:	89.65%	87.65%
Benefit per 1000:	2.9 (SD 2.6)	1.8 (SD 2.8)

Mononitrate:	22 131	16 523
Placebo:	22 078	16 543

Figure 16.7   Effect of mononitrate for 1 month on mortality in ISIS-4. The results were not significant. (Reproduced with permission from Ref. 49.)

randomized to intravenous TNG or control for 24 hours, followed by transdermal patches for 6 weeks of treatment.[81] When results from the two trials were combined, mortality in the nearly 80 000 patients at 5 or 6 weeks was 7.14% in treated patients and 6.87% in control patients, a nonsignificant reduction of 2.8 ± 1.9 per 1000 patients.[49] No particular subgroups appeared to derive special benefit, and no interaction was seen with other study medications (magnesium and captopril in ISIS-4,[49] and lisinopril in GISSI-3[81]).

One limitation of these trials is the fact that nontrial nitrates were administered to 54% and 57% of patients in ISIS-4 and GISSI-3, respectively. This administration may have diluted a possible treatment effect and contributed to the negative findings. However, no treatment effect was seen in countries with low nitrate use, and the baseline characteristics of patients receiving and not receiving nontrial nitrates were similar.[49]

An additional explanation for the discrepancy between the positive meta-analysis of the earlier trials and the more recent studies is concomitant use of aspirin (four-fifths), thrombolytics (one-third to two-thirds), and intravenous beta-blockers (one-tenth to one-third) in ISIS-4 and GISSI-3, respectively. Indeed, when nitrates have been considered in other recent, but smaller, trials, the results were similarly disappointing. Morris and others randomized 316 patients to intravenous isosorbide dinitrate or placebo for 24–48 hours and found no effect on infarct size measured by creatine kinase (CK) release or ST-segment resolution.[82] Another study conducted collaboratively in Europe and Russia between 1990 and 1992 evaluated molsidomine, a nitric oxide donor with similar properties to TNG, against placebo control. In the 4017 patients enrolled, no difference was found in short- or long-term mortality.[83] In this latter study, the majority of patients received aspirin, heparin, and beta-blockers, and 20% received thrombolytics. Thus, concomitant effective therapy may render nitrates less beneficial when other agents have already reduced blood pressure or lowered afterload. The meta-analysis consisted of studies conducted before the deployment of other treatments, so nitrates were assessed essentially in isolation. An additional possibility is that the earlier trials combined in the meta-analysis, while a statistically sound process, may not have been inclusive of unpublished or obscure negative studies, or may have simply reflected a type 1 error.

Across the trials, nitrates were found to be largely safe, with a minimum of adverse events attributable to active treatment. In ISIS-4, hypotension, requiring termination of study treatment, was seen in 14.4% of control patients and was significantly higher (17.4%) in patients receiving mononitrate. There was also a more than five-fold excess of headache and a slight excess of dizziness. Earlier concerns about the reduction of coronary perfusion pressure extending or reinitiating infarction were not borne out.[49]

Role of Nitrates based on Trial Evidence

The critical role of nitric oxide as an endogenous mediator of vascular tone is emerging,[84] and may form the strongest biological hypothesis yet favoring the use of nitrates in acute infarction. However, clinical trial evidence is also now conclusive as to their lack of benefit to patients. Although nitrates may be useful to treat anginal symptoms and perhaps acute heart failure,[85] and have been shown to be safe and well tolerated, there is no basis for their routine use in uncomplicated infarction. If nitrates are used early in infarction, then the cheaper oral preparations should be favored over the more expensive intravenous route, unless precise control over borderline blood pressure is required.

Summary and Conclusions

Of the four treatments in this chapter, RCTs have unambiguously shown efficacy only for beta-blocker treatment during and after acute myocardial infarction. Calcium blocking agents have no proven efficacy acutely, and in the case of short-acting nifedipine and the rate-slowing agents verapamil and diltiazem in the setting of heart failure, may be harmful. Magnesium, while relatively safe and very inexpensive, did not reduce mortality in a trial of unprecedented size, and nitrates, long the mainstay of the coronary care unit, did not reduce mortality when evaluated in the contemporary context of other effective therapies such as thrombolytic, aspirin, and beta-blocker.

The evaluation of these four treatments has spanned the past two decades during a time of evolving therapy for acute myocardial infarction. As mortality has fallen, due in part to treatments evaluated in RCTs and perhaps to other unknown factors,[69] the size of trials has grown as a necessary consequence of the requirement of statistical power in the setting of modest benefit and low event rates. The advent of the 'mega-trial' has raised questions about the cost and effort that may be required to evaluate new therapies.

As effective treatments are developed and proven in RCTs, one troubling finding is delayed[66] and incomplete[86] deployment. Specialists tend to recognize and apply RCT results in their own field better than do generalists,[28] but even in the USA, where acute myocardial infarction management is largely the province of the cardiologist, revascularization (which has received comparatively little evaluation in RCTs) may be preferred without complete use of medical treatments which have clearly shown mortality benefit in RCTs of tens of thousands of patients.[87]

As practitioners have attempted to grapple with increasing masses of data, evaluating growing numbers of clearly or potentially effective therapies, techniques such as meta-analysis have attempted to restore order to a disorganized literature of small and diverse RCTs. However, given the discrepancy between the RCT and meta-analysis in two of the examples in this chapter (see *Figure 16.6*), the proper role of meta-analysis is not as a substitute for an RCT, but rather as a prelude to one, since meta-analyses are not experiments themselves. RCTs, on the other hand, are inherently hypothesis-testing and, as such, will continue to define the management of the acute myocardial infarction patient.

References

1. Mitchell JRA. But will it help my patients with myocardial infarction? The implication of recent trials for every day countryfolk. *Br Med J* 1982; **285**: 1140–8.
2. The Coronary Drug Project Research Group. The Coronary Drug Project: initial findings leading to modifications of its research protocol. *JAMA* 1970; **214**: 1303–6.
3. Aspirin Myocardial Infarction Study Research Group. A randomized, controlled trial of aspirin in persons recovered from myocardial infarction. *JAMA* 1980; **243**: 661–9.
4. IMPACT Research Group. International mexiletine and placebo antiarrhythmic coronary trial. I. Report on arrhythmia and other findings. *J Am Coll Cardiol* 1984; **4**: 1148–63.
5. Cardiac Arrhythmia Suppression Trial (CAST) Investigators. Preliminary report: effect of encainide and flecainide on mortality in a randomized trial of arrhythmia suppression after myocardial infarction. *N Engl J Med* 1989; **321**: 406–12.
6. The MIAMI Trial Research Group. Metoprolol in acute myocardial infarction (MIAMI). A randomised placebo-controlled international trial. *Eur Heart J* 1985; **6**: 199–226.
7. ISIS-I (First International Study of Infarct Survival) Collaborative Group. Mechanisms for the early mortality reduction produced by beta-blockade started early in acute myocardial infarction: ISIS-I. *Lancet* 1988; **i**: 921–3.
8. Ahlquist RP. A study of the adrenoptropic receptors. *Am J Physiol* 1948; **153**: 586–600.
9. Black JW, Stephenson JS. Pharmacology of a new adrenergic beta-receptor-blocking compound (nethalide). *Lancet* 1962; **ii**: 311–14.
10. Norwegian Multicenter Study Group. Six-year follow-up of the Norwegian Multicenter Study on timolol after acute myocardial infarction. *N Engl J Med* 1985; **313**: 1055–8.
11. Beta Blocker Heart Attack Trial Research Group. A randomized trial of propranolol in patients with acute myocardial infarction: 1. Mortality results. *JAMA* 1982; **247**: 1701–14.
12. Beta-Blocker Heart Attack Trial Research Group. Beta-blocker heart attack trial: design, methods, and baseline results. *Controlled Clin Trials* 1984; **5**: 382–437.
13. CASS Principal Investigators and their Associates. Coronary Artery Surgery Study (CASS): a randomized trial of coronary artery bypass surgery. Comparability of entry characteristics and survival in randomized patients and nonrandomized patients meeting randomization criteria. *J Am Coll Cardiol* 1984; **3**: 114–28.
14. Beta Blocker Heart Attack Trial Research Group. A randomized trial of propranolol in patients with acute myocardial infarction. *JAMA* 1983; **250**: 2814–19.
15. Gheorghiade M, Schultz L, Tilley B, Kao W, Goldstein S. Effects of propranolol in non-Q-wave acute myocardial infarction in the Beta Blocker Heart Attack Trial. *Am J Cardiol* 1990; **66**: 129–33.
16. Pederson TR, and the Norwegian Multicenter Study Group. Six-year follow-up of the Norwegian Multicenter Study of Timolol after acute myocardial infarction. *N Engl J Med* 1985; **313**: 1055–8.
17. Friedman LM, Byington RP, Capone RJ, Fuberg CD, Goldstein S, Lichstein E. Effect of propranolol in patients with myocardial infarction and ventricular arrhythmia. *J Am Coll Cardiol* 1986; **7**: 1–8.
18. Chadda K, Goldstein S, Byington R, *et al*. Effect of propranolol after acute myocardial infarction in patients with congestive heart failure. *Circulation* 1986; **73**: 503–10.
19. Cruickshank JM. *β*-Blockers, plasma lipids, and coronary heart disease. *Circulation* 1990; **82**(Suppl II): 60–5.
20. Australian and Swedish Pindolol Study Group. The effect of pindolol on the two years' mortality after myocardial infarction. *Eur Heart J* 1983; **4**: 367–75.
21. Taylor SH, Silke B, Ebbutt A, *et al*. A long-term prevention study with oxprenalol in coronary heart disease. *N Engl J Med* 1982; **307**: 1293–301.
22. Boissel J-P, Leizorovicz A, Picolet H, *et al*. Efficacy of acebutolol after acute myocardial infarction. *Am J Cardiol* 1990; **66**: 24C–31C.
23. Hjalmarson Å, Herlitz J, Málek I, *et al*. Effect on mortality of metoprolol in acute myocardial infarction. *Lancet* 1981; **2**: 823–7.
24. The MIAMI Trial Research Group. Metoprolol in Acute Myocardial Infarction (MIAMI): A randomised placebo-controlled international trial. *Eur Heart J* 1985; **6**: 199–226.
25. TIMI Investigators. Immediate versus deferred *β*-blockade following thrombolytic therapy in patients with acute myocardial infarction. Results of the Thrombolysis in Myocardial Infarction (TIMI) II-B Study. *Circulation* 1991; **83**: 422–37.

26. Rogers WJ, Bowlby LJ, Chandra NC, *et al*. Treatment of myocardial infarction in the United States (1990 to 1993). Observations from the national registry of myocardial infarction. *Circulation* 1994; **90**: 2103–14.
27. Kennedy HL, Rosenson RS. Physician use of beta-adrenergic blocking therapy: a changing perspective. *J Am Coll Cardiol* 1995; **26**(2): 547–52.
28. Ayanian JZ, Hauptman PJ, Guadagnoli E, *et al*. Knowledge and practices of generalist and specialist physicians regarding drug therapy for acute myocardial infarction. *N Engl J Med* 1994; **331**: 1136–42.
29. Viskin S, Kitzis I, Lev E, *et al*. Treatment with beta-adrenergic blocking agents after myocardial infarction: from randomized trials to clinical practice. *J Am Coll Cardiol* 1995; **25**: 1327–32.
30. Kjekshus J, Gilpin E, Cali G, Blackey AR, Henning H, Ross Jr J. Diabetic patients and beta-blockers after acute myocardial infarction. *Eur Heart J* 1990; **11**: 43–50.
31. Thadani U. *β*-Adrenergic blockers and intermittent claudication. Time for reappraisal. *Arch Intern Med* 1991; **151**: 1705–7.
32. Montague TJ, Ikuta RM, Wong RY, Bay KS, Teo KK, Davies NJ. Comparison of risk and patterns of practice in patients older and younger than 70 years with acute myocardial infarction in a two year period (1987–1989). *Am J Cardiol* 1991; **68**: 843–7.
33. Smith SC, Gilpin E, Ahnve S, *et al*. Outlook after acute myocardial infarction in the very elderly compared to that in patients aged 65 to 75 years. *J Am Coll Cardiol* 1990; **16**: 784–92.
34. Kjekshus JK. Importance of heart rate in determining beta blocker efficacy in acute and long term myocardial infarction trials. *Am J Cardiol* 1986; **57**: 43F–9F.
35. Muller JE, Morrison J, Stone PH, *et al*. Nifedipine therapy for patients with threatened and acute myocardial infarction: a randomized double-blind, placebo-controlled comparison. *Circulation* 1984; **69**: 740–7.
36. Sirnes PA, Overskeid K, Pedersen TR, *et al*. Evaluation of infarct size during the early use of nifedipine in patients with acute myocardial infarction: The Norwegian Nifedipine Multicenter Trial. *Circulation* 1984; **70**: 638–44.
37. Wilcox RG, Hampton JR, Banks BC, *et al*. Trial of early nifedipine in acute myocardial infarction: the TRENT study. *Br Med J* 1986; **293**: 1204–8.
38. The Israeli SPRINT Study Group. Secondary Prevention Reinfarction Israeli Nifedipine Trial (SPRINT). A randomized intervention trial of nifedipine in patients with acute myocardial infarction. *Eur Heart J* 1988; **9**: 354–64.
39. Goldbourt U, Behar S, Reicher-Reiss H, *et al*. for the SPRINT Study Group. Early administration of nifedipine in suspected acute myocardial infarction. The Secondary Prevention Reinfarction Israel Nifedipine Trial 2 Study. *Arch Intern Med* 1993; **153**: 345–53.
40. The Danish Study Group on Verapamil in Myocardial Infarction. Verapamil in acute myocardial infarction. *Eur Heart J* 1984; **5**: 516–28.
41. The Danish Study Group on Verapamil in Myocardial Infarction. Effect of verapamil on mortality and major events after acute myocardial infarction (The Danish Verapamil Infarction Trial II – DAVIT II). *Am J Cardiol* 1990; **66**: 779–85.
42. The Multicenter Diltiazem Postinfarction Trial Research Group. The effect of diltiazem on mortality and reinfarction after myocardial infarction. *N Engl J Med* 1988; **319**: 335–92.
43. Gibson RS, Boden WF, Therous P, *et al*. Diltiazem and reinfarction in patients with non-Q-wave myocardial infarction. Results of a double-blind, randomized, multicenter trial. *N Engl J Med* 1986; **315**: 423–9.
44. Report of the Holland Interuniversity Nifedipine/Metoprolol Trial (HINT) Research Group. Early treatment of unstable angina in the coronary care unit: a randomised, double blind, placebo controlled comparison of recurrent ischaemia in patients treated with nifedipine or metoprolol or both. *Br Heart J* 1986; **56**: 400–13.
45. Lamas GA, Pfeffer MA, Hamm P, *et al*., for the SAVE Investigators. Do the results of randomized clinical trials of cardiovascular drugs influence medical practice? *N Engl J Med* 1992; **327**: 241–7.
46. Waters D. Proischemic complications of dihydropyridine calcium channel blockers. *Circulation* 1991; **84**: 2598–600.
47. Teo KK, Yusuf S, Collins R, Held PH, Peto R. Effects on intravenous magnesium suspected acute myocardial infarction: overview of randomised trials. *Br Med J* 1991; **303**: 1499–503.
48. Woods KL, Fletcher S, Roffe C, Haider Y. Intravenous magnesium sulphate in suspected acute myocardial infarction: results of the second Leicester Intravenous Magnesium Intervention Trial (LIMIT-2). *Lancet* 1992; **339**: 1553–8.
49. ISIS-4. A randomised factorial trial assessing early oral captopril, oral mononitrate, and intravenous magnesium sulphate in 58 050 patients with suspected acute myocardial infarction. *Lancet* 1995; **345**: 669–85.
50. Woods KL. Mega-trials and management of acute myocardial infarction. *Lancet* 1995; **346**: 611–14.
51. Yusuf S, Flather M. Magnesium in acute myocardial infarction. ISIS 4 provides no grounds for its routine use. *Br Med J* 1995; **310**: 751–2.
52. Egger M, Smith GD. Misleading meta-analysis. Lessons from 'an effective, safe, simple' intervention that wasn't. *Br Med J* 1995; **310**: 752–4.
53. Hlatky M. Commentary on 'Captopril but not mononitrate or intravenous magnesium reduced short-term mortality after suspected myocardial infarction'. ACPJ Club. 1995 Sept–Oct. (*Ann Intern Med* **123**(Suppl 2): 44). Comment on: ISIS-4. *Lancet* 1995; **348**: 669–82.
54. Antman EM. Randomized trials of magnesium in acute myocardial infarction: big numbers do not tell the whole story. *Am J Cardiol* 1995; **75**: 391–3.
55. Antman EM. Magnesium in acute MI. Timing is critical. *Circulation* 1995; **92**: 2367–72.
56. Woods KL. Possible pharmacological actions of magnesium in acute myocardial infarction. *Br J Clin Pharmacol* 1991; **32**: 3–10.
57. Arsenian MA. Magnesium and cardiovascular disease. *Prog Cardiovasc Dis* 1993; **35**(4): 271–310.

58. MacMahon S, Collins R, Peto R, Koster RW, Yusuf S. Effects of prophylactic lidocaine in suspected acute myocardial infarction: an overview of results from the randomized, controlled trials. *J Am Med Assoc* 1988; **260**: 1910–16.
59. Tzrioni D, Banai S, Schuger C, *et al*. Treatment of torsades de pointes with magnesium sulfate. *Circulation* 1988; **77**: 372–7.
60. Bailie DS, Inone H, Kaseder S, *et al*. Magnesium suppression of early afterdepolarization and ventricular tachy-arrhythmias induced by cesium in dogs. *Circulation* 1988; **77**: 1395–402.
61. Horner SM. Efficacy of intravenous magnesium in acute myocardial infarction in reducing arrhythmias and mortality. Meta analysis of magnesium in acute myocardial infarction. *Circulation* 1992; **86**: 774–9.
62. Woods KL, Fletcher S. Long-term outcome after intravenous magnesium sulphate in suspected acute myocardial infarction: the second Leicester Intravenous Magnesium Intervention Trial (LIMIT-2). *Lancet* 1994; **343**: 816–19.
63. ISIS-4 Collaborative Group. Fourth International Study of Infarct Survival: protocol for a large, simple study of the effects of oral mononitrate, of oral captopril, and of intravenous magnesium. *Am J Cardiol* 1991; **68**: 87D–100D.
64. Yusuf S, Teo K, Woods K. Intravenous magnesium in acute myocardial infarction. An effective, safe, simple, and inexpensive intervention. *Circulation* 1993; **87**(6): 2043–6.
65. Casscells R. Magnesium and myocardial infarction. *Lancet* 1994; **343**: 807–9.
66. Antman EM, Lau K, Kupelnick B, Mosteller F, Chalmers TC. A comparison of results of meta-analyses of randomized control trials and recommendations of clinical experts. Treatments for myocardial infarction. *JAMA* 1992; **268**: 240–8.
67. Borzak S, Ridker PM. Discordance between meta-analyses and large-scale randomized, controlled trials. Examples from the management of acute myocardial infarction. *Ann Intern Med* 1995; **123**: 873–7.
68. Ridker PM, Buring JE, Hennekens CH. Meta-analysis in cardiovascular disease: strengths and limitations. In: Braunwald E (ed.), *Heart Disease: A Textbook of Cardiovascular Medicine*, 4th edn. Philadelphia: WB Saunders, 1992; Vol. 3: 54–64.
69. Gheorghiade M, Ruzumna P, Borzak S, Havstad S, Ali A, Goldstein S. Decline in the hospital mortality from acute myocardial infarction: impact of changing management strategies. *Am Heart J* 1996; **131**: 250–6.
70. Murrell W. Nitro-glycerine as a remedy for angina pectoris. *Lancet* 1879; **i**: 151–2.
71. Forrester JS, Diamond G, Chatterjee K, Swan HJC. Medical therapy of acute myocardial infarction by application of hemodynamic subsets. *N Engl J Med* 1976; **295**: 1356–62.
72. Yusuf S, Collins R, MacMahon S, Peto R. Effect of intravenous nitrates on mortality in acute myocardial infarction: an overview of the randomised trials. *Lancet* 1988; **i**: 1088–92.
73. Jugdutt BI, Warnica JW. Intravenous nitroglycerin therapy to limit myocardial infarct size, expansion, and complications. *Circulation* 1988; **78**: 906–19.
74. Come PC, Pitt B. Nitroglycerin-induced severe hypotension and bradycardia in patients with acute myocardial infarction. *Circulation* 1976; **54**(4): 624–8.
75. Berk SI, Grunwald A, Pal S, Bodenheimer MM. Effect of intravenous nitroglycerin on heparin dosage requirements in coronary artery disease. *Am J Cardiol* 1993; **72**: 393–6.
76. Romeo F, Rosano GMC, Martuscelli E, *et al*. Concurrent nitroglycerin administration reduces the efficacy of recombinant tissue-type plasminogen activator in patients with acute anterior wall myocardial infarction. *Am Heart J* 1995; **130**: 692–7.
77. Nicolini FA, Ferrini D, Ottani F, *et al*. Concurrent nitroglycerin therapy impairs tissue-type plasminogen activator-induced thrombolysis in patients with acute myocardial infarction. *Am J Cardiol* 1994; **74**: 662–6.
78. Stamler J, Cunningham M, Lascalzo J. Reduced thiols and the effect of intravenous nitroglycerin on platelet aggregation. *Am J Cardiol* 1988; **62**: 377–80.
79. Diodati J, Théroux P, Latour J-G, Lacoste L, Lam JYT, Waters D. Effects of nitroglycerin at therapeutic doses on platelet aggregation in unstable angina pectoris and acute myocardial infarction. *Am J Cardiol* 1990; **66**: 683–8.
80. Parker JD, Farrell B, Fenton T, Cohanim M, Parker JO. Counter-regulatory responses to continuous and intermittent therapy with nitroglycerin. *Circulation* 1991; **84**: 2336–45.
81. GISSI-3 Collaborators. GISSI-3: effects of lisinopril and transdermal glyceryl trinitrate singly and together on 6-week mortality and ventricular function after acute myocardial infarction. *Lancet* 1994; **343**: 1115–22.
82. Morris JL, Zaman AG, Smyllie JH, Cowan JC. Nitrates in myocardial infarction: influence on infarct size, reperfusion, and ventricular remodelling. *Br Heart J* 1995; **73**: 310–19.
83. European Study of Prevention of Infarct with Molsidomine (ESPRIM) Group. The ESPRIM trial: short-term treatment of acute myocardial infarction with molsidomine. *Lancet* 1994; **344**: 91–7.
84. Harrison DG, Bates JN. The nitrovasodilators. New ideas about old drugs. *Circulation* 1993; **87**: 1461–7.
85. Verma SP, Silke B, Reynolds GW, Richmond A, Taylor SH. Nitrate therapy for left ventricular failure complicating acute myocardial infarction: a haemodynamic comparison of intravenous, buccal, and transdermal delivery systems. *J Cardiovasc Pharmacol* 1989; **14**: 756–62.
86. Ketley D, Woods KL. Impact of clinical trials on clinical practice: example of thrombolysis for acute myocardial infarction. *Lancet* 1993; **342**: 891–4.
87. Krumholz HM, Radford MJ, Ellerbeck EF, *et al*. Aspirin for secondary prevention after acute myocardial infarction in the elderly: prescribed use and outcomes. *Ann Intern Med* 1996; **124**: 292–8.

17

Antiarrhythmic Treatment Strategies

Lars Wilhelmsen

Introduction

Over just a few years, an estimated 50 000 people died from taking drugs intended to prevent cardiac arrest. After hundreds of thousands of patients routinely took these drugs, a definitive medical experiment proved they did not prevent cardiac arrest as doctors had believed. ... The results of this single medical misjudgment about the properties of these drugs produced a death toll larger than the United States combat losses in wars such as Korea and Vietnam.

This quotation is taken from the book *Deadly Medicine*, by Thomas J. Moore.[1]

The field of antiarrhythmic drug use emphasizes the importance of conducting well-designed and appropriately powered clinical trials before drugs are put to wide use. It is clearly demonstrated that apparently logical pathophysiological reasoning with use of surrogate endpoints may lead to erroneous conclusions.

Ventricular Arrhythmias and Cardiovascular Death

Left ventricular function is the most important determinant of survival following myocardial infarction, at least during the first several years of follow-up. Ventricular arrhythmias are related to infarct size – the larger the infarct, the greater is the risk of subsequent ventricular arrhythmias.[2,3] However, the presence of ventricular arrhythmias adds independent risk information[4,5] (*Figure 17.1*). This is logical, as about 50% of those who die after a myocardial infarction die suddenly owing to ventricular arrhythmias.

Early findings of hospital mortality in myocardial infarction being related to ventricular fibrillation led to the development of coronary care units to detect and treat fibrillation as early as possible and to prevent it occurring, i.e. to treat more benign ventricular arrhythmias. There is evidence for a nearly exponential decline in mortality, and notably in arrhythmic deaths, after the first days of the event. However, sudden death, presumably caused by ventricular arrhythmias, is also a major cause of death later in many postinfarction victims. Long-term detection and treatment with the hope of preventing such deaths has thus quite naturally also been of major concern in postinfarction management. Early

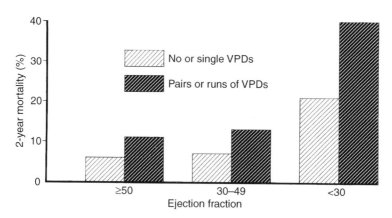

Figure 17.1   Relationships between left ventricular dysfunction, ventricular premature depolarizations (VPD) and 2-year mortality in infarct patients ($n = 766$).[4]

treatment can use both peroral and injectable drugs, whereas nonhospital treatment usually has to rely on peroral medication.

In addition to the use of Holter monitoring to assess the presence of ventricular arrhythmias, one can use methods such as signal-averaged electrocardiogram (ECG) analysis to detect evidence of delayed or slowed conduction, the substrate for sustained re-entrant ventricular arrhythmias. Kuchar et al.[6] and Gomes et al.[7] found late potentials to be associated with increased incidence of sudden death among postinfarction patients, this information being independent of indices of infarct size.

Similarly, programmed stimulation with the induction of ventricular tachycardia predicts increased risk of death or spontaneous tachycardia or fibrillation.[8] Kleiger et al.[9] also demonstrated that decreased heart-rate variability is an important indicator of postinfarction prognosis, and Farell et al.[10] found that decreased heart-rate variability was more predictive of arrhythmic events than are late potentials. Heart-rate variability reflects the influence of the parasympathetic nervous system on the heart, which may point to an important pathway through which arrhythmias may be affected.

Another way of analyzing the effects of the autonomous nervous system is to measure baroreceptor sensitivity. It has been shown in an experimental model that the lowest levels of vagal influence in association with myocardial ischemia are associated with an increased susceptibility to sudden death.[11]

Similar to the findings in postinfarction patients, it has been demonstrated that indices of impaired left ventricular function as well as ventricular arrhythmia are determinants of the prognosis and the risk of sudden cardiac death in patients with dilated or hypertrophic cardiomyopathies.[12–15] It has also been found that sudden death is common among patients in congestive heart failure, and patients with this disorder who also have ventricular arrhythmias are at particular risk of fatal cardiovascular events.[16,17] However, in the absence of structural heart disease, frequent or unsustained complex ventricular ectopy or unsustained ventricular tachycardia is not associated with a significant incidence of serious or life-threatening ventricular arrhythmia.[18]

It is easy to draw the conclusion that a reduction in the potentially lethal arrhythmias would cause a reduction in sudden deaths among postinfarction victims, who are believed to be at high risk of sudden death owing to their proneness to arrhythmia (the arrhythmia suppression hypothesis).

Methods

The present overview is particularly concerned with the mortality results of trials that have studied both effects on ventricular arrhythmias and effects on mortality.

Owing to the above-mentioned risk of arrhythmias being particularly high in post-infarction patients, most trials have been conducted among this group of patients, but a few have been conducted in patients with supraventricular arrhythmias and in cardiac failure. It is of considerable importance that publication bias is excluded, especially as it is known that 'negative' and inconclusive studies tend to remain unpublished. However, previous overviews, for example the recent one by Teo *et al.*,[19] have tried to overcome this bias. A careful MEDLINE search has not revealed any earlier studies that were undetected by those authors. A few recently published trials have been added. No other attempts to find previously unpublished trials have been made. With the exception of some ongoing unpublished studies, primarily concerning implantable defibrillators, the conclusions drawn in the present analysis would not differ materially if single unpublished studies have been missed.

The Vaughan Williams classification[20] of arrhythmias has been used in the present overview, even though there are some doubts as to the proper classification of certain antiarrhythmic drugs. According to this classification beta-blockers and calcium blockers belong to classes II and IV, respectively. These drugs have been dealt with in Chapter 16 and thus the results concerning them are only commented on very briefly here.

The statistical method is now the accepted methodology, according to Yusuf and Peto,[21,22] of combining estimates of odds ratios. Odds ratios and the associated 95% confidence intervals (CIs) are given in all tables. Results are described for each agent and subclass of agents according to the classification mentioned above. It should be emphasized, however, that drugs may have different effects on mortality and morbidity even if they belong to the same class of drugs according to the Vaughan Williams classification. It should be emphasized at the start that many of the studies done, particularly the early ones, had a low statistical power.

Class IA Antiarrhythmics

The drugs that have been tested and the number of trials done on each of the subgroups are listed in *Table 17.1*. The mortality in trials of class IA agents is summarized in *Table 17.2*.

Quinidine

Quinidine and procainamide have the longest history of all the antiarrhythmic drugs. Quinidine came into use early in the twentieth century, principally for the re-establishment and maintenance of sinus rhythm after atrial fibrillation. Six trials reporting the effects of quinidine on these arrhythmias as well as on mortality have been published.[23–28]

All the trials were very small. The blinding in the earlier trials may be questioned, but this may be of limited importance in regard to total mortality, which is reported here. In the meta-analysis published by Coplen *et al.*,[29] the pooled findings were a significantly improved prevalence of patients in sinus rhythm after 3, 6, and 12 months of cardioversion with 69%, 58%, and 50% in sinus rhythm in the quinidine group compared with 45%, 33%, and 25%, respectively, in the placebo groups ($P < 0.0001$ at all time intervals). There were 12 deaths in the quinidine groups and 3 in the placebo groups, i.e. there was an increased

Table 17.1 Summary of trials of class IA antiarrhythmic agents

Agent	No. of trials	No. of patients
Quinidine:		
Atrial fibrillation[23–28]	6	800
Myocardial infarction[30,31]	2	207
Procainamide[33–37]	5	364
Imipramine[38]	1	202
Disopyramide[39–45]	7	2912
Moricizine[38,46]	3	2897

Table 17.2 Mortality in trials of class IA antiarrhythmic agents

Agent	No. deaths/Total No. patients		Odds ratio (95% CI)	P
	Active	Control		
Quinidine:				
Atrial fibrillation	12/413	3/387	2.98 (1.07–8.33)	0.05
Myocardial infarction	10/94	6/113	2.05 (0.73–5.78)	0.17
Procainamide	15/182	19/182	0.77 (0.38–1.56)	0.46
Disopyramide	104/1460	98/1452	1.06 (0.80–1.41)	0.68
Imipramine	7/102	6/100	1.15 (0.38–3.54)	0.80
Moricizine	117/1454	88/1443	1.39 (1.04–1.87)	0.02
Total	265/3705	220/3677	1.22 (1.01–1.47)	0.02

mortality in the quinidine-treated groups (odds ratio (OR) 2.98; $P < 0.05$) (Table 17.2). Deaths were usually due to various cardiovascular causes, there being no clear tendency for any specific cause.

Quinidine has also been effective in the treatment of ventricular arrhythmias, and this effect logically led to its use in the prevention of these arrhythmias after myocardial infarction. Two controlled trials reporting on mortality in this condition have been published.[30,31] The first of these trials (104 infarction patients) could not definitely determine whether quinidine had an effect on ventricular arrhythmias, whereas the second one (103 infarction patients) found a significantly lower incidence of ventricular tachycardia with quinidine. However, mortality in the first mentioned study[30] was non-significantly higher in patients receiving quinidine (9/49 versus 4/55), whereas there was a slightly lower mortality on quinidine in the second study (4/45 and 6/58, respectively). The pooled results of these two trials gave a nonsignificant doubling of mortality in the quinidine treated group (Table 17.2).

Morganroth and Goin[32] compared results from four trials in which quinidine had been compared with other antiarrhythmic drugs in a total of 1009 patients. Quinidine ($n = 502$) was compared to flecainide ($n = 141$), mexilitine ($n = 246$), tocainide ($n = 67$), and propafenone ($n = 53$); there were 12 deaths with quinidine compared to 4 with the other drugs ($P = 0.05$).

Procainamide

Procainamide also has a rather long history, and has a similar use to that of quinidine. Five trials reporting its effect and associated mortality in myocardial infarction have been published.[33-37] In the hospital-based study of acute infarctions by Koch-Weser et al.,[33] the percentage of patients with ventricular tachycardia and fibrillation was 38% in the placebo group and 19% in the actively treated group ($P < 0.01$). The mortality experience seemed to be positive: three deaths in the placebo group, none in the procainamide group. The other hospital trial in acute myocardial infarction[35] found no effect of procainamide on ventricular fibrillation or on mortality in 106 patients.

The three long-term trials[34,36,37] tended to show fewer major arrhythmias and a nonsignificant trend towards lower mortality on active treatment (*Table 17.2*). The pooled mortality results of all five trials showed a tendency to lower mortality for the actively treated versus placebo groups ($P = 0.46$). However, procainamide was not widely used owing to the high incidence of toxic reactions; in the study by Kosowsky et al.,[37] after 6 months, 50% of the patients had stopped taking the drug because of side-effects. Arthralgia was the commonest subjective side-effect, and in that trial all patients who took the drug for 1 year or longer had a positive antinuclear factor test.

Imipramine

Imipramine has been tested only in one small randomized controlled trial ($n = 202$),[38] which showed a nonsignificant effect on mortality, less efficacy regarding arrhythmias, and more side-effects with imipramine than with the other antiarrhythmics tested. Imipramine was thus not accepted for inclusion in the Cardiac Arrhythmia Suppression Trial (CAST) (see below).

Disopyramide

Disopyramide has been compared against placebo in seven randomized controlled trials.[39-45] Six studies included patients in the acute phase of myocardial infarction. In total, more patients ($n = 2912$) were studied in these trials than in any of the others discussed so far. The effects of disopyramide were positive on the incidence of ventricular arrhythmias, but mixed with regard to mortality; a significant reduction in mortality ($P = 0.0025$) was found by Zainal et al.,[41] but a nonsignificant tendency towards increased mortality was found when the results of all studies were combined (OR 1.06, 95% CI 0.80–1.41).

Moricizine

Moricizine was used in the Cardiac Arrhythmia Pilot Study (CAPS)[38] and the CAST trial.[46] The drug had an acceptable effect on ventricular arrhythmias according to CAPS, but in CAST it showed an increased mortality in the 14-day period: 17/665 of the moricizine patients died or had cardiac arrest as compared with 3/660 patients on placebo. In the long-term phase there was a tendency in the same direction, with 49 versus 42 deaths in the moricizine and placebo groups, respectively ($P = 0.40$). The CAST trial will be elaborated in more detail later in this chapter.

Conclusions

When all trials of class IA agents are pooled, a significantly increased mortality emerges (OR 1.22, 95% CI 1.01–1.47).

Class IB Antiarrhythmics

The drugs that have been tested and the number of trials done are listed in *Table 17.3*. The results on mortality are given in *Table 17.4*.

Lidocaine

Of the Class IB antiarrhythmics, lidocaine has been the most frequently used and studied in the acute phase of a myocardial infarction. Originally, so-called 'warning arrhythmias' were considered to be highly sensitive and specific in predicting ventricular fibrillation, but this concept was later questioned. It was found that ventricular ectopic beats occurred in only half of patients who developed primary ventricular fibrillation and with similar frequency among those who did not. In fact, lidocaine was routinely used as prophylaxis for ventricular fibrillation for several years in many coronary care units based on the concept of monitoring and treating 'warning arrhythmias', and its use was also recommended in several editorials[47,48] and reviews.[49,50] The recommendations were, however, not based on strong, conclusive evidence from randomized controlled trials.

Ten trials analyzed intravenous administration[51–60] and seven studied intramuscular administration.[61–67] One of the trials was single-blind, three were open, and the rest were double-blind trials. All were short-term, the total time of drug treatment not exceeding 48 hours.

Table 17.3 Summary of trials of class IB antiarrhythmic agents

Agent	No. of trials	No. of patients
Lidocaine[51–67]	17	10 115
Tocainide[68–72]	6	1446
Phenytoin[73,74]	2	718
Mexiletine[34,75–80]	7	1734

Table 17.4 Mortality in trials of class IB antiarrhythmic agents

Agent	No. deaths/Total No. patients		Odds ratio (95% CI)	P
	Active	Control		
Lidocaine	156/5116	123/4999	1.25 (0.97–1.60)	0.07
Tocainide	20/721	23/725	0.87 (0.47–1.60)	0.66
Phenytoin	41/359	40/359	1.04 (0.65–1.65)	0.88
Mexiletine	89/872	89/862	0.99 (0.72–1.36)	0.94
Total	306/7068	275/6945	1.06 (0.89–1.26)	0.50

Various exclusion criteria were used, such as previous ventricular fibrillation or tachycardia, congestive heart failure, cardiogenic shock, hypotension, and bradycardia. In some trials patients were only eligible if they presented within 6 hours of onset of symptoms. In several trials patients were randomized before a diagnosis of myocardial infarction had been confirmed, and outcome data were often only reported for patients with definite infarctions. However, because the incidence of ventricular fibrillation and death was very low in the noninfarction patients, these exclusions will not materially affect the conclusions drawn here.

The overall result of these trials was a decrease in incidence of about one-third in ventricular fibrillation in the lidocaine groups, the decrease being of borderline significance ($P = 0.04$), and a nonsignificant trend toward excess mortality for lidocaine compared with controls (OR 1.25, 95% CI 0.97–1.60; $P = 0.07$) (*Table 17.4*). However, only in one trial[64] was the reduction in ventricular fibrillation significant, and this trial contributed substantially to the overall result on ventricular fibrillation. In fact the result of this trial was significantly different from the results on ventricular fibrillation obtained in the trials overall.

A major problem with lidocaine prophylaxis was the high incidence of adverse reactions. Central nervous system disturbances were common; these were usually of mild nature, but convulsions and syncope occurred in 2% of patients.[55]

Tocainide

Tocainide is a structural analog of lidocaine with high oral availability and a long half-life. It can also be given intravenously. It was a logical step in the light of the arrhythmia suppression hypothesis to try this drug in the long-term follow-up of postinfarction patients owing to their high rate of sudden, arrhythmia-associated deaths. The drug has been tested in six trials, of which four were short-term and two were long-term.[68–72] A total of 1446 patients were included in these randomized trials. Although some authors reported reductions in ventricular ectopic beats with the drug, there was no established effect on the serious arrhythmias, such as ventricular tachycardia or fibrillation. None of the studies reported a significant effect of tocainide on mortality, and the overview shows 20/721 deaths for the active drug as compared to 23/725 deaths with placebo (OR 0.87, 95% CI 0.47–1.60). The effect of the drug during long-term follow-up could not be evaluated owing to few events. Central nervous system side-effects were uncommon.

Phenytoin

Phenytoin was one of the very early drugs tested to reduce the incidence of ventricular arrhythmias. Two controlled trials with a total of 718 patients and planned for a 1–2 year follow-up have been conducted.[73,74] Neither trial showed any significant effect on mortality, and the combined effect was zero: 41/359 deaths on active treatment and 40/359 in controls. Owing to great variations in plasma concentrations between patients the drug is difficult to monitor, and never became widely used.

Mexiletine

Mexiletine has been tested in seven trials, of which six started early after an acute randomized. Patient groups were stratified according to clinic center, ejection fraction, and time after myocardial infarction.

The primary endpoint was death from arrhythmia, which included witnessed instantaneous death in the absence of severe congestive heart failure or shock, unwitnessed death with no preceding change in symptoms and for which no other cause could be ascribed, and cardiac arrest.

CAST was designed as a one-tailed statistical test and was intended to assess whether drug therapy was beneficial or had no beneficial effect, with an α value of 0.025 and a power of approximately 0.85. The study was not designed to prove that the antiarrhythmic drug could cause harm. It was projected that the incidence of the primary endpoint in the placebo group would be 11% during 3 years of follow-up, and active treatment would reduce this incidence by 30%. The estimated required sample size was 4400 patients. The data and safety monitoring board for the trial projected meetings twice yearly to monitor the data. A monitoring protocol and stopping rules were set up before the board started its monitoring work. The boundaries were designed to be adaptable to the number of arrhythmic events expected by the planned end of the study. This number was initially estimated to be 425. The board received endpoint data by group, but was blinded with regard to which of the groups were given placebo or active drug.

On March 30, 1989, a total of 2309 patients had been recruited and had completed or were undergoing open-label titration. Suppression of arrhythmias had been achieved in 1727 patients, and 1455 had been assigned to encainide, flecainide, or placebo, and 272 to moricizine or placebo. The board met on April 16–17, 1989, and found that the actively treated group as a whole had crossed the boundary for harm (set boundary $Z = -3.11$; observed $Z = -3.22$). Additional subgroup analysis revealed that this adverse finding was limited to encainide and flecainide. Thus, the study was recommended to be stopped for these two drugs but to continue for moricizine, with the investigators remaining blinded to the effects of moricizine.

The baseline characteristics of the actively treated group were very similar to those of the placebo group in all relevant variables. The mortality in the two groups is shown in *Table 17.7*. Deaths from arrhythmia, nonarrhythmic cardiac events and total mortality were all higher among patients assigned to encainide/flecainide, than to placebo, and no significant differences were found between encainide and flecainide. Subgroup analyses of baseline covariates revealed a remarkable consistency of drug effect, that is encainide/flecainide were harmful or could not be evaluated because of a lack of endpoints.

Thus, this study clearly demonstrated that suppression of ventricular arrhythmias after myocardial infarction did not confer any benefit; on the contrary, it increased mortality with the drugs tested. The adverse experience also with moricizine, a class IA drug, points

Table 17.7 Events in patients randomized to encainide/flecainide or placebo in CAST[46]

Variable	Encainide/flecainide ($n = 730$)	Placebo ($n = 725$)
Average exposure (days)	293	300
Arrhythmia/sudden death	33	9
Other cardiac death	14	6
Noncardiac/unclassified cause	9	7
Total deaths and cardiac arrests	56	22

towards a more general effect of the class I antiarrhythmic agents, and not merely to a toxicity of the specific drugs. According to CAPS these drugs had shown outstanding suppression of arrhythmia. Other drugs had been reviewed and had been excluded from testing because other studies had suggested they were less effective in suppressing arrhythmias or had adverse effects that made them unsuitable for long-term use. For some newer drugs, there was not sufficient experience in their use to include them in the trial.

The study was started on the assumption that arrhythmia suppression would be beneficial, and that the initial open-label phase was safe. The later experience with moricizine, which was discussed earlier in this chapter, indicates that this assumption was probably wrong. As the open-label phase was not randomized between encainide/ flecainide and placebo it can never be revealed whether there was also already an increased mortality in this phase, as was shown in the continuation of the trial with moricizine.

In summary, this trial has clearly demonstrated the risk of relying on a surrogate endpoint such as ventricular arrhythmias, as well as the importance of planning trials with well-designed protocols, strong statistical power, and clear guidelines for the data and monitoring board. Blinding of the board with regard to treatment allocation may be hazardous, especially if the cause-specific, drug-induced mortality is of similar pattern as the usual mortality in the disease under study.

Explanatory analyses to elucidate the mechanisms of the adverse drug effects and several studies of predictors of mortality have been performed.[84,85] The vast majority of excess deaths appeared to be the result of an increase in arrhythmia events without any protective effect of the drug.

Class II Antiarrhythmics

This class contains the beta-blockers, which have been dealt with in Chapter 16. Several overviews have shown positive effects of these drugs on total mortality, due to a reduction in sudden deaths as well as the effects on nonfatal recurrences.[19,86] According to the overview by Teo *et al.*[19] based on 1464 deaths among 26 973 patients in the beta-blocker groups versus 1727 deaths among 26 295 patients in the placebo groups, the odds ratio for mortality was 0.81 (95% CI 0.75–0.87; $P = 0.00001$). Thus, the effects found in trials of beta-blockers in postinfarction patients are very convincing. It has been shown in postinfarction studies based on nonselected patients from the general population in Sweden that about 70% of patients do not have contraindications to this treatment, and presumably benefit from it.[87]

Beta-blockers are not particularly effective on ventricular premature contractions in general, and thus their ability to reduce myocardial ischemia and their possible effects on the sympathetic nervous system in the brain by increasing vagal tone[88] are probably the most important mechanisms for their beneficial effects in reducing ventricular fibrillation and sudden death.

Class III Antiarrhythmics

This group contains only one drug, namely amiodarone. Twelve placebo-controlled trials have been published[89–102] (*Table 17.8*).

The 12 trials were conducted both in patients after myocardial infarction and in cardiac arrest are randomized to amiodarone or implantable defibrillator, with a recruitment goal of 400 patients, to be followed for 1 year each.

The Antiarrhythmics Versus Implantable Defibrillators (AVID) study compares a defibrillator approach with treatment with either amiodarone or sotalol.[115] A pilot study with 200 patients was completed in 1994, and an additional 1000 patients will be enrolled until March 1997 and followed until September 1998.

General Comments

It is evident from this overview that a reduction in ventricular ectopic beats, despite their documented increased risk for sudden (arrhythmic) death, does not uniformly lead to reduced mortality. On the contrary, class I antiarrhythmic drugs have a strong tendency to increase mortality. It is evident that none of the single studies, except for the CAST studies, showed a statistically adverse outcome for the active drug versus placebo. However, homogeneity testing performed by several researchers has not shown any significant variation between the results of these drugs, which all act through similar mechanisms.

Class II drugs (beta-blockers) have been subjected to many trials, and the overview results are convincingly positive. They have become used routinely in many patients.

At present class III contains only one drug, amiodarone. The summary results are presently positive.

Class IV drugs (calcium blockers) do not show a uniform trend to either positive or negative treatment effects. Those that increase heart rate tend to increase mortality ($P = 0.06$), whereas those that reduce heart rate might have a beneficial effect; however, the data on this difference are far from significant ($P = 0.46$).

The mode of action of antiarrhythmic drugs, and thus the possibility of preventing sudden death, is apparently much more complicated than was appreciated when these drugs first become available. For many years drugs that have not been adequately tested in randomized controlled trials have been widely used until they were found to increase mortality in spite of beneficial effects on the surrogate endpoint, ventricular ectopic beats. This experience shows us the importance of conducting well-designed, adequately large, statistically high-powered trials before treatment is distributed to a large number of patients. In the area of arrhythmias, such trials also must be performed on the implantable cardioverter defibrillator as well as with any new antiarrhythmic drug that may give hopes of benefit.

References

1. Moore TJ. Why tens of thousands of heart patients died in America's worst drug disaster. In: Moore TJ (ed.), *Deadly Medicine*. New York: Simon & Schuster, 1995.
2. Roberts R, Husain A, Ambos HD, Oliver GC, Cox Jr JR, Sobel BE. Relation between infarct size and ventricular arrhythmia. *Br Heart J* 1975; **37**: 1169–75.
3. Califf RM, McKinnis RA, Burks J, *et al.* Prognostic implications of ventricular arrhythmias during 24-hour ambulatory monitoring in patients undergoing cardiac catheterization for coronary artery disease. *Am J Cardiol* 1982; **50**: 23–31.
4. Bigger Jr JT, Fleiss JL, Kleiger R, *et al.*, and the Multicenter Post-Infarction Research Group. The relationship among ventricular arrhythmias, left ventricular dysfunction, and mortality in the 2 years after myocardial infarction. *Circulation* 1984; **69**: 250–8.
5. Mukharji J, Rude RE, Poole WK, *et al.*, and the MILIS Study Group. Risk factors for sudden death after acute myocardial infarction: two-year follow-up. *Am J Cardiol* 1984; **54**: 31–6.
6. Kuchar DL, Thorburn CW, Sammel NL. Prediction of serious arrhythmic events after myocardial infarction: signal-averaged electrocardiogram, Holter monitoring and radionuclide ventriculography. *J Am Coll Cardiol* 1987; **9**: 531–8.
7. Gomes JA, Winters SL, Martinson M, Machac J, Stewart D, Targonski A. The prognostic significance of quantitative

signal-averaged variables relative to clinical variables, site of myocardial infarction, ejection fraction and ventricular beats: a prospective study. *J Am Coll Cardiol* 1989; **13**: 377–84.

8. Denniss AR, Richards DA, Cody DV, *et al*. Prognostic significance of ventricular tachycardia and fibrillation induced at programmed stimulation and delayed potentials detected on the signal-averaged electrocardiograms of survivors of acute myocardial infarction. *Circulation* 1986; **74**: 731–45.

9. Kleiger RE, Miller JP, Bigger JT, Moss AJ. The Multicenter Post-Infarction Research Group. Decreased heart rate variability and its association with increased mortality after acute myocardial infarction. *Am J Cardiol* 1987; **59**: 256–62.

10. Farrell TG, Bashir Y, Cripps T, *et al*. Risk stratification for arrhythmic events in post-infarction patients based on heart rate variability, ambulatory electrocardiographic variables and the signal-averaged electrocardiogram. *J Am Coll Cardiol* 1991; **18**: 687–97.

11. Schwartz PJ, La Rovere MT, Vanoli E. Autonomic nervous system and sudden cardiac death: experimental basis and clinical observations for post-myocardial infarction risk stratification. *Circulation* 1992; **85**: 177–91.

12. Surgrue DD, Rodeheffer RJ, Codd MB, Ballard DJ, Fuster V, Gersh BJ. The clinical course of idiopatic dilated cardiomyopathy: a population-based study. *Ann Intern Med* 1992; **117**: 117–23.

13. Wilson JR, Schwartz JS, St John Sutton M, *et al*. Prognosis in severe heart failure: relation to hemodynamic measurements and ventricular ectopic activity. *J Am Coll Cardiol* 1983; **21**: 403–10.

14. Francis GS. Development of arrhythmias in the patient with congestive heart failure: pathophysiology, prevalence and prognosis. *Am J Cardiol* 1986; **57**: 3B–7B.

15. McKenna WJ, Chetty S, Oakley CM. Exercise electrocardiographic and 48-hour ambulatory electrocardiographic monitor assessment of arrhythmia on and off beta-blocker therapy in hypertrophic cardiomyopathy. *Am J Cardiol* 1979; **43**: 420 (abstract).

16. Meinertz TE, Hoffman T, Kasper W. *et al*. Significance of ventricular arrhythmias in idiopathic dilated cardiomyopathy. *Am J Cardiol* 1984; **53**: 902–7.

17. Unverferth DV, Magorien RD, Moeschberger ML, Baker PB, Fetters JK, Leier CV. Factors influencing one-year mortality of dilated cardiomyopathy. *Am J Cardiol* 1984; **54**: 147–52.

18. Kennedy HL, Whitlock JA, Sprague MK, Kennedy LJ, Buckingham TA, Goldberg RJ. Long-term follow-up of asymptomatic healthy subjects with frequent and complex ventricular ectopy. *N Engl J Med* 1985; **312**: 193–7.

19. Teo KT, Yusuf S, Furberg C. Effects of prophylactic antiarrhythmic drug therapy in acute myocardial infarction. An overview of results from randomized controlled trials. *JAMA* 1993; **270**: 1589–95.

20. Vaughan Williams EM. Classification of antiarrhythmic drugs. In: Sandöe E, Flensted-Jensen E, Olesen K (eds), *Cardiac Arrhythmias*. Södertälje, Sweden: AB Astra, 1981: 449–72.

21. Yusuf S, Peto R, Lewis J, Sleight P. Beta-blockade during and after myocardial infarction: an overview of the randomized trials. *Prog Cardiovasc Dis* 1985; **17**: 335–71.

22. Early Breast Cancer Trialists' Collaborative Group. Effects of adjuvant tamoxifen and of cytotoxic therapy on mortality in early breast cancer. *N Engl J Med* 1988; **319**: 1681–92.

23. Hartel G, Vouhija A, Konttinen A, Halonen PI. Value of quinidine in maintenance of sinus rhythm after electrical conversion of atrial fibrillation. *Br Heart J* 1970; **32**: 57–60.

24. Byrne-Quinn E, Wing AJ. Maintenance of sinus rhythm after DC reversion of atrial fibrillation. A double-blind controlled trial of quinidine bisulphate. *Br Heart J* 1970; **32**: 370–6.

25. Hillestad L, Bjerkelund C, Dale J, Maltau J, Storstein O. Quinidine in maintenance of sinus rhythm after electroconversion of chronic atrial fibrillation: a controlled clinical study. *Br Heart J* 1971; **33**: 518–21.

26. Södermark T, Jonsson B, Olsson A, *et al*. Effect of quinidine on maintaining sinus rhythm after conversion of atrial fibrillation or flutter: a multicentre study from Stockholm. *Br Heart J* 1975; **37**: 486–92.

27. Boissel JP, Wolf E, Gillet J, *et al*. Controlled trial of a long-acting quinidine for maintenance of sinus rhythm after conversion of sustained atrial fibrillation. *Eur Heart J* 1981; **2**: 49–55.

28. Lloyd EA, Gersh BJ, Forman R. The efficacy of quinidine and disopyramide in the maintenance of sinus rhythm after electroconversion from atrial fibrillation. *S Afr Med J* 1984; **65**: 367–9.

29. Coplen SE, Antman EM, Berlin JA, Hewitt P, Chalmers TC. Efficacy and safety of quidine therapy for maintenance of sinus rhythm after cardioversion. A meta-analysis of randomized control trials. *Circulation* 1990; **82**: 1106–16.

30. Holmberg S, Bergman H. Prophylactic quinidine treatment in myocardial infarction. A double blind study. *Acta Med Scand* 1967; **181**: 297–304.

31. Jones DT, Kostuk WJ, Gunton RW. Prophylactic quinidine for the prevention of arrhythmias after acute myocardial infarction. *Am J Cardiol* 1974; **33**: 655–60.

32. Morganroth J, Goin JE. Quinidine-related mortality in the short- to medium-term treatment of ventricular arrhythmias. A meta-analysis. *Circulation* 1991; **84**: 1977–83.

33. Koch-Weser J, Klein SW, Foo-Canto LL, Kastor JA, DeSanctis RW. Antiarrhythmic prophylaxis with procainamide in acute myocardial infarction. *N Engl J Med* 1969; **281**: 1253–60.

34. Campbell RWF, Dolder MA, Prescott LF, Talbot RG, Murray A, Julian DG. Comparison of procainamide and mexiletine in prevention of ventricular arrhythmias after acute myocardial infarction. *Lancet* 1975; **i**: 1257–9.

35. Reynell PC. Prophylactic procaine amide in myocardial infarction. *Br Heart J* 1961; **23**: 421–4.

36. Nielsen BL, Clausen J, Nielsen JS. Can procainamide improve the prognosis of patients with ventricular arrhythmias after myocardial infarction? *Dan Med Bull* 1978; **25**: 121–5.

96. Cosin J, Bayés de Luna A, Navarro F, Guindo J, Murrugat J, on behalf of the Spanish Trial on Sudden Death. Spanish Trial on Sudden Death: follow-up of 382 patients. *Circulation* 1991; **84**(Suppl): II-348 (abstract).

97. Singh SN, Fletcher RD, Fisher SG, *et al.*, for the Survival Trial of Antiarrhythmic Therapy in Congestive Heart Failure. Amiodarone in patients with congestive heart failure and asymptomatic ventricular arrhythmia. *N Engl J Med* 1995; **333**: 77–82.

98. Doval HC, Nul DR, Grancelli HO, Perrone SV, Bortman GR, Curiel R. Randomised trial of low-dose amiodarone in severe congestive heart failure. *Lancet* 1994; **344**: 493–8.

99. Camm AJ, Julian D, Janse G, *et al.*, on behalf of the EMIAT Investigators. The European Myocardial Infarct Amiodarone Trial (EMIAT). *Am J Cardiol* 1993; **72**: 95F–8F.

100. Julian DG, Camm AJ, Frangin G, *et al.*, on behalf of the EMIAT Investigators. Randomised trial of effect of amiodarone on mortality in patients with left-ventricular dysfunction after recent myocardial infarction: EMIAT. *Lancet* 1997; **349**: 667–74.

101. Cairns JA, Connolly SJ, Roberts R, Gent M, on behalf of the CAMIAT Investigators. Canadian Amiodarone Myocardial Infarction Arrhythmia Trial (CAMIAT): rationale and protocol. *Am J Cardiol* 1993; **72**: 87F–94F.

102. Cairns JA, Connolly SJ, Roberts R, Gent M, on behalf of the CAMIAT Investigators. Randomised trial of outcome after myocardial infarction in patients with frequent or repetitive ventricular premature depolarisations: CAMIAT. *Lancet* 1995; **349**: 675–82.

103. Breithardt G. Amiodarone in patients with heart failure. *Lancet* 1995; **333**: 121–2.

104. Held PH, Yusuf S, Furberg CD. Calcium channel blockers in acute myocardial infarction and unstable angina: an overview. *Br Med J* 1989; **299**: 1187–92.

105. Yusuf S, Held P, Furberg CD. Update of effects of calcium antagonists in myocardial infarction or angina in light of the Second Danish Verapamil Infarction Trial (DAVIT-II) and other recent studies. *Am J Cardiol* 1991; **67**: 1295–7.

106. Mirowski M, Reid PR, Mower MM, *et al.* Termination of malignant ventricular arrhythmias with an implanted automatic defibrillator in human beings. *N Engl J Med* 1980; **303**: 322–4.

107. Zipes DP, Heger JJ, Miles WM, *et al.* Early experience with an implantable cardioverter. *N Engl J Med* 1984; **311**: 485–90.

108. Lehmann MH, Saksena S. Implantable cardioverter defibrillators in cardiovascular practice: report of the policy conference of the North American Society of Pacing and Electrophysiology. *PACE* 1991; **14**: 969–79.

109. Newman D, Sauve MJ, Herre J, *et al.* Survival after implantation of the cardioverter defibrillator. *Am J Cardiol* 1992; **69**: 899–903.

110. Connolly SJ, Yusuf S. Evaluation of the implantable cardioverter defibrillator in survivors of cardiac arrest: the need for randomized trials. *Am J Cardiol* 1992; **69**: 959–62.

111. Yusuf S, Teo KK. Approaches to prevention of sudden death: need for fundamental reevaluation. *J Cardiovasc Electrophysiol* 1991; **2**: S233–9.

112. Moss AJ, Hall WJ, Cannom DS, *et al.*, for the Multicenter Automatic Defibrillator Implantation Trial Investigators. Improved survival with an implemented defibrillator in patients with coronary disease at high risk for ventricular arrhythmia. *N Engl J Med* 1996; **335**: 1933–40.

113. Siebels J, Cappato R, Rüppel R, Schneider MAE, Kuck KH, and the CASH investigators. Preliminary results of the Cardiac Arrest Study Hamburg (CASH). *Am J Cardiol* 1993; **72**: 109F–13F.

114. Connolly SJ, Gent M, Roberts RS, *et al.*, on behalf of the CIDS Co-Investigators. Canadian Implantable Defibrillator Study (CIDS): study design and organization. *Am J Cardiol* 1993; **72**: 103F–8F.

115. The AVID Investigators. Antiarrhythmics versus implantable defibrillators (AVID) – rationale, design, and methods. *Am J Cardiol* 1995; **75**: 470–5.

18

Heart Failure

John G. F. Cleland

Introduction

The first large double-blind placebo-controlled trial in heart failure was reported in 1986.[1] Such studies have proliferated over the ensuing 10 years, driven not only by the need to find new treatments for a condition associated with such a poor prognosis, but also the feasibility of conducting trials of short duration because of the high morbid event rate associated with heart failure.

Despite the burden of symptoms and the high morbidity and mortality associated with heart failure, treatment was very much an art rather than a science until the late 1980s. An undue emphasis was placed on vasodilator therapy during the period 1940–1980, a concept that had been developed in the previous century[2] and was reinforced by the development of technology to measure hemodynamics. Demonstration of short-term improvements in hemodynamics led to the licensing of drugs such as prazosin for heart failure, now generally held to be useless or harmful in heart failure.

The first multicenter study of the benefits of treatment with an angiotensin converting enzyme (ACE) inhibitor was reported in 1983.[3] The demonstration that cardiologists could work together to provide a critical mass of patients rapidly led to a move away from measuring surrogate endpoints, such as hemodynamics, exercise performance, and ejection fraction, and towards measuring endpoints that really matter to those who suffer from heart failure (*Table 18.1*). For this change we are indebted not only to our US, Canadian and Scandinavian colleagues, but also to the pharmaceutical industry, which supported the trials, the US Veterans organization, and the US National Heart, Lung, and Blood Institute.

Clinical trials are imperfect, but continue to evolve. Trials conducted in one country may not accurately reflect the impact of the same drug in another owing to differences in etiology of disease, background therapy, or cultural differences in such things as the readiness to hospitalize a patient (physician and institutional remuneration can put a heavy positive or negative bias on such endpoints). Recent trials have adapted to these criticisms by becoming much more international in their recruitment. It is to be hoped that this trend will continue.

It can also be argued that clinical trials in heart failure have become obsessed with large numbers. Although large numbers are required to show differences in mortality in mild heart failure, a trial that *requires* several hundred patients to show an improvement in symptoms suggests that any benefit is weak, uncertain, and of dubious clinical value.

Only trials addressing mortality as a part or the whole of the primary endpoint are

Table 18.1   Goals of treatment in congestive heart failure

- Reduce mortality
- Improve or maintain the quality of life:
  - by reducing symptoms of disease
  - by avoiding side-effects of drugs and procedures
  - by preventing morbidity (e.g. myocardial infarction, hospitalization)

reported here, with the exception of trials of digoxin as, at the time of writing, the results of the Digoxin Investigators Group (DIG) trial were not fully in the public domain. Also, at the time of writing several trials had not been formally published; these are indicated as it is recognized that data in preliminary and final reports may differ slightly owing to an incomplete database at the time of the initial report. All the trials reported in this chapter were analyzed on an intention-to-treat basis, were conducted double-blind and were placebo controlled, with seven exceptions. The Randomized Trial of Low-Dose Amiodarone in Severe Congestive Heart Failure (GESICA)[4] and Accupril Congestive Heart Failure Investigation and Economic Variable Evaluation (ACHIEVE)[5] are randomized open-label studies but were, or will be, analyzed on an intention-to-treat basis; thus mortality, at least, remains a valid outcome unlikely to have been biased by knowledge of treatment. The Veterans Affairs Cooperative Study on Vasodilator Therapy of Heart Failure[11] (V-HeFT-II)[6] compared the combination of hydralazine plus nitrate with enalapril, and lacked a placebo control. The Assessment of Treatment with Lisinopril and Survival (ATLAS), a Triple Blind, Parallel Group Study of the Effects of Enalapril Dose on Incidence of Hospitalisation and Mortality in Patients with Symptomatic Heart Failure[11] (NETWORK), and ACHIEVE studies[5] compare different doses of lisinopril, enalapril, and quinapril, respectively, and did not have a placebo control. The primary analysis of the captopril plus digoxin multicenter trial[7] was for patients remaining on treatment, although an intention-to-treat analysis was also performed. The comparative trial of digoxin and captopril by Just *et al.*[8] had no placebo control. All the trials reported here can be considered of high quality, and have had an impact on clinical research and practice.

Controlled Trials of ACE Inhibitors against Placebo or another 'Active' Agent

The demography, comparisons, and results of the four trials that established the mortality benefit of ACE inhibitors are shown in *Tables 18.2* and *18.3*.[6,9–11]

Entry Criteria and Study Populations

The Cooperative North Scandinavian Enalapril Survival Study (CONSENSUS)[9] required only a clinical diagnosis of heart failure. Although it is clear that most patients did have an echocardiogram as part of their evaluation,[12] objective evidence of cardiac dysfunction at entry was not required.

Patients could be entered into the V-HeFT-II study[6] if they met one of three criteria for cardiac dysfunction combined with a peak oxygen consumption of <25 ml kg^{-1} min^{-1}. The criteria for cardiac dysfunction were either a cardiothoracic ratio of >0.55 on chest X-ray, an echocardiographic left ventricular end-diastolic dimension (LVEDD) of >2.7 cm m^2, or a radionuclide ejection fraction (EF) of $<45\%$. It should be noted that a large adult

Table 18.2 Baseline characteristics of patients in trials comparing ACE inhibitors with placebo or another 'active' agent

	CONSENSUS	V-HeFT-II	SOLVD Treatment	SOLVD Prevention
No. Randomized	253	804	2569	4228
No. screened (% excluded)	Not given	2741 (71%)	55069 (T + P) (88%)	
Age (years)	71	61	61	59
Follow-up (years)	0.5	2.5	3.5	3.1
Gender (%F/%M)	29/71	0/100	20/80	11/89
NYHA I + II/III/IV	All grade IV	57/43/0	68/30/2	100/0/0
Current angina (%)	Not given	Not given	38	34
CAD (%)	73	53	71	83
DCM (%)	15	Not given	18	9
Hypertension (%)	22	48	42	37
Diabetes (%)	23	20	26	15
Atrial fibrillation (%)	50	14	10	4
Heart rate (bpm)	80	78	80	75
Systolic BP (mmHg)	120	126	125	125
EF (%)	Not given	29	25	28
Diuretics (%)	100 (98 loop)	100?	85 (75 loop)	18 (7 loop)
Digoxin (%)	93	100?	67	12
Other vasodilator (%)	52	61	51	47
Beta-blocker/calcium antagonist (%)	3/?	Not given	8/31	24/35
Aspirin/warfarin (%)	??/34	30/15[a]	33/16	54/12

BP, Blood pressure; CAD, coronary artery disease; DCM dilated cardiomyopathy; EF, ejection fraction; NYHA, New York Heart Association.
[a]Percentage of the duration of the study treated either with warfarin or aspirin.

man would have a body surface area (BSA) of around 2 m^2 and thus the qualifying left ventricular diastolic dimension would have been only 54 mm (i.e. within the normal range for many laboratories), although the mean LVEDD was 68 mm.

Patients could be entered into the Studies of Left Ventricular Dysfunction (SOLVD) if they had an EF of <35% and were <80 years of age.[10,11,13–16] In 68% of patients the EF was measured by radionuclide ventriculography, in 21% by echocardiography, and in 11% by contrast angiography. No attempt was made to substantiate the quality of the EF measurements using any of the above methods. It is clear that there are large differences in the measurement of EF between methods and between centers, and the reproducibility of EF even in the same patient at the same center is limited. The <35% entry criterion in SOLVD should be interpreted merely as evidence of substantial impairment of left ventricular systolic function.

Patients in SOLVD were subdivided into those with evidence of heart failure requiring treatment (SOLVD–treatment[11]) for that condition, and those without evidence of heart failure and not receiving treatment for heart failure (SOLVD–prevention[10]). It is likely that some protocol violation took place at this stage, accounting for the 7% of patients in SOLVD–prevention taking loop diuretics and the higher number of patients taking digoxin than had atrial fibrillation.[15] About 25% of patients in SOLVD–treatment were not taking loop diuretics, indicating that many patients had rather mild heart failure.

Patients with recent myocardial infarction, severe or unstable angina, major pulmonary or renal dysfunction, or standard contraindications to ACE inhibitors were excluded from all three studies. Patients with angina limiting exercise were excluded from V-HeFT-II, but more than one-third of patients in the SOLVD trials had angina.

Table 18.3 Comparisons in and results of trials comparing ACE inhibitors with placebo or another 'active agent'

Trial	Comparison and target dose	Dose achieved	Withdrawals (%)	Myocardial infarction, n (%)	Worsening CHF	Hospitalizations, n (%)		Total mortality, n (%)	Mortality/ annum[a]
						Total	CHF		
CONSENSUS	Enalapril 20 mg b.d. (n = 127)	9.2 mg b.d.	17	One withdrawal in each group due to MI	??	102 (80)[c]	??	50 (39) RRR 27%; P < 0.001	36
	vs								
	Placebo (n = 126)	'13.7 mg b.d.' (P < 0.001)	14 (NS)		??	108 (86)[c]	??	68 (54)[d]	52
V-HeFT-II	Enalapril 10 mg b.d. (n = 403)	7.5 mg b.d.	22	20	??	183 (45) (NS)	76 (19) (NS)	132 (33) (RRR 13%; P = 0.08)	13
	vs								
	Hydralazine 75 mg q.i.d. + Nitrate 40 mg q.i.d. (n = 401)	50 mg q.i.d. + 25 mg q.i.d.	29/31	22	??	185 (46)	78 (19)	153 (38)[d]	15
SOLVD: treatment	Enalapril 10 mg b.d. (n = 1285)	8.4 mg b.d.[b] 49% Top dose	33	127 (10) (RRR 23%, P = 0.02)	182[c] (14) (RRR 44%; P < 0.01)	893 (69) (RRR 7%; P < 0.01)	332 (26) (RRR 30%; P < 0.0001)	452 (35) (RRR 16%; P < 0.005)	10
	vs								
	Placebo (n = 1284)	'9.0 mg b.d.' 49% Top dose	42	158 (12)	320 (25)	950 (74)	470 (37)	510 (40)	11
SOLVD: prevention	Enalapril 10 mg b.d. (n = 2111)	8.4 mg b.d.[b]	24	161 (8) (RRR 24%, P = 0.01)	102 (5) (RRR 50, P < 0.01)	1167 (55) (NS)	184 (9) (RRR 31%; P < 0.001)	313 (15) (RRR 8%; NS)	4.8
	vs								
	Placebo (n = 2117)	Not reported	27	204 (9)	218 (10)	1202 (57)	273 (13)	334 (16)	5.1

b.d., twice daily; CHF, congestive heart failure; q.i.d., four times daily; RRR, relative risk reduction.

[a]Crude average rate (i.e. total mortality/duration) except in the case of the CONSENSUS study (mean duration 0.5 years) where actual 1-year mortality is given. The values listed can be used to calculate the numbers of lives saved by treating 100 patients for 1 year (Active% − Placebo% = Lives saved/100 treated).

[b]Of those taking medicine.

[c]Patients randomized to placebo spent 3696 days in hospital versus 3818 randomized to enalapril. Owing to the improved survival, this represented 19.6% of study days on placebo, but only 15.0% of days on enalapril.

[d]Data given here are for total mortality. This was not the primary endpoint of CONSENSUS or V-HeFT-II. RRR in mortality for the primary endpoint at 6 months in CONSENSUS was 40% (P = 0.002) and in V-HeFT-II at 2 years was 28% (P = 0.016).

The CONSENSUS study did not report how many patients were screened, but as only patients with New York Heart Association (NYHA) grade IV heart failure could be enrolled this was a very selected group. The V-HeFT-II and SOLVD trials excluded 70–90% of patients who had already met the basic entry criteria of age and the prespecified entry criteria for cardiac dysfunction. Thus, SOLVD and V-HeFT-II were also much more highly selective studies than their entry criteria might suggest.

Patients in the V-HeFT-II and SOLVD trials were over a decade younger than the average age of patients with heart failure in the community.[17] This may reflect the origin of the patients in V-HeFT-II and the age limit imposed in the SOLVD trials. It is also possible that the EF criteria in SOLVD excluded many older patients, many of whom appear to have heart failure in the absence of a severely depressed EF. The mean age of patients in the CONSENSUS trial, which did not have an EF entry criterion, comes close to that observed in the community. The trials generally show a larger proportion of patients with dilated cardiomyopathy than is observed in community studies. This may reflect better work-up of patients in clinical trials or more guesswork; community studies of dilated cardiomyopathy show that many patients are given this label without a coronary angiogram which, if done, frequently shows coronary disease.[18] The community studies have got round this problem by categorizing about a third of patients with heart failure as 'cause uncertain', to which 'an educated guess' can be added as a subscript.[17,19,20] The proportion of patients with atrial filbrillation and diabetes appear appropriate to the population under study. Digoxin use in the V-HeFT-II and SOLVD treatments was relatively high.

Endpoint Definitions

A primary endpoint of all four trials was all-cause mortality, prespecified as the mortality at 6 months in CONSENSUS, and at 2 years and overall in V-HeFT-II. An additional primary endpoint in CONSENSUS was the 'cause of death'.

The V-HeFT-II trials censored patients from further analysis if they underwent transplantation, an appropriate method of handling this issue, at least if more patients are dying on the transplant waiting list than are being transplanted.

Although all the trials described a classification of the mode or cause of death, only CONSENSUS gave any sort of definition, and in no trial can the definitions be considered satisfactory.[21,22] This was partially overcome in V-HeFT-II and CONSENSUS by the use of an endpoints committee, but the definition was left to the investigator in SOLVD.[22]

All the trials reported hospitalization for heart failure and for all causes. However, only in SOLVD was heart-failure-related hospitalization a prespecified outcome.

A number of subsequent reports from the CONSENSUS study described long-term outcome, effects on renal function, general tolerability, and the influence of neuroendocrine factors.[12,23–26]

Other secondary outcome measures in V-HeFT-II included quality-of-life questionnaires, EF, exercise performance, and plasma noradrenaline.[27–41] Additional secondary-outcome measures in SOLVD were myocardial infarction (although originally included as a check on safety because of predicted harm, and therefore has to be treated with some circumspection) and quality of life. A number of substudies investigated exercise tolerance, ventricular function, neuroendocrine function, and arrhythmias.[13–16,42–64] The SOLVD-prevention trial had the onset of heart failure as an additional outcome.

Treatment Compliance

Compliance with study medication appeared good in CONSENSUS, partly because of the short duration of follow-up. In the V-HeFT-II and SOLVD treatment trials, around 25% of patients withdrew from enalapril, 42% from placebo, and about 30% from hydralazine and/or nitrates. A reduction in worsening heart failure appears to account for most of the better compliance with ACE inhibitor than with placebo. About one-half of patients tolerated the full dose of 10 mg twice daily in SOLVD. In CONSENSUS 22% of patients were titrated to the top dose of enalapril (20 mg b.d.), but only 45% to the notional top dose of placebo, indicating a reluctance of investigators to use high doses, regardless of drug effect.

Hypotension was the major reported reason for withdrawal in CONSENSUS. The reasons for withdrawal in V-HeFT-II are not clear, except that headache and palpitation were more frequently reported as the cause for those receiving hydralizine plus nitrates. Only a few patients assigned to either treatment regimen subsequently received the alternative open-label treatment. In SOLVD–treatment more than half the patients withdrawn were subsequently placed on an open-label ACE inhibitor for worsening heart failure. About one-third ($n = 218$) of patients withdrawing from placebo in the SOLVD–prevention trial did so because of worsening heart failure and 19% ($n = 396$) of patients initially randomized to placebo subsequently received an open-label ACE inhibitor.

The high crossover rates in the long-term ACE inhibitor trials greatly reduces the apparent effect of enalapril on mortality on an intention-to-treat analysis. Withdrawal of patients from enalapril, who were not infrequently treated subsequently with an open-label ACE inhibitor, will have had little effect. Treating patients randomized to placebo with an ACE inhibitor may have markedly reduced the placebo mortality, not only because of a general beneficial effect of ACE inhibitors, but also because it was probably those patients at greatest risk of dying, that is those who were deteriorating, who were targeted for open-label ACE inhibitor treatment. A retrospective comparison of V-HeFT-I and -II data supports this view;[6] ACE inhibitors were not considered routine treatment during the V-HeFT-I study. The true impact of an ACE inhibitor may be to reduce mortality by up to 50%, even in mild to moderate heart failure, rather than by the 16% suggested by SOLVD.

What the Studies Showed: Primary Endpoints

The CONSENSUS study showed a 40% relative risk reduction (RRR) in mortality at 6 months (22 lives saved out of 126 treated; $P = 0.002$). All the benefit could be attributed to a reduction in mortality due to a progression of heart failure.

The V-HeFT-II showed a 28% RRR in mortality at 2 years (about 27 lives saved of 403 treated; $P = 0.016$) and 11% overall (21 lives saved of 403 treated; $P = 0.08$).

The SOLVD–treatment trial showed a 16% RRR in mortality over 3.5 years (about 58 lives saved of 1284 treated; $P = 0.0036$), and the SOLVD prevention trial an 8% RRR over 3.1 years (21 lives saved of 2117 treated; NS).

Thus the overall results of V-HeFT-II and SOLVD–treatment are in close agreement for the direction and magnitude of effect with enalapril. The CONSENSUS study indicates that a much larger absolute treatment effect can be expected in a sicker population with a higher event rate, but also suggests that the relative mortality benefit may be greater. However, the mortality at 1 year in CONSENSUS, even among those patients randomized to enalapril, was 39%, which is still unacceptably high and indicates the need for better and/or earlier treatment of heart failure. Almost all patients in CONSENSUS were taking substantial doses of loop diuretics, while only 75% were in SOLVD–treatment and only 7% in SOLVD–prevention. Loop diuretics activate the renin–angiotensin system, and this activation has been shown to augur a bad prognosis[26,36,40] and is also a marker of greater benefit with ACE inhibitors.[26,36,40] Thus, diuretic use may account for the apparently greater relative benefit in CONSENSUS compared to SOLVD. Of some concern is the observation that low-dose aspirin appeared entirely to negate the mortality benefits and attenuate the morbidity benefits of enalapril in SOLVD.[65–67] There is some evidence that aspirin may be harmful to patients with heart failure, even when this is due to coronary disease.[67]

With regard to the primary endpoint, the SOLVD–prevention study must be regarded as negative. However, the frequency of the endpoint of development of heart failure, whether requiring therapy or hospitalization, was reduced by enalapril (RRR 37–44%; all P <0.001). A reduction in the need for hospitalization is not only laudable, as it reflects a reduction in patient morbidity, but also may result in important cost savings.[68] Patients with worsening heart failure were twice as likely to die and many times more likely to die from conditions that enalapril could alter favorably. The fact that many of these patients were withdrawn from placebo and placed on an open-label ACE inhibitor confounded the mortality result of the SOLVD–prevention study. Nonetheless, it does suggest that a policy of withholding an ACE inhibitor until evidence of heart failure appears (i.e. the need for diuretics) may be as effective as treatment in anticipation of symptoms, at least in patients with only moderate impairment of left ventricular function.[69,70] It does appear that mortality was reduced in the tercile of patients with the lowest EF, suggesting that patients with severe left ventricular dysfunction might best be treated with an ACE inhibitor, regardless of the presence of symptoms. Evidence indicating a mortality benefit from ACE inhibitors even prior to the onset of heart failure in patients with major ventricular dysfunction is supported by data from the Survival and Ventricular Enlargement (SAVE) study.[71]

What the Studies Showed: Secondary Endpoints

Ventricular Function

A CONSENSUS substudy suggested little or no reduction in mortality among patients with well-preserved left ventricular function.[12]

A report from the V-HeFT-I and -II studies suggested that patients with an EF above 35% had a better prognosis than did those with a lower EF.[69] There was no evidence of a mortality benefit in this subgroup of patients with any therapeutic regimen in V-HeFT-I. However, in V-HeFT-II 18 of 103 patients with an EF >35% died, versus 31 of 115 randomized to hydralazine plus nitrate ($P = 0.035$). This benefit was mostly due to a reduction in sudden death. Arrhythmias were also reduced. This is the only reasonably good evidence that treating patients with milder degrees of ventricular dysfunction with an ACE inhibitor may have a mortality benefit.

Nonetheless, the V-HeFT studies indicate that the EF may be one of the best predictors of prognosis in heart failure.[33,37,39,40,73] The V-HeFT-II study suggested that the EF increased by around 2% during treatment with enalapril. This is in close agreement with the effect of captopril in the Captopril-Digoxin Multi-centre Research Group (CDMRG) study,[7] which had a placebo control. The increase in EF with hydralizine plus nitrate in V-HeFT-II was 3–4%, which is in close agreement with the effect observed in V-HeFT-I.[1] The inconsistency between the effect on EF and mortality between regimens in V-HeFT-II suggest that changes in EF may not be a good surrogate marker for mortality.

The SOLVD radionuclide substudy incorporated only a small number of patients; reports suggested that ACE inhibitors could attentuate left ventricular dilatation and increase EF, but that they reduced left ventricular compliance.[53,56,59] Effects were less prominent among SOLVD–prevention patients. The larger echocardiographic substudy showed that enalapril could attenuate the increases in ventricular volumes and mass observed in the placebo group and reduce E-wave velocities, and thereby E/A ratios.[45] The observed changes in E/A ratio may reflect reduced filling pressure or reduced ventricular compliance (most likely the former).

Exercise Performance

Exercise performance is also a predictor of prognosis, as was confirmed in both the V-HeFT and SOLVD studies.[37,40,54] However, as with EF, it is not clear that an improvement in exercise capacity with therapy will result in improved prognosis. The data from V-HeFT-II would suggest not, showing that hydralazine plus nitrate exerted a greater effect on exercise capacity, but enalapril had a greater effect on mortality. Exercise performance as measured by oxygen consumption increased only in the hydralazine plus nitrate group in V-HeFT-II by 0.6–0.8 ml kg^{-1} min^{-1}, which was significantly more ($P < 0.02$ or greater) at three of the five time points tested compared with enalapril.[31] In SOLVD, peak oxygen uptake was reduced in patients with EF $<35\%$ but without symptons,[47] and in this group of patients enalapril increased peak oxygen consumption by 1–2 ml kg^{-1} min^{-1} ($P = 0.02$).[61] Trends to an improvement in exercise testing were not significant in this substudy of 188 patients.

Neuroendocrine Measurements

The CONSENSUS study showed that baseline plasma concentrations of angiotensin II, aldosterone, noradrenaline, and atrial natriuretic peptide (ANP) could predict prognosis, and that enalapril could reduce all of these.[26] The extent of the reduction in angiotensin II and aldosterone during treatment with enalapril also tended to indicate a better prognosis, those with more complete suppression having a lower mortality.[26] This may reflect the patients' ability to take larger and possibly more effective doses. The SOLVD studies reported that RAAS activation was essentially confined to patients taking diuretics,[49,55,74] providing further circumstantial evidence that the major benefit of ACE inhibition is to be found among those patients taking diuretics, at least in the setting of chronic heart failure. In contrast plasma concentrations of noradrenaline,[63,74] ANP and antidiuretic hormone (ADH) were elevated even among patients with asymptomatic left ventricular dysfunction. The SOLVD–treatment trial also showed that enalapril could reduce plasma concentrations of noradrenaline and atrial natriuretic peptide, a guide to atrial pressures.[44] No significant effect of enalapril was observed in SOLVD–prevention. Baseline plasma renin activity and noradrenaline predicted outcome in V-HeFT-II.[36,40] The V-HeFT-II study also showed that enalapril could attenuate the increase in noradrenaline to a greater extent than could hydralazine plus nitrate.

Hospitalization

The CONSENSUS study showed a reduction in the average number of admissions to hospital from 10.1 to 7.3 per 1000 days at risk, and the percentage of study days in hospital from 19.6% to 15%.[24] Both SOLVD studies showed a reduction in heart-failure-related hospitalization[10,11] and hospitalization for primarily cardiac reasons ($P = 0.006$ or greater). In addition, the SOLVD–treatment, but not SOLVD–prevention, trial showed a reduction in hospitalization for all causes ($P = 0.006$). The V-HeFT trials failed to show a reduction in total or heart-failure-related hospitalization.[31] Altogether, the SOLVD trials showed a reduction in patients hospitalized from 2152 on placebo to 2060 on enalapril, an absolute difference of 92 and an RRR of 4%. The total number of hospitalizations was reduced from 5672 (2833 and 2839 in treatment and prevention, respectively) on placebo to 5041 (2396 and 2645, respectively) on enalapril, an overall difference of 631 and an RRR of 11%. A recent report from the SOLVD study suggested that enalapril is a highly cost-effective treatment for heart failure.[68] Only the CONSENSUS study has reported the effect on the overall duration of admission, such data being necessary if the effects of ACE inhibitor treatment on the costs of hospital treatment are to be calculated accurately. The reduction in total hospitalizations with enalapril, although small, is remarkable considering that enalapril improved survival. Dead patients cannot be rehospitalized!

Quality of Life

Both SOLVD and V-HeFT studies found that quality-of-life scores were highly reproducible and that there was a modest relationship between functional capacity and quality-of-life scores at baseline.[32,48,57] However, there was a poor relationship between quality-of-life score and the severity of ventricular dysfunction.[57] The relationship between quality-of-life score and prognosis has also been reported.[126]

The SOLVD study showed improvements in 6 of 14 aspects of quality of life at some point in the trial.[50] However, in only 2 of 14 aspects was the improvement observed consistently in consecutive time periods. No consistent improvement in any aspect of quality of life was noted in SOLVD–prevention. The differences observed in the treatment trial are difficult to quantify but, at least superficially, appear small. It is not clear whether the disappointment should be directed at the possible inadequacy of the quality-of-life scales to show improvement, or at a lack of effect of treatment. However, NYHA class, usually considered a crude measure, clearly improved with enalapril, suggesting that quality-of-life instruments need to be interpreted with care. The V-HeFT-II study found no difference in quality-of-life scores when hydralazine plus nitrate was compared to enalapril.[32]

In the overall SOLVD program, 28.1% of patients on enalapril and 16.0% of patients on placebo reported side-effects ($P < 0.0001$). Hypotension (14.8% versus 7.1%), uremia (3.8% versus 1.6%), cough (5.0% versus 2.0%), fatigue (5.8% versus 3.5%), hyperkalemia (1.2% versus 0.4%), and angioedema (0.4% versus 0.1%) were all significantly more common with enalapril. Side-effects resulted in discontinuation of blinded therapy in 15.2% of patients on enalapril but only in 8.6% of patients on placebo ($P < 0.0001$).

Myocardial Infarction

The V-HeFT and CONSENSUS studies found no effect of enalapril on the incidence of myocardial infarction, while the SOLVD studies noted a reduction in the risk of myocardial infarction.[58] The data were collected as safety rather than outcome data in SOLVD, and the presence of myocardial infarction was reclassified by a committee after code breaking, which has led to some criticism of the acceptance of the results. However, as long-term trials of ACE inhibitors postinfarction have consistently shown significant reductions in infarction or trends in that direction, the SOLVD report is almost certainly correct.[70,75,76] Trials are underway to see if ACE inhibitors can reduce the risk of infarction in patients without evidence of ventricular dysfunction.

Mode of Death

The CONSENSUS and SOLVD studies suggest that the predominant effect of ACE inhibitors is to delay progressive heart failure death. The V-HeFT-II study found no effect of enalapril on progressive heart failure death, in agreement with a series of smaller studies.[38,76] Much of the conflict between the V-HeFT-II and SOLVD results rests with the lack of an endpoints committee in SOLVD,[22] the assumption that sudden death is arrhythmic rather than vascular, and the lumping together of 'progressive heart failure death' along with 'death due to arrhythmia with worsening heart failure' in SOLVD. The data from SOLVD and V-HeFT-II, as well as the long-term postinfarction studies, are consistent with the concept that the predominant effect of ACE inhibitors is to prevent sudden death in the setting of worsening heart failure.[76] Newer classifications of the mode of death in future studies will hopefully help avoid further confusion.[21]

Arrhythmias

The V-HeFT-II study showed a reduction in ventricular arrhythmias with enalapril, while the SOLVD study did not.[35,43] However, it is notable that in the SOLVD arrhythmia substudy, in contrast to the main study, all the benefit of enalapril was in reducing sudden death. Trends to a reduced frequency of admission with arrhythmia were noted. Earlier small studies showing a reduction in arrhythmias generally excluded the use of potassium-sparing diuretics, and consequently many patients were hypokalemic on placebo.[77,78] Correction of hypokalemia could be the principal mode of action of ACE inhibitors on arrhythmias.

What the Studies did not Show

The V-HeFT-II, CONSENSUS, and SOLVD studies all show that patients with better preserved ventricular function have a better prognosis, and little evidence of a mortality benefit with an ACE inhibitor, apparently even if symptoms of heart failure are severe.[12] Only the V-HeFT-II study has suggested that a mortality benefit may occur in those with less severe ventricular dysfunction (mean EF 43%).[72] There is no clear indication to treat patients with so-called 'diastolic' heart failure with an ACE inhibitor; ACE inhibitors have not been shown to improve symptoms in such patients, and their use may induce hypotension.

The SOLVD prevention study did not show that it was better to treat patients with asymptomatic left ventricular dysfunction with an ACE inhibitor early, rather than wait for the appearance of symptoms, instituting the ACE inhibitor and diuretic concurrently.[69,70] However, as discussed above, a case could be made for early treatment of severe asymptomatic left ventricular dysfunction.

The studies effectively excluded the large number of elderly patients (75–80 years and over) with mild to moderately severe heart failure. As these patients have poorer renal function, are more likely to have vascular disease in the renal and carotid territories, and may be more prone to problems such as symptomatic hypotension, it cannot be assumed that the benefits observed in younger patients will also be seen in the elderly.[69]

Trials of ACE Inhibitors Comparing Doses

The landmark trials of ACE inhibition all used relatively high doses of ACE inhibitors in twice-daily dosing regimens. ACE inhibitors are commonly used once daily in much smaller doses. Such a strategy may minimize the side-effects of treatment and its cost, but may be clinically ineffective and thus a false economy. Three studies have been set up to address this issue: NETWORK, ATLAS and ACHIEVE.[5,79] The doses of enalapril compared in NETWORK were 2.5, 5, and 10 mg twice daily, double-blind. Patients in ATLAS received 30 mg of lisinopril or placebo on top of open-label background therapy of 2.5–5.0 mg. ACHIEVE compared 2.5 mg and 20 mg twice daily of quinapril (open-label).

Entry Criteria and Study Populations

The demography and comparisons in the two major trials that have completed recruitment (ATLAS and NETWORK) are shown in *Table 18.4*. The results of NETWORK, the only study to have reported, are shown in *Table 18.5*. All studies excluded patients with standard contraindications to ACE inhibitors. NETWORK and ATLAS were double-blind studies.

The NETWORK study solicited patients with heart failure being looked after by primary-care physicians, but also recruited patients from hospital practice; the eventual split was about 40:60. Patients had to show symptoms of heart failure (NYHA II–IV), be aged 18–85 years, and to receive treatment for heart failure other than an ACE inhibitor. Patients already on an ACE inhibitor were excluded, preventing criticism that some patients may have been taken off effective doses of ACE inhibitors and randomized to a low dose, or that the study was only conducted on patients who had already been shown to tolerate ACE inhibitors. All patients had to have an echocardiogram with evidence of

Table 18.4 Baseline characteristics of patients in dose ranging studies with ACE inhibitors

	NETWORK	ATLAS
No. randomized	1532	3164
No. screened	2481	
Age (years)	70	
Duration of follow-up	6 months	3 years (minimum)
Gender (%F/%M)	36/64	
NYHA I + II/III/IV	65/33/2	
Current angina (%)	31	
CAD (%)	71	
DCM (%)	9	
Hypertension (%)	10	
Diabetes (%)	11	
Atrial fibrillation (%)	24	
Heart rate (bpm)	79	
Systolic BP (mmHg)	139	
EF (%)	Not given	
Diuretics (%)	94	
Digoxin (%)	24	
Other vasodilator (%)	27 (Nitrates)	
Beta-blocker/calcium antagonist (%)	10/27	
Aspirin/warfarin (%)	41	

BP, blood pressure; CAD, coronary artery disease; DCM, dilated cardiomyopathy; EF, ejection fraction.

Table 18.5   Results of the NETWORK dose ranging study

Comparison and target dose	Achieving target dose (%)	Withdrawals (%)	Myocardial infarction	Hospitalization for CHF only, n (%)	Total mortality, n (%)	Mortality annual[a] (%)
Enalapril 2.5 mg b.d. (n = 506)	99	20	?	26 (5)	21 (4.2)	8.4
vs						
Enalapril 5 mg b.d. (n = 510)	90	19	?	28 (6)	17 (3.3)	6.6
vs						
Enalapril 10 mg b.d. (n = 516)	71% on 10 mg b.d., 86% on 5 or 10 mg b.d. (P < 0.01)	26 (NS)	?	36 (7) (NS)	15 (2.9) (NS)	5.8

b.d., twice daily.
[a] Crude average annualized rate.

cardiac dysfunction supporting a diagnosis of heart failure (no specific criteria were set, and patients believed to have diastolic dysfunction could be entered). Treatment was only for 6 months. Classification of events was by an endpoints committee.

About one-third of patients screened from the community were randomized into the study. The reasons for failing to randomize referred patients included an inability to substantiate the diagnosis at the hospital, or the discovery of important valve disease or causes of heart failure requiring treatment other than with an ACE inhibitor. Some centers refused to randomize patients with 'diastolic' heart failure on the grounds that ACE inhibitors were not of proven benefit in this group.

The characteristics of the NETWORK population suggest that it may reflect the general population with heart failure more closely than any of the other studies of ACE inhibitors.

The ATLAS study recruited patients with NYHA III–IV heart failure from hospital clinics with an EF <30% (by echocardiography, radionuclide ventriculography, or angiography). Patients with NYHA II heart failure could also be included, but only if they had received emergency treatment or had been hospitalized for heart failure within the previous 6 months. All patients should have received diuretics for at least 60 days before entering the study. Patients also had to be able to tolerate 12.5–15 mg of lisinopril during the run-in period. This prevented patients who could not tolerate a substantial dose of lisinopril being randomized. Classification of events was by an endpoints committee.

The ATLAS study population is rather similar to the population recruited into the other landmark studies of ACE inhibitors in heart failure.

The ACHIEVE study is recruiting patients from primary-care physicians. The entry criteria are similar to those in the NETWORK study, i.e. a clinical diagnosis of heart failure, absence of contraindications to an ACE inhibitor, and treatment with a diuretic. However, no echocardiographic confirmation of left ventricular dysfunction is required. Randomization is open-label by telephone after baseline criteria have been logged.

Endpoint Definitions

The primary outcome in the NETWORK study was the combined endpoint of all-cause mortality, worsening heart failure, and heart-failure-related hospitalization. If a patient reached more than one of these endpoints, only the first event contributed to the primary outcome. Worsening heart failure was defined as a report to that effect from the investigator, but only if this was associated with a substantial increase in therapy for heart failure. Heart-failure-related hospitalization was defined as hospitalization for heart failure or for complications related to the treatment of heart failure. As syncope could be due to heart-failure treatment or an arrhythmia, all falls were assumed to be heart-failure related unless there was clear evidence to the contrary. Secondary outcomes included myocardial infarction and stroke.

The primary outcome in the ATLAS study is all-cause mortality. The main secondary outcomes include cardiovascular mortality, hospitalization for a nonfatal cardiovascular cause, and myocardial infarction.

Treatment Compliance

Only data from the NETWORK study are available so far. Compliance with the 10 mg twice daily dose in NETWORK and SOLVD treatment were similar at similar time points. There was a trend for more withdrawals among patients with higher compared to lower doses. The commonest side-effects reported were dizziness, cough, fatigue, and renal dysfunction. Apart from a trend to more fatigue with higher doses, the incidence of side-effects, including symptomatic hypotension, was similar across the three groups. Enalapril 10 mg twice daily was well tolerated by the majority of patients.

Outcome

Only the primary outcome and its components have been reported so far from the NETWORK study. Two of the components (mortality and heart-failure-related hospitalization) of the primary outcome are given in *Table 18.5*. Sixty-two (12%) patients in the 2.5 mg twice daily dose regimen, 65 (13%) in the 5 mg twice daily group, and 72 (14%) in the 10 mg twice daily group reached a primary endpoint (NS). The trend to more events in the high-dose group was entirely due to a higher rate of heart-failure-related hospitalization; there were no differences in the incidence of worsening heart failure. Although there was a 25% reduction in mortality with the high dose in this study, this did not achieve statistical significance owing to the overall low mortality.

The event rate, based on the 6-month outcome in SOLVD, for the 10 mg twice daily dose was exactly as predicted. It was the fewer than expected events with the 2.5 mg twice daily dose that resulted in a failure to find the anticipated difference between the 2.5 and 10 mg twice daily doses. The confidence intervals around the result do not exclude a 17% benefit with the higher dose. The ATLAS study is powered to identify a 15% difference in mortality between doses. For these reasons it would be premature to assume that there are no important differences between doses of ACE inhibitors.

However, there was no evidence that higher doses of enalapril exerted greater symptomatic benefit in this group of patients with predominantly rather mild heart failure.

Trials Comparing Non-ACE, Non-calcium Antagonist Vasodilators with Placebo

Three large trials have reported on the effects of non-ACE inhibitor, non-calcium-antagonist vasodilators on mortality, but only one of these has reported its results in

Table 18.6   Baseline characteristics of patients[a] in trials comparing non-ACE, non-calcium-antagonist vasodilators with placebo

	V-HeFT-I	PROFILE[b]	FIRST[b]
No. randomized	642	2304	471
No. screened (% excluded)	Not given	Not available	Not given
Age (years)	58	65	
Follow-up (years)	2.3	0.68	
Gender (%F/%M)	0/100[c]	21/79	
NYHA I + II/III/IV	Not available	0/88/12	Class III or IV
Current angina (%)	Limiting angina excluded	Not available	
CAD (%)	44	Not available	
DCM (%)	Not available		
Hypertension (%)	41		
Diabetes (%)	20		
Atrial fibrillation (%)	16		
Heart rate (bpm)	82		
Systolic BP (mmHg)	119		
EF (%)	30		<25%[c]
Diuretics (%)	100[c]	100[c]	
Digoxin (%)	100[c]	100[c]	
ACE inhibitors (%)	Prohibited[c]	100[c]	
Other vasodilator (%)	Prohibited[c]		
Beta-blocker/calcium antagonist (%)	Prohibited[c]		
Aspirin/warfarin (%)	13/14[d]		

BP, blood pressure; CAD, coronary artery disease; DCM, dilated cardiomyopathy, EF, ejection fraction.
[a]Around 40% of patients had a past history of excessive alcohol intake.
[b]Provisional data.
[c]By protocol.
[d]Percentage of time receiving each of the above.

detail.[1] The Prospective Randomised Flosequinan Longevity Evaluation (PROFILE) study with flosequinan and the Flolan International Randomised Survival Trials (FIRST) study with epoprostenol[80,127] both showed trends to excess mortality with the active agent and this was also associated with an increase in morbid events. These results, combined with the lack of benefit of prazosin and the borderline statistical significance[1] of the benefits demonstrated with hydralazine plus nitrate combination, might suggest that the vasodilator hypothesis has been disproved and that the benefits of ACE inhibitors are unique among vasodilators. The combination of hydralazine plus nitrate has an antiaggregatory effect on platelets and may have antioxidant effects, which could account for benefit by means other than vasodilation.[81] However, it is possible that flosequinan has inotropic properties at therapeutic concentrations; epoprostenol had to be given by continuous central venous infusion; and both flosequinan and prazosin increase plasma concentrations of noradrenaline.[82] Thus, the failure of most vasodilator trials to support the vasodilator hypothesis could reflect the peculiarities of the vasodilators used.

The demography, comparisons made and results of the only major trial of a non-ACE inhibitor, non-calcium-antagonist vasodilator are given in *Tables 18.6* and *18.7*. At the time of writing, full reports on the major trials of flosequinan (PROFILE) and epoprostenol (FIRST) had not been published. Available interim data are provided in the tables but, as neither agent is likely to enter widespread clinical use and full reports are not available, these trials are not discussed further.

Table 18.7 Comparisons in and results of trials comparing non-ACE, non-calcium-antagonist vasodilators with placebo

Trial	Comparison and target dose	Dose achieved	Withdrawals, n (%)	Myocardial infarction	Worsening CHF (%)	Hospitalization: Total/CHF n (%)	Total mortality, n (%)	Mortality/ annum[a] (%)
V-HeFT-I	Hydralazine 75 mg q.i.d. + nitrate 40 mg q.i.d. (n = 186)	68 mg q.i.d. + 34 mg q.i.d. 55% Top dose	51 (27), 69 (37)[a]	No data	No data	109 (59)/45 (24) (NS)	72 (39) (RRR 12%; P = 0.09)	16.8
	vs							
	Placebo (n = 273)	83% Top dose	60 (22)			166 (61)/65 (24)	120 (44)	19.1
	vs							
	Prazosin 5 mg q.i.d. (n = 183)	4.7 mg q.i.d. 75% Top dose	50 (27)			116 (63)/54 (30) (NS)	91 (50) (RER 13%; NS)	21.6
PROFILE	Flosequinan 75–100 mg	18%: 75 mg, 82%: 100 mg	Data not available	Data not available	Data not available	Data not available	(20.8) (RER 41%; P < 0.01)	19.7 27.0
	vs							
	Placebo	20%: 75 mg, 80%: 100 mg					? (14.7)	19.1 19.4
FIRST	Epoprostenol		Data not available	Data not available	56	Data not available	53% (at 6 months) (RER 29%; P < 0.01)	100
	vs							
	Control				56		41% (at 6 months)	82

CHF, congestive heart failure; q.i.d., four times daily; RER, relative excess risk; RRR, relative risk reduction.
[a] Recalculated.

Entry Criteria and Study Populations

The entry criteria for V-HeFT-I[1] were identical to those of the V-HeFT-II study. In general, the characteristics of the patients in V-HeFT-I and -II were similar. All the patients were men and the mean age was about 15 years lower than in community studies of heart failure.

The V-HeFT-I study is the only mortality study to exclude ACE inhibitor therapy, as such treatment had not been proven beneficial at the time of recruitment.

Endpoint Definition

All-cause mortality.

Withdrawals

In contrast to the studies with ACE inhibitors, more patients discontinued treatment from active treatment in V-HeFT-I. The nitrate plus hydralazine combination, in the intended doses, was particularly poorly tolerated, and barely half of patients were prescribed full doses. There was no difference in withdrawal for worsening heart failure among the three groups. Side-effects were the reason for more withdrawals among those on active treatment.

Outcome

Prazosin exerted no effect on mortality. At 1 year there was a 38% RRR with hydralazine plus nitrate, at 2 years a 25% reduction, and at 3 years a 23% reduction. However, overall this did not reach conventional levels of statistical significance ($P = 0.093$ on a log rank test and P not less than 0.05 on the Wilcoxon statistic after adjustment for multiple tests).

Systolic and diastolic blood pressure were reduced by prazosin at 1 year by 5 and 3 mmHg, respectively, changes very similar to those observed with enalapril in the SOLVD studies. Blood pressure was not altered by the hydralazine plus nitrate combination at 1 year. The EF increased significantly only in the hydralazine plus nitrate group by a mean of 4%. None of the treatments had an effect on rates of hospitalization.[31] The combination of hydralazine and nitrate increased exercise performance ($P < 0.04$ at 1 year), but prazosin did not.[34]

In summary, some doubt must remain whether the combination of hydralazine and nitrate is effective in reducing mortality, especially in view of the failure of other vasodilator regimens. The high side-effect profile and the inability to modify withdrawal due to worsening heart failure or hospitalization suggest that this treatment may not reduce the morbidity associated with heart failure. There is a paucity of evidence for symptomatic benefit with hydralazine or nitrates in heart failure alone or in combination or when added to an ACE inhibitor.[2,83] However, the combination of hydralazine and nitrate improved exercise performance consistently in the V-HeFT trials. Further trials are required to establish the place of this therapeutic regimen in current treatment, although among patients who are intolerant to ACE inhibitors and other therapies it should be considered.

Calcium Antagonists

Several studies with short-acting preparations of nifedipine, diltiazem, and verapamil in heart failure and after myocardial infarction suggested that such treatments worsen symptoms and increase morbidity and/or mortality.[84,85] Three large trials of newer and/or longer acting calcium antagonists have been set up to address the safety or efficacy of calcium antagonists in heart failure. Preliminary reports are available from two of these studies at the time of writing (Prospective Randomised Amlodipine Survival Evaluation Study Group (PRAISE)[86,87] and V-HeFT-III[87,88]), and recruitment has been completed in a third (MACH-1).[87] Data on the PRAISE and V-HeFT-III trials are given in *Tables 18.8* and *18.9.*

Entry Criteria and Study Populations

The PRAISE study recruited patients with EF < 30% and NYHA IIIB–IV heart failure despite optimal treatment with ACE inhibitors, diuretics, and digoxin. Thus the PRAISE study recruited severely ill patients with a high mortality, with the intention of demonstrating the safety rather than efficacy of amlodipine, a new-generation long-acting calcium antagonist. Demonstration of safety in this group of patients would suggest that it might be used for the management of hypertension or angina with confidence in patients with poor ventricular function.

V-HeFT-III recruited men with NYHA II/III heart failure with objective evidence of

Table 18.8   Baseline characteristics of patients randomized in trials of calcium antagonists

	PRAISE	V-HeFT-III
No. randomized	1153	675
No. screened (% excluded)	Not reported	Not reported
Age (years)	65	63
Follow-up (months)	13.8	18
Gender (%F/%M)	24/76	0/100
NYHA I + II/III/IV	0/81%/19%	
Current angina (%)	Not reported	
CAD (%)	63	52
DCM (%)	Not reported	
Hypertension (%)	56 (history of)	
Diabetes (%)	Not reported	
Atrial fibrillation (%)	Not reported	
Heart rate (bpm)	83	
Systolic BP (mmHg)	118	
EF (%)	21 (<30%[a])	30
Diuretics (%)	100	
Digoxin (%)	99	
ACE inhibitor (%)	99	
Other vasodilator (%)	Not reported	
Beta-blocker/calcium antagonist (%)	Not reported	
Aspirin/warfarin (%)	Not reported	

BP, blood pressure; CAD, coronary artery disease; DCM, dilated cardiomyopathy; EF, ejection fraction.
[a]By protocol.

Table 18.9 Comparisons in and results of trials of calcium antagonists

Trial	Comparison and target dose	Dose achieved (mean at 1 month)	Withdrawals	Myocardial infarction	Hospitalization		Total mortality	Mortality/annum[a] (%)
					Total	CVS		
PRAISE	Amlodipine 5 mg daily (n = 571)	8.8 mg	82 (40 for worsening CHF)	16 (3%)	Not reported	62 (10.9%) (RER 17%)	190 (33%) (RRR 16%; P = 0.07)	28.9
	vs							
	Placebo (n = 582)	8.9 mg	94 (32 for worsening CHF)	18 (3%)		54 (9.3%)	223 (38%)	33.3
V-HeFT-III (abstract only)	Felodipine 5 mg b.d.	Not reported	Not reported	Not reported	Not reported	Not reported	I/IIa: 9.1% IIb/III: 16.2%	6.1 10.8
	vs							
	Placebo						I/IIa: 10.2% IIb/III: 13.7% (NS)	6.8 9.1

b.d., twice daily; CVS, cardiovascular; RER, relative excess risk; RRR, relative risk reduction.
[a]Recalculated.

cardiac dysfunction (criteria as for V-HeFT-I and -II). Patients in V-HeFT-II had milder heart failure than in PRAISE.

The philosophy behind MACH-1,[87] using mibefradil, was similar to that behind PRAISE.

Endpoints

The primary endpoint in PRAISE was a combined one of all-cause mortality or cardiovascular hospitalization. The primary endpoint in V-HeFT-III was exercise tolerance, and that in MACH-1 ($n = 2000$) is all-cause mortality. An exercise substudy is being conducted in MACH-1.

Withdrawals

There were significantly more episodes of pulmonary (85 versus 58) and peripheral (155 versus 103) edema recorded in patients on amlodipine. However, similar overall numbers of patients were withdrawn from amlodipine and placebo in the PRAISE study.

Outcome

The PRAISE study showed no overall effect on the primary (combined) endpoint but there was a trend for a small reduction in mortality that just failed ($P = 0.07$) to achieve a conventional level of statistical significance. The PRAISE study suggested an interaction between etiology of heart failure and the primary outcome ($P = 0.04$) that was even stronger for mortality alone ($P = 0.004$). All the benefit in the primary outcome occurred among patients not known to have ischemic heart disease (IHD) (inevitably this will be a group with very diverse etiologies for their heart failure). There was also a highly significant reduction in mortality in the group without IHD (absolute reduction in mortality 13%, RRR 38%; $P = 0.001$). The outcome in patients in whom IHD was the known cause of heart failure was entirely neutral. Currently it is not clear if amlodipine is beneficial in all cases of ventricular dysfunction but that the benefit is lost in a subset of patients with IHD due to, for instance, a coronary steal phenomenon. Studies with amiodarone and possibly beta-blockers suggest that it may be easier to modify favorably the prognosis of patients with heart failure due to causes other than IHD. Unfortunately, it is patients with IHD as the cause of heart failure who have a particularly poor prognosis, and IHD is the more common cause of heart failure.[89] Amlodipine had as great, or a greater, effect on sudden death as death due to circulatory failure.[86] The PRAISE-2 study has been set up to determine prospectively whether amlodipine reduces mortality in patients with heart failure but not known to have IHD.

The V-HeFT-III study suggests a neutral outcome with felodipine, although the event rate was much lower than in PRAISE and the confidence intervals around the result much wider. V-HeFT-III did not observe a trend to greater benefit among those without IHD as the cause of heart failure.

Currently, it would appear that amlodipine is safe to use in heart failure and may be used when there is an additional reason, such as angina or hypertension, to prescribe such an agent. However, currently, there is a lack of data on the efficacy of calcium antagonists for the reduction of angina or hypertension in the setting of heart failure. There is insufficient evidence to support their use for the treatment of heart failure itself, either to reduce symptoms of heart failure or to reduce mortality in any subgroup of patients. Relief of angina and improvement of reversible ischemic ventricular dysfunction could improve breathlessness. Improved control of hypertension could also improve heart-failure symptoms. Both these hypotheses remain to be proved. It would appear that the PRAISE trial contained few such patients. It is not yet clear if the safety of amlodipine represents a class effect of long-acting calcium antagonists.

Digoxin

Details of the four studies reported so far with the largest populations of patients on digoxin are shown in *Tables 18.10* and *18.11*. The Digoxin Investigators Group (DIG) trial was reported recently; data for the main study and the ancillary study of patients with ejection fraction >45% is given here.[90]

Table 18.10   Baseline characteristics of patients randomized in trials of digoxin

	CDMRG	CADS	RADIANCE	DIG
No. randomized	300	222	178	6800[b]
No. screened (% excluded)	464 (35)	Not given	216 (18)	Not available
Age (years)	57	Not given	60	64
Follow-up	6 months	2 years	12 weeks	37 months
Gender (%F/%M)	27/83	Not given	24/76	78/22
NYHA I + II/III/IV	77/13/0	100/0/0[a]	73/27/0	67/31/2
Current angina (%)	Limiting angina excluded	Limiting angina excluded	Limiting angina excluded	27
CAD (%)	62	100[a]	60	71
DCM (%)	32	0	38	15
Hypertension (%)	Not given	Not given	Not given	45
Diabetes (%)	Not given	Not given	Not given	28
Atrial fibrillation (%)	0[a]	Not given	0[a]	Excluded
Heart rate (bpm)	Not given	Not given	78	Not given
Systolic BP (mmHg)	Not given	Not given	126	Not given
EF (%)	25 (<40[a])	Not given	27 (<35[a])	28 (⩽45%[a]) Ancillary study >45%[b]
Diuretics (%)	84	None[a]	100[a]	82
Digoxin (%)	65 (withdrawn 10 days prior to randomization)	None[a]	100[a] (at baseline)	41 (at screening)
ACE inhibitor (%)	7 (withdrawn 10 days prior to randomization)	None[a]	100[a] Captopril: 74 mg day^{-1}/Enalapril: 15 mg day^{-1}	94
Other vasodilator (%)	Prohibited	None[a]	33	43
Beta-blocker/ calcium antagonist (%)	Prohibited	Allowed	Not reported	Not given
Aspirin/warfarin	Not given	Allowed	Not reported	Not given

BP, blood pressure; CAD, coronary artery disease; DCM, dilated cardiomyopathy; EF, ejection fraction; IHD, ischemic heart disease.
[a]By protocol.
[b]A further 988 patients were recruited to a parallel study of patients with heart failure and EF > 45%.

Table 18.11 Comparisons in and results of trials of digoxin

	Comparison and target dose	Dose achieved	Withdrawals (%)	Myocardial infarction n (%)	Worsening CHF	Hospitalization for CHF only, n (%)	Total mortality, n (%)	Mortality/annum (%)
CDMRG	Digoxin 0.125–0.375 mg daily (n = 96)	Not given	8[a]	Not given	4[b]	8 (8) (RRR 58%; P < 0.05)	7 (7) (NS)	14.6
	vs							
	Placebo (n = 100)	Not given	15[a]	Not given	15[b]	19 (19)	6 (6)	12.0
	vs							
	Captopril 50 mg t.i.d. (n = 104)	Not given	11[a]	Not given	6[b]	10 (10) (RRR 47%; P < 0.05)	8 (8) (NS)	15.4
CADS	Digoxin 0.125 mg b.d. (n = 67)	Not given	~5	Not given	Not given	?	2	?
	vs							
	Placebo (n = 66)	Not given	~9	Not given	Not given	?	2	?
	vs							
	Captopril 25 mg b.d. (n = 63)	Not given	~4	Not given	Not given	?	0	?
RADIANCE	Digoxin continued (target 0.9–2.0 ng ml^{-1} (n = 85)	0.38 mg (1.2 ng ml^{-1})	14 (n = 12)	2	4 (5%) (RRR 80%; P < 0.001)	2 (2) (RRR 85%; P = 0.02)	3 (4) (NS)	15.3
	vs							
	Withdrawal to placebo (n = 93)		37 (n = 34)	0	23 (25%)	12 (13)	1 (1)	4.7
DIG	Digoxin (n = 3397)	18% on 0.125 mg, 71% on 0.25 mg, 11% on >0.25 mg day^{-1}	71% of survivors	Fatal only 143 (3.7) (RER 28%; NS)	Not reported	910 (26.8) (RRR 23%; P < 0.001)	1181 (34.8)	11.3
	vs							
	Placebo (n = 3403)	Placebo 'doses' similar to above		113 (2.9)	Not reported	1180 (34.7)	1194 (35.1)	11.4
DIG Ancillary (EF >45%)	Digoxin (n = 492)	Not reported	Not reported	Not reported	Not reported	Nonsignificant reduction	115 (23.4)	7.6
	Digoxin (n = 496)						116 (23.4)	7.6

b.d., twice daily; CHF, congestive heart failure; RER, relative excess risk; RRR, relative risk reduction; t.i.d., three times daily.
[a]Withdrawals for treatment failure + withdrawals for adverse reactions + withdrawals after test dose.
[b]Withdrawals for treatment failure.

Study Design

Most of the studies with digoxin have adopted a withdrawal study design. Withdrawal studies have several inherent flaws. Firstly, only patients who tolerate the therapy can be withdrawn from it; withdrawal trials will underestimate the side-effects and toxicity associated with active treatment. Secondly, some substances (e.g. alcohol and, possibly, phosphodiesterase inhibitors) are harmful but produce alarming reactions when withdrawn. Continuation of treatment obscures the very problem it causes; withdrawal appears deleterious, but so may initiation.

Study Inclusion Criteria

The Captopril-Digoxin Multicentre Research Group (CDMRG) study recruited patients <75 years old who had an EF < 40% and moderately, though not severely, impaired exercise tolerance due to symptoms compatible with heart failure.[7] Of the patients in this study 65% were receiving digoxin prior to entry, although digoxin was withdrawn for an unspecified period prior to baseline evaluation.

The Captopril Digoxin Study (CADS)[8] included patients <75 years old with a prior history (>2 months) of myocardial infarction, abnormal ventricular function by echocardiography or angiography, and symptoms of heart failure (NYHA II) after withdrawal from all heart-failure medication. The proportion of patients withdrawn from digoxin was not stated.

The Randomised Assessment of the Effect of Digoxin on Inhibitors of the Angiotensin Converting Enzyme (RADIANCE) study[91] recruited patients with an EF < 35%, an echocardiographic left ventricular end-diastolic dimension of >60 mm (or 34 mm m^{-2}), impaired exercise tolerance despite optimal treatment with an ACE inhibitor, digoxin and diuretics, and in NYHA class II to III. The RADIANCE study, in common with most other studies of digoxin, is a withdrawal study.

The DIG study recruited patients with clinical heart failure in sinus rhythm. For the main study patients were required to have an ejection fraction ≤45%, but an ancillary study of 988 patients with ejection fractions >45% was also recruited. All grades of heart failure could be included. Patients had to be in sinus rhythm but could have stable angina. The vast majority of patients were taking ACE inhibitors and diuretics at baseline and 41% were taking digoxin. Thus about half the randomized population were being randomized to digoxin withdrawal and the other half to digoxin initiation. However, it made no difference to the study outcome whether or not the patient was receiving digoxin at baseline.

Primary Endpoints

The primary endpoints in CDMRG were exercise duration, NYHA class, EF, and ventricular ectopic beats. Endpoints were only counted while the patient continued on blinded therapy. Thus CDMRG deviates from the intention-to-treat principle. The primary endpoints in CADS were exercise time and quality of life. The primary endpoints in RADIANCE were the rate and timing of withdrawal from randomized medication and the change in exercise tolerance. The primary endpoint in the DIG study was all-cause mortality.

Unplanned Withdrawals from Assigned Medication

In the CDMRG study withdrawal rates were significantly higher from placebo than either digoxin or captopril, although there was no difference in withdrawal rates between the two active treatments. The withdrawal rate in CADS was 12% at 1 year, with no difference reported between groups. Patients were almost three times more likely to 'withdraw' from placebo than digoxin in the RADIANCE study. In the DIG trial, slightly more of the digoxin-treated group remained on blinded medication compared to placebo (70.8% versus 67.9%). At 1 year, 3.0% of those randomized to digoxin had withdrawn for worsening heart failure versus 6.4% of those on placebo. The figures at the end of the study were 6.7% versus 11.0%. Discontinuation for atrial fibrillation was also reduced (2.8% versus 3.4%) by digoxin at study end.

Outcome

In the CDMRG study, compared to placebo, digoxin increased the EF by 4.4% but had no effect on other primary endpoints. Captopril improved NYHA class (intention-to-treat, or by-protocol) and exercise time (per-protocol analysis only) compared to placebo, and reduced the frequency of ectopics compared to digoxin (per-protocol analysis only). The number of patients requiring an increase in diuretics ($P < 0.005$) or admission to hospital or assessment in a hospital emergency department ($P < 0.05$) was greater on placebo than either active regimen.

The CADS study reported a significant improvement in NYHA class with digoxin ($P < 0.05$ versus placebo). Symptom scores improved to a greater extent on digoxin than on placebo or captopril ($P < 0.05$ at least). More patients developed worsening angina ($P < 0.02$) on captopril (24%) than on digoxin (8%) or placebo (15%). There was no difference in exercise capacity between the three groups after 1 or 2 years of follow-up.

The RADIANCE study showed that patients who stayed on digoxin were less likely to withdraw for worsening heart failure ($P < 0.001$), or to require hospital admission or an emergency department visit ($P = 0.02$). Patients remaining on digoxin were more likely to maintain their maximal ($P < 0.05$) and submaximal ($P = 0.01$) exercise capacity. NYHA score ($P < 0.02$) and patient self-assessment ($P < 0.01$) favored digoxin maintenance. Heart rate ($P < 0.001$), body weight ($P < 0.001$), and left ventricular end-diastolic dimension ($P < 0.04$) all increased after digoxin withdrawal, while the EF decreased by about 4% ($P < 0.001$).

The DIG study showed no overall effect on mortality, a reduction in death due to progressive heart failure ($P = 0.03$) being balanced by an increase in death due to myocardial infarction and sudden death. The main DIG study showed a reduction in cardiovascular hospitalizations ($P < 0.01$) and the total number of patients hospitalized (2184 versus 2282; $P = 0.006$). The reduction in hospitalization was predominantly for worsening heart failure. Effects on hospitalization for arrhythmias or myocardial infarction were minimal. There were only 67 admissions for suspected digoxin toxicity in those randomized to digoxin, versus 31 of those randomized to placebo. How much of the latter was due to false diagnosis and how much was due to open-label treatment with digoxin is unclear. Preliminary (unconfirmed) reports have also indicated that there may be a relationship between mortality and serum digoxin concentration within the therapeutic range. Thus, doses of digoxin that have been shown to be clinically effective may have an adverse effect on survival, whereas serum levels that are currently considered sub-therapeutic, as observed in the DIG study, may be safe or even reduce mortality. This scenario appears uncannily similar to that observed with other inotropic agents. More evidence that low-dose digoxin is clinically effective is now required.[62]

Preliminary reports from the DIG study have indicated that digoxin is also safe in patients with heart failure and well preserved systolic function, and that treatment is associated with a reduction in hospitalization for worsening heart failure, although perhaps not for overall hospitalization.

In summary, digoxin exerts no important effect on overall mortality. There is powerful evidence that digoxin can reduce episodes of decompensation of heart failure and should be considered for patients who have demonstrated such a propensity. In general, patients with advanced heart failure are most prone to recurrent decompensation and admission. As up to 50% of patients with severe heart failure are already in atrial fibrillation, the use of digoxin, as viewed in the above context, may decline. However, as most patients, even with mild heart failure, remain quite symptomatic, the demonstration that digoxin is safe may lead to increased use. However, we still do not know what is a *safe and effective* dose of this agent. It would appear that the DIG study has advanced our understanding of digoxin, but that the 200-year-old controversy over who to treat is set to continue for somewhat longer.

Other Inotropic Agents

The full results of two large trials (Prospective Randomised Milrinone Survival Evaluation (PROMISE)[92] and vesnarinone[93]) of inotropic agents other than digoxin were available at the time of writing, with preliminary data from two others (VEST and PRIME-II[94]) (*Tables 18.12* and *18.13*). Although novel inotropic agents are being increasingly treated with suspicion because of perceived adverse effects on mortality, overall the results are no worse than trials of vasodilator agents. Indeed, some would regard milrinone (a phosphodiesterase inhibitor) and ibopamine (a dopamine analog), two unsuccessful inotropic agents, more as vasodilator than inotropic agents.

The inotropic agents are a diverse group and it is those agents that act throught cAMP (either by stimulating its formation, e.g. dobutamine, or by preventing its breakdown, e.g. the PDE III inhibitors) for which there is most evidence of a deleterious effect on survival. This makes sense in that increased sympathetic activity also stimulates cAMP and is associated with a worse prognosis, while adrenergic receptor antagonists are associated with improved survival in heart failure.

Vesnarinone is the only example of a nonvasodilating, largely non-cAMP-mediated inotropic agent. Although the first large trial of vesnarinone looked promising, a subsequent trial (VEST) also showed an increase in mortality.

Entry Criteria and Study Populations

The PROMISE study[92] recruited patients with a radionuclide EF $< 35\%$ who remained in NYHA class III–IV despite optimal medical therapy with diuretics, digoxin, and ACE inhibitors for at least 4 weeks. The PROMISE study recruited a high percentage of patients with dilated cardiomyopathy and with severe heart failure.

The vesnarinone trial[93] recruited patients with a radionuclide EF $< 30\%$ who had symptoms of heart failure despite conventional therapy. As vesnarinone may cause serious neutropenia, patients at risk of this condition were excluded. Similarly to the PROMISE trial there was a high proportion of patients with dilated cardiomyopathy,

Table 18.12 Baseline characteristics of patients randomized in trials of inotropic agents other than digoxin

	PROMISE	Vesnarinone	PRIME-II
No. randomized	1088	477[a]	1906
No. screened (% excluded)	Not given	Not given	Not given
Age (years)	64	58	65
Follow-up	6 months	6 months	~3 years
Gender (%F/%M)	22/78	23/87	20/80
NYHA I + II/II/IV	0/58/42	19/70/11	0/60/32IIIb/8
Current angina (%)	27	Not given	34
CAD (%)	54	52	59
DCM (%)	40	42 (nonischemic)	31
Hypertension (%)	Not given	Not given	Not given
Diabetes (%)	Not given	Not given	20
Atrial fibrillation (%)	Not given	Not given	81
Heart rate (bpm)	84	Not given	81
Systolic BP (mmHg)	115	Not given	122
EF (%)	21	20 ($<30\%$[b])	26 (<30[b])
Serum sodium (mmol l^{-1})	139	137	
Diuretics (%)	100[b]	Not given	99[b]
Digoxin (%)	100[b]	87	64
ACE inhibitors (%)	100[b]	90	90
Other vasodilator (%)	58	Not given	Not given
Beta-blocker/calcium antagonist (%)	Not given	Not given	14
Aspirin/warfarin (%)	Not given	Not given	Not given

BP, blood pressure; CAD, coronary artery disease; DCM, dilated cardiomyopathy; EF, ejection fraction.
[a]Baseline characteristics of 87 patients allocated to vesnarinone 120 mg daily not given.
[b]By protocol.

probably reflecting the large number of transplant centers involved, and severity of ventricular dysfunction, although the NYHA class was somewhat less severe in the vesnarinone trial. Despite these similarities, the mortality in the placebo group of PROMISE was almost double that in the vesnarinone trial.

PRIME-II recruited patients with EF < 30% (measured by various techniques) or a LVEDD >60 mm with a fractional shortening of <20% or cardiothoracic >50%, NYHA III–IV and treated with diuretic and ACE inhibitors, unless contraindicated.

Endpoints

The primary endpoint in PROMISE was all-cause mortality. Secondary endpoints included cardiovascular mortality, hospitalization, addition of vasodilators because of worsening heart failure, symptons, and adverse reactions.

The primary endpoint of the vesnarinone trial was a combined one of all-cause mortality or admission to hospital for the treatment of heart failure with intravenous inotropic agents for at least 4 hours. The secondary endpoint was all-cause mortality. Classification of deaths was by an endpoints committee. Data on 19 patients (13 on placebo) who had transplants during the study were censored at the date of operation.

The primary endpoint in PRIME-II was all-cause mortality. Secondary endpoints were the mode of death, need for transplantation, hospitalization, and quality of life.

Table 18.13 Comparisons in and results of trials of inotropic agents other than digoxin

	Comparison and target dose	Dose achieved	Withdrawals, n (%)	Myocardial infarction, n	Worsening CHF, n (%)	Hospitalization (total CHF), n (%)	Deaths no. studied, n (%)	Annualized mortality[a] (%)
PROMISE	Milrinone 10–15 mg q.i.d. (n = 561)	37 mg daily	71 (13) (P = 0.04)	Not given	168 (30) (NS)	247 (44) (RER 13%; P < 0.05)	168 (30) (RER 28%; P < 0.04)	60
	vs							
	Placebo (n = 527)	38 mg daily	46 (9)		153 (29)	205 (39)	127 (24)	48
Vesnarinone	Vesnarinone 60 mg daily (n = 239)	? Patients who did not withdraw took full dose	21	6	18 (8) (RRR 46%; P < 0.01)	Not given	13 (5) (RRR 62%; P < 0.01)	10.9
	vs							
	Vesnarinone 120 mg daily (n = 87)		6	1	Not given	Not given	16 (18) Placebo mortality ~8% at same time point (RER 125%; P = 0.01)	
	vs							
	Placebo n = 238		12	6	33 (14)	Not given	33 (14)	27.7
PRIME-II	Ibopamine (n = 953)	No data	No data	No data	No data	No data	232 (24) (RER 20%; P = 0.017)	
	vs							
	Placebo (n = 953)						193 (20)	

CHF, coronary heart failure; q.i.d., four times daily; RER, relative excess risk; RRR, relative risk reduction.
[a] 800 mg daily for the first 14 days, then 400 mg daily for the rest of the first year, then 300 mg daily.

The primary endpoint of VEST was all-cause mortality.

Withdrawals

The rate of withdrawal from milrinone in the PROMISE study was relatively low, although the rate from placebo was lower still ($P < 0.05$). The rates of withdrawal in the vesnarinone study showed a similar pattern. Data from PRIME-II are not yet published.

Outcome

The PROMISE trial showed a relative excess risk (RER) of 28% in all-cause mortality ($P < 0.05$), a 34% RER of cardiovascular death ($P < 0.02$), and an excess of hospitalization ($P < 0.05$), hypotension ($P < 0.01$), palpitation ($P < 0.05$), and syncope ($P < 0.01$), as well as a series of more minor problems such as headache and diarrhea. Patients in NYHA class IV had a 53% RER in mortality versus only a 3% RER in those in NYHA III. No subgroup had a reduction in risk with milrinone. An equal number of patients on milrinone and placebo showed an improvement or worsening of NYHA class.

As neither symptoms nor mortality improved, this study suggests that there is no clinical role for the use of oral milrinone in heart failure. The lack of a significant excess mortality in patients with NYHA class III heart failure suggests that milrinone may be less harmful in this group and does not exclude the possibility of benefit. However, as many patients will eventually deteriorate from class III into class IV, it would still be difficult to know how to use such an agent.

The 120 mg daily arm of the vesnarinone trial was discontinued early owing to an excess mortality. The 60 mg daily dose in the vesnarinone trial showed a 50% RRR ($P = 0.003$) in the primary outcome and a 62% RRR ($P = 0.002$) in all-cause mortality. The reduction in mortality was due equally to a reduction in sudden death (43% of all deaths) and death due to worsening heart failure (54% of all deaths). Vesnarinone did not improve EF or NYHA class, but did improve a broad range of quality-of-life scores (P at least < 0.02). The incidence of neutropenia was 2.5%.

The vesnarinone study presents several difficulties in interpretation. First, there is some controversy as to whether the 60 mg daily dose has an inotropic or hemodynamic effect. No increase in EF was observed in this trial. It is possible that vesnarinone is working by some other mechanism, possibly an effect on cytokines.[95,96] Secondly, the therapeutic to toxic dose range may be low, although doses of vesnarinone < 60 mg daily could be effective. It is unlikely that an 80-kg 50-year-old man and 75-year-old 60-kg woman will require the same dose.

The Vesnarinone Survival Trial (VEST) showed a significant increase ($P = 0.016$) in mortality when vesnarinone 60 mg daily and placebo were compared; a trend to increased mortality was also observed with 30 mg daily. The excess mortality was attributed entirely to an increase in sudden death. No subgroup has yet been identified in which vesnarinone did not increase mortality. It is unlikely that the development of vesnarinone will be pursued further.

The PRIME-II study showed a significant increase in all-cause mortality ($P = 0.017$). Publication of the full data is awaited.

At least one design feature of both the PROMISE and the vesnarinone trials is odd. All of the patients in the first study and 87% in the latter study were taking another inotropic agent, digoxin. Although the vesnarinone study did not suggest any interaction between digoxin and vesnarinone, such an interaction cannot be excluded in PROMISE. An adverse interaction between flosequinan and digoxin has been verbally reported in the PROFILE study.

Antiarrhythmic Agents

The Cardiac Arrhythmia Suppression Trial (CAST) is included in this section.[97–102] Although considered a postinfarction trial, patients could be included up to 2 years after the index event, and about one-third were receiving digoxin and/or diuretics and half had an EF < 40%. Two large trials of amiodarone have been reported in heart failure in addition to some observational studies[4,89,103,104] (Tables 18.14 and 18.15).

Entry Criteria and Study Populations

Patients in the CAST study could be entered between 6 days and 2 years after a myocardial infarction. Patients had to have 6 or more ventricular ectopic beats per hour on at least 18 hours of Holter monitoring. If the qualifying Holter was performed more than 90 days after the index infarction the EF had to be less than 40%. Patients with symptomatic arrhythmias or with nonsustained ventricular tachycardia of more than 15 beats were

Table 18.14 Baseline characteristics of patients randomized in trials of antiarrhythmic drugs

	CAST	GESICA	CHF-STAT
No. randomized	1498	516	674
No. screened (% excluded)	2309	?	1303 (48)
Age (years)	61	59	66
Follow-up	10 months	13 months	3.8 years
Gender (%F/%M)	18/82	19/81	1/99
NYHA I + II/III/IV	13% had overt CHF	21/48/31	57/43 (III or IV)
Current angina (%)	19	?	?
CAD (%)	100[a]	39 (MI)	72
DCM (%)	0	21 (+ 9% Chagas')	28 (nonischemic)
Hypertension (%)	32	40	?
Diabetes (%)	20	13	?
Atrial fibrillation (%)	3	29	15
Heart rate (bpm)	74	90	80
Systolic BP (mmHg)	126	117	127
EF (%)	40	20 (<35[a])	<30–67% 30–40–33% (<40[a])
Diuretics (%)	32	92	83 (on loop; mean 78 mg frusemide)
Digoxin (%)	20	76	70
ACE inhibitors (%)	?	90 (enalapril)	78 (captopril 78 mg daily)[b]
Other vasodilator (%)	Nitrate: 46	Nitrate: 35	14
Beta-blocker/calcium antagonist (%)	32/51	?	4/?
Aspirin/warfarin (%)	?	?/31	?

BP, blood pressure; CAD, coronary artery disease; CHF, coronary heart failure; DCM, dilated cardiomyopathy; EF, ejection fraction; MI, myocardial infarction.
[a]By protocol.
[b]Captopril accounted for over 80% of ACE inhibitor use in this study.

Table 18.15 Comparisons in and results of trials of antiarrhythmic drugs

	Comparison and target dose	Dose achieved	Withdrawals, n (%)	Myocardial infarction, n (%)	Worsening CHF, n (%)	Hospitalization for CHF	Total mortality, n (%)	Mortality, per annum (%)
CAST	Flecainide 100–150 mg b.d.	>90% compliance in 70% of patients	(8.4)	19 (2.5) (RRR 43%; P = 0.058)	57 (7.5) (NS)	?	61 (8.1)[c] (RER 131%; P < 0.001)	10
	Encainide 35–50 mg t.i.d. (n = 755)							
	vs							
	Placebo (n = 743)		8.6	33 (4.4)	51 (6.9)		26 (3.5)	4.2
GESICA	Amiodarone 300 mg daily[a] (n = 260)	?	15 (6)	Not given	Not given. More patients on amiodarone improved NYHA class	32 (not including hospital deaths) (NS)	87 (33.5) (RRR 28%; P = 0.024)	30.9
	vs							
	Control (n = 256)		? None			43	106 (41.4)	38.2
CHF-STAT	Amiodarone 300 mg daily[b] (n = 336)	?	136 (40)	Not given	Not given	Not given	131 (39) (RRR 7%; NS)	10.3
	vs							
	Placebo (n = 338)		110 (33)				143 (42)	11.1

CHF, coronary heart failure; b.d., twice daily; t.i.d., three times daily; RER, relative excess risk.

[a]600 mg daily for 14 days, then 300 mg daily.

[b]800 mg daily for the first 14 days, then 400 mg daily for the rest of the first year, then 300 mg daily.

[c]There were two further cases with succesful resuscitation from cardiac arrest who contributed to the primary endpoint.

excluded. The age and concomitant diseases were similar to those observed in the large trials of ACE inhibitors in heart failure, although the mean EF was somewhat higher. Patients had to demonstrate an at least 80% suppression of ventricular ectopic beats and no evidence of a proarrhythmic effect during an initial open-label titration phase. Patients with EF < 30% were not allocated to flecainide because of concern about its negative inotropic effect.

The GESICA trial[4] included patients with 'advanced' NYHA class II or class III–IV chronic heart failure adequately treated with standard therapies and who had a marked impairment in left ventricular systolic function (EF < 35%, cardiothoracic ratio > 55% or echocardiographic LVEDD > 32 mm m^{-2}). Patients receiving antiarrhythmic agents, those with symptomatic ventricular arrhythmias or nonsustained ventricular tachycardia for > 10 beats, and those with atrioventricular conduction defects were excluded, as were patients with standard contraindications to amiodarone. The study population was somewhat different from that observed in CHF-STAT; about 10% of patients had Chagas' disease, the prevalence of ischemic heart disease was lower, and the prevalence of hypertension (40%), alcoholism (33%), and trial fibrillation (29%) were higher.

The Congestive Heart Failure: Survival Trial of Antiarrhythic Therapy (CHF-STAT)[104] recruited patients with a clinical diagnosis of heart failure and an EF < 40% who had at least 10 ventricular extrasystoles per hour without symptoms of arrhythmia. Patients also had to have an echocardiographic LVEDD > 55 mm or a cardiothoracic ratio of > 50%. Of patients in the trial, 99% were men; the trial was from the US Veterans organization. The population was slightly older than in the major trials of ACE inhibitors and the prevalence of atrial fibrillation was slightly higher (although how much of this was detected by Holter monitoring is unclear), but the EF and diuretic and digoxin use were similar to those in the SOLVD trial. Most patients were taking an ACE inhibitor.

Endpoints

The primary endpoint of the CAST study was a combined endpoint of death due to arrhythmia or resuscitation from an arrhythmic cardiac death. Arrhythmic death was defined as witnessed and instantaneous, witnessed and preceded by symptoms of myocardial ischemia provided cardiogenic shock or NYHA class IV heart failure were not present, witnessed and preceded by syncope or near syncope, or unwitnessed but without evidence of another cause. Death was also not classified as arrhythmic if death due to heart failure appeared likely within 4 months of a fatal episode. Endpoints were ratified by a committee. The committee agreed with the investigators' decision as to mode of death in 86% of cases. A large number of secondary endpoints were also defined, including the development of heart failure.

Endpoints in the GESICA study were all-cause mortality, cardiopulmonary resuscitation, and symptomatic sustained ventricular tachycardia. Preplanned subgroup analyses by gender, NYHA class, and the presence or absence of nonsustained ventricular tachycardia were preplanned. An analysis of death due to progressive heart failure (not defined) versus sudden death (defined as death within 1 hour of presentation of new symptoms) was also planned.

The primary endpoint of the CHF-STAT trial was all-cause mortality. Secondary endpoints were sudden cardiac death, effect on EF, and suppression of arrhythmias. Randomization was stratified by etiology of heart failure (ischemic versus other) and by EF (above or below 40%). Endpoints were reviewed by a committee.

Withdrawals

In CAST, 70% of patients achieved a compliance, according to tablet counts, of greater than 90%. Of the active and placebo groups, 5% withdrew because of adverse effects; the small difference between groups was due to the development of more cases of heart failure in the active treatment group.

In GESICA, the data were censored at the time of transplantation or surgery in 11 patients receiving amiodarone and a similar number of controls. A total of 15 patients (6%) withdrew from open-label amiodarone. As there was no placebo group, no comparative control withdrawal rate is available.

In CHF-STAT, patients who developed symptomatic ventricular tachycardia or episodes of asymptomatic ventricular tachycardia lasting >30 seconds were withdrawn according to the protocol, although follow-up was continued by the intention-to-treat principle. Altogether, 41% of patients withdrew from amiodarone and 35% from placebo. This was due to intolerable side-effects in 27% and 23% of patients, respectively (NS). Gait disturbance and pulmonary toxicity were the main reasons for the small excess of events in the amiodarone group.

Outcome

Despite an attempt to identify a group of patients with a high risk of arrhythmic death, but without proarrhythmic risk, the annual mortality in the placebo group of CAST was <5%. The CAST study showed a marked increase in all-cause mortality in patients randomized to active treatment. There were 63 primary endpoints in the active treatment groups versus 26 in the placebo group ($P < 0.0001$). The apparently better outcome with flecainide compared to encainide reflected the exclusion of high-risk patients with a low EF. It has been argued that the CAST study shows that an antiarrhythmic drug is harmful in patients at low risk of arrhythmia, and therefore should not be extrapolated too far into clinical practice. However, subgroups, such as those with EF < 30% or those using a diuretic or digoxin at baseline (i.e. those likely to have heart failure) could be identified with a >5% annual mortality. Active therapy increased mortality in these groups three- to fourfold. Patients with heart failure appear to have constituted 50% or more of all deaths in CAST. In no subgroup was a reduction in mortality observed. Active treatment neither reduced nor increased nonlethal arrhythmic events, leading to some confusion about how active treatment increased the risk of sudden death.[102] In conclusion, the CAST study emphasizes the dangers of using class I antiarrhythmic agents in heart failure,[105,106] and demonstrates the risk of assuming that treatment that is good for surrogate endpoints for mortality is necessarily good for the patient. Patients excluded from the trial because of proarrhythmia had a particularly poor prognosis, even when class I drugs were not used.

The GESICA study showed a 28% RRR in all-cause mortality ($P = 0.024$). The reduction in mortality appeared to be due equally to a reduction in sudden and progressive heart failure deaths (though neither individual effect was statistically significant). 59% of the control group died or were admitted to hospital, versus 46% of the amiodarone group (31% RRR; $P < 0.01$). Female patients, patients with nonsustained ventricular tachycardia at baseline, and those in NYHA class II tended to have a better outcome, although no subgroup difference was statistically significant. Patients on amiodarone were more likely to improve and/or less likely to worsen their NYHA class than the control group. However, endpoints other than all-cause mortality must be treated with suspicion in view of the lack of blinding in this study.

The CHF-STAT study failed to confirm the findings of GESICA. There was no reduction in overall mortality, and the trend towards a reduction in sudden death were nonsignificant. The CHF-STAT study suggested that patients with heart failure due to causes other than ischemic heart disease may benefit in terms of survival. No good explanation for this difference is apparent. Amiodarone reduced the mean frequency of ectopic beats from 279 to 44 per hour ($P < 0.001$), and halved the number of patients with nonsustained ventricular tachycardia ($P < 0.001$). Baseline EFs were about 25% in both groups, but had increased to 35% in the amiodarone group versus 30% in the placebo group ($P < 0.001$) by 3 years. Some of this apparent increase in EF in both groups may have been due to selective loss of patients with low EFs, but the difference between placebo and amiodarone is probably a real effect. Patients with a lower EF had a worse prognosis, but there was no interaction with the effect of amiodarone. However, the increase in EF did not translate into clinical improvement, reduced diuretic requirement, or fewer hospitalizations.[107]

There are many reasons for the differences in outcome between CHF-STAT and GESICA.[103] The annual mortality in GESICA was 3–4 times that of CHF-STAT, GESICA having one of the highest annual mortality rates of any heart-failure study. Patients in CHF-STAT had milder heart failure, but it was NYHA II patients that showed particular benefit in GESICA. Although women showed more benefit in GESICA than men, the numbers of women in the two studies was small. The withdrawal rate from CHF-STAT appears much higher but, as the median duration of CHF-STAT was four times longer, the annualized withdrawal rates are similar. As CHF-STAT was the larger study, had a longer follow-up, and was placebo controlled, it must be taken as the best available evidence. However, CHF-STAT and GESICA do show that amiodarone is safe in patients with arrhythmias and ventricular dysfunction and should be considered the first-line antiarrhythmic treatment for symptomatic arrhythymias requiring treatment.

Preliminary results from two substantial postinfarction trials with amidodarone were announced at the American College of Cardiology in March 1996: the European Myocardial Infarction Amiodarone Trial (EMIAT), and the Canadian Acute Myocardial Infarction Amiodarone Trial (CAMIAT). Patients in EMIAT were identified as high risk by the presence of substantial ventricular dysfunction, and in CAMIAT by the presence of frequent, but asymptomatic and nonsustained, arrhythmias. Neither trial showed a reduction in overall mortality. These studies lend weight to the CHF-STAT results indicating that amiodarone is probably the safest antiarrhythmic agent around (digoxin and beta-blockers excluded), but that it has little to offer except in patients with symptoms or possibly those with very high-grade arrhythmias.

In conclusion, the trials of antiarrhythmic agents in heart failure are disappointing, given that 50% or more of patients with heart failure will die suddenly.[21] This suggests either that currently used antiarrhythmic agents are ineffective, or that sudden death in heart failure is not predominantly due to arrhythmias and could be due primarily, for instance, to coronary vascular occlusion. The failure of two classes of agents to reduce mortality supports the hypothesis that sudden death may not generally be arrhythmic in origin. However, the potential of beta-blockers to reduce arrhythmias (see below) must be kept in mind.

Beta-blockers

Although some have advocated the use of beta-blockers in heart failure for over 20 years, until now they have generally been considered contraindicated in heart failure.[108] Five substantial trials have been conducted (*Tables 18.16* and *18.17*).

Table 18.16 Baseline characteristics of patients randomized in trials of beta-blockers

	Xamoterol	MDC	CIBIS	ANZ	US carvedilol
No. randomized	516 (2:1)	383	641	415	1094
No. screened (% excluded)	Not given	417 (92)	Not given	442	
Age (years)	62	49	60	67	58
Follow-up (years)	0.24	≥1	1.9	1.5	0.5
Gender (%F/%M)	26/74	27/73	17/83	20/80	23/77
NYHA I+II/III/IV	0/76/24	47/49/4	0/95/5	84/16/0	53/44/3
Current angina (%)	Limiting angina excluded	–	37?	25 (on exercise test)	?
CAD (%)	61	–	55	100	48
DCM (%)	30	100	36	0	52
Hypertension (%)	16	–	6	?	?
Diabetes (%)	Not given	–	?	?	
Atrial fibrillation (%)	22	?	13	14	?
Heart rate (bpm)	84	91	83	76	84
Systolic BP (mmHg)	122	118	127	129	116
EF (%)	25	22 (<40[a])	25 (<40)	29 (<45)	23 (<35)
Diuretics (%)	100,[a] 91% frusemide	76% on frusemide	100[a]	75	95
Digoxin (%)	49	79	57	38	91
ACE inhibitor (%)	100[a]	80	90	85	95
Other vasodilator (%)	52	14 (nitrates only)	48		32
Beta-blocker/calcium antagonist (%)	0[a]/14	0[a]/?	0[a]/8	0[a]/?	0[a]/2
Aspirin/warfarin (%)	Not given	Not given	26/40	?	?

BP, blood pressure; CAD, coronary artery disease; DCM, dilated cardiomyopathy; EF, ejection fraction.
[a]By protocol.

Entry Criteria and Study Populations

The study of xamoterol in severe heart failure[107] should be considered as a trial of a beta-blocker because, despite its beta-agonist properties, it clearly reduced heart rate (suggesting more beta-antagonist than beta-agonist properties) in this population. Patients had to be in NYHA class III–IV, despite treatment with an ACE inhibitor and diuretic for at least 2 months. A clinical diagnosis of heart failure had to be confirmed by a cardiothoracic ratio of >55%, a left ventricular fractional shortening on M-mode echocardiography of <20%, an LVEDD >60 mm, or an EF <35%.

The Metoprolol in Dilated Cardiomyopathy Trial (MDC)[110] recruited only patients with dilated cardiomyopathy, EF < 40% (technique not specified), and age < 75 years. Patients with a >50% obstruction of a coronary artery were excluded, but the incidental finding of coronary disease in patients believed to have dilated cardiomyopathy did not automatically preclude recruitment. Patients consuming >700 g alcohol per week and those with a heart rate of <45 bpm, insulin-dependent diabetes, or other contraindication to beta-blockers were excluded. Most patients were already receiving digoxin, ACE inhibitors, and/or diuretics. The mean age of this population was only 49 years.

The Cardiac Insufficiency Bisoprolol Study (CIBIS)[111] recruited patients in NYHA class III–IV, EF < 40% (measured by various techniques), and <75 years old. Patients had to be ambulatory and not awaiting heart transplantation. All patients had to be receiving a diuretic and a vasodilator (this could include an ACE inhibitor). Patients with a resting

Table 18.17 Comparison in and results of trials of beta blockers

	Comparison and target dose	Dose achieved	Withdrawals, n (%)	Myocardial infarction, n (%)	Worsening CHF, n (%)	Hospitalization, n (%)		Total mortality, n (%)	Mortality per annum (%)
						Total	CHF		
Xamoterol	Xamoterol 200 mg daily (n = 327)	?	69 (19)	?	?	?	?	32 (9.2) (RER 149%; P = 0.02)	37
	vs Placebo (n = 150)	?	19 (12)	?	?	?	?	6 (3.7)	15
MDC	Metoprolol 50 mg b.d.–t.i.d. (n = 194)	108 mg daily	23	? None	19[c] (P < 0.0001)	?	37 (51[d])	23 (12) (RER 20%; NS)	~10
	vs Placebo (n = 189)	115 mg daily	31	? None	2[c]	?	49 (83[d])	19 (10)	~8
CIBIS	Bisoprolol 5 mg daily (n = 320)	3.8 mg daily (59% on top dose)	75 (23)	3	41 (13) (NS)	?	61 (P < 0.01)	53 (17) (RRR 20%; NS)	8.7
	vs Placebo (n = 321)	4.5 mg daily (82% on top dose)	82 (26)	2	35 (11)	?	90	67 (21)	11.0
ANZ	Carvedilol 25 mg b.d. (n = 207)	41 mg daily (56% on top dose) (NS)	30 (14) (P = 0.01[a])	30 (14) (RRR 33%; P = 0.068[b])	82 (40) (NS)	99 (48) (RRR 17%; P = 0.052)		20 (9.7) (RRR 25%; NS)	6.5
	vs Placebo (n = 208)	46 mg daily	13 (6)	44 (21)	85 (41)	120 (58)		26 (12.5)	8.3
US carvedilol	Carvedilol 25–50 mg b.d. (n = 696)	(66% reached target dose)	11	3 (NS)	Reduced	CVS only (14)	(5)	22 (3.2) (RRR 65%; P < 0.0001)	6.4
	vs Placebo (n = 398)		17 P = 0.002	4		(20)	(10)	31 (7.8)	15.6

b.d., twice daily; CHF, coronary heart failure; CVS, cardiovascular; t.i.d., three times daily.

[a] Data at 6 months.

[b] Combined endpoint of myocardial infarction, unstable angina, or need for revascularization.

[c] Defined as need for transplantation.

[d] Total number of admissions as opposed to number of patients with one or more admission.

heart rate of <65 bpm or another standard contraindication to a beta-blocker were excluded.

The Australia–New Zealand Heart Failure Research Collaborative Group (ANZ) trial[112,113] recruited only patients with documented ischemic heart disease who had EF < 45% and NYHA I–III heart failure, although NYHA I patients had to have previously had a worse functional class. Patients with a heart rate of <50 bpm were excluded, as were insulin-dependent diabetics and those with standard contraindications to beta-blockers.

The US carvedilol trials[108,114] selected patients with a clinical diagnosis of heart failure and an EF < 35% who had evidence of exercise impairment on a corridor walk test (i.e. were not able to walk 550 m in 6 minutes). Patients, after undergoing a common entry protocol, were then randomized into a series of smaller studies with specific goals, including the assessment of the effects on symptoms, quality of life, EF, heart-failure-related hospitalization, and mortality. A dose-ranging study was also performed. A common data and safety monitoring board was formed to assess any increase or decrease in mortality.

The populations recruited into the beta-blocker trials are generally similar to those recruited into the large trials of ACE inhibitors, except that patients in the xamoterol trial and CIBIS had more severe symptoms and all the trials except the ANZ trial recruited a much higher proportion of patients with dilated cardiomyopathy.

Endpoints

The primary endpoint of the xamoterol study was exercise duration. Mortality and morbidity data were collected as adverse events. Other endpoints were symptoms and Holter monitoring.

The primary objective of the MDC trial was a combined one of all-cause mortality and clinical deterioration to the point where heart transplantation was recommended. Set criteria were laid down by which a patient should be referred for transplantation; as these included a fall in EF by >10%, an outcome less likely with a beta-blocker, this could have biased the trial result. Functional class, quality of life, hemodynamics, and EF were also measured.

One primary outcome in the CIBIS trial was all-cause mortality. The secondary outcome was the number of withdrawals from treatment. The mode of death was subclassified, functional class followed up, and several subgroup analyses were perspecified (including NYHA class, history of myocardial infarction, and etiology of heart failure). The primary outcome at 18 months in the ANZ trial was all-cause mortality or hospitalization combined. NYHA class, EF, and exercise performance were evaluated at interim periods.

The overall US carvedilol trials program was monitored to determine the safety of carvedilol. In particular, the data safety and monitoring board was charged with the responsibility of monitoring mortality, not just to make sure that no harm was done, but also to recognize the possibility that carvedilol might reduce mortality. A number of studies formed the component parts of the overall program (see entry criteria above).

Screening and Titration Phases

In common with the SOLVD study of ACE inhibition, many of the beta-blocker studies involved an open-label run-in period. The MDC trial had a 2–7 day test period of 5 mg metoprolol twice daily, the ANZ trial had open-label dosing with carvedilol for 2–3 weeks at doses of 3.125–6.25 mg twice daily, and the US carvedilol trials had a 2 week open-label treatment with carvedilol 6.25 mg twice daily.

This is of some concern, as withdrawal of the beta-blocker could be associated with a period of adrenergic hypersensitivity and increased risk in the placebo group. A screening phase enhances the apparent safety of randomized treatment and makes sure that a large number of patients in the randomized trial are likely to be taking their allocated treatment. On the other hand, a large number of dropouts during the screening phase would also mean that the study did not reflect the more general population.

However, the long treatment periods and lack of an early increase in placebo mortality make it unlikely that there was a deleterious withdrawal effect in the placebo group. In general, about 5% of patients did not tolerate the test dose period. Although this percentage may decline with greater physician experience, it is likely to be higher in the general population, who are less well investigated and selected for treatment than in a trial setting, and in older populations with more concomitant disease.

The mortality during the 2-week, open-label active run-in of the US carvedilol trials was higher (0.6%) than in the 1-week open-label active treatment phase of the SOLVD trials (0.0006%; 4 deaths out of 6797 patients), but the latter included prevention trial data in asymptomatic patients. In the US trials, there was a 1.7% mortality in the 3 weeks preceding the open-label carvedilol challenge compared to a 0.005% mortality in the SOLVD combined placebo run-in phase. These data suggest no excess mortality with carvedilol in the run-in period that could have biased the study.

Apart from the xamoterol study, all trials had a phase where doses were titrated upwards gradually, generally at 1- to 2-week intervals. Maintenance doses were achieved after about 6 weeks.

Withdrawals

The percentage of withdrawals after randomization was similar, with active and placebo groups in most of the beta-blocker trials, although there were trends to less withdrawals for progressive heart failure. Treatment failure and intercurrent events such as stroke, cardiac surgery, etc., led to the majority of withdrawals in CIBIS. In the first month 4% and 6% of patients withdrew from placebo and bisoprolol, respectively. In the ANZ trial 14% of patients withdrew from carvedilol versus 6% from placebo in the first 6 months of the trial ($P = 0.01$). Patient preference without known adverse effect accounted for the majority of withdrawals. In contrast, more patients withdrew from placebo than carvedilol in the US trials: 89% of patients were receiving or had completed treatment with carvedilol compared to only 83% of those randomized to placebo ($P = 0.002$).

Outcomes

The xamoterol trial showed a 149% relative excess risk for mortality with an increase in both sudden death and death from progressive heart failure ($P = 0.02$). Symptom scores showed a reduction in breathlessness with xamoterol ($P < 0.02$), but exercise tolerance did not improve. Holter monitoring showed a reduction in average daytime but not night-time heart rate. Assuming that beta-blockers are indeed beneficial in heart failure, as suggested in later studies, there are at least two possible reasons why xamoterol increased mortality. First, the beta-agonist properties of xamoterol could have been deleterious. Alternatively, the xamoterol study is the only one of this group of studies that did not include a titration phase. It is quite possible that other beta-blockers would have fared similarly with a similar study design.

The MDC trial achieved a borderline result on the primary endpoint ($P = 0.058$) with 38% (20%) events on placebo and 25 (13%) on metoprolol (RRR 34%). The mortality component of the combined endpoint tended in the opposite direction, all the benefit being in a reduction in the need for transplantation (19 versus 2; $P < 0.0001$). However, as metoprolol increased the EF by about 6%, and this was one of the criteria for referral for transplantation, the result, in isolation, has to be treated with circumspection. Metoprolol tended to have a favorable effect on hemodynamics, although the increase in systolic blood pressure and stroke work index could be attributed directly to a reduction in heart rate; cardiac output and vascular resistances did not change. NYHA class ($P = 0.01$), symptoms ($P = 0.01$), and exercise capacity ($P < 0.001$) improved.

The CIBIS trial showed no effect on overall mortality and no difference in withdrawal rates (primary and secondary endpoints). The mortality rate was similar to that in the SOLVD–treatment study, suggesting that the patients were closer to NYHA class II in severity than to class III-IV, and only half the patients reached the target dose of 5 mg daily. One or both of the above may account for the lack of a significant reduction in mortality in the CIBIS study. Patients taking bisoprolol had fewer episodes of heart failure decompensation (19% versus 28%; $P < 0.01$) and NYHA class was more likely to improve on bisoprolol (21% versus 15%; $P < 0.03$). Arryhthmic events were few, but were reduced by bisoprolol ($P = 0.03$). Trends to a greater benefit in patients with NYHA class IV heart failure were not significant, but the reduction in mortality in patients who had not suffered a prior myocardial infarction was ($P = 0.01$), a result that appeared significantly different ($P = 0.034$) from patients with prior infarction. This was largely, but not entirely, due to a reduction in mortality among patients with dilated cardiomyopathy.

The ANZ trial showed a 41% RRR in the primary endpoint at 18 months ($P < 0.02$). This was predominantly due to a reduction in hospitalizations (RRR 33%; $P = 0.052$). Overall mortality was low at 11% over 18 months, which is consistent with mild heart failure; the 25% RRR in mortality was not significant. There was no reduction in worsening heart failure, but a borderline significant ($P = 0.068$; RRR 37%) reduction in major cardiac events, including myocardial infarction, unstable angina, or a need for revascularization, occurred. Carvedilol did not improve exercise performance or symptoms, but did improve EF from about 29% to 34% ($P < 0.0001$). The failure to improve symptoms may reflect the difficulty of showing improvements in a population with mild heart failure.

The US carvedilol trials showed a 65% RRR ($P < 0.001$) in all-cause mortality. Reduction in mortality appeared due to a reduction in sudden death and death due to progressive heart failure. Within the various substudies,[108] reductions in hospital admissions for worsening heart failure, improvements in functional status, and an improvement in EF by about 6% were also noted. Exercise performance, maximal or submaximal, was generally not improved, and improvement in quality-of-life scores was inconsistent. Patients and doctors both showed consistent preference for carvedilol.

Overall, there is conclusive evidence that beta-blockers are safe and reduce morbidity in patients with heart failure. Carvedilol, at least, and possibly other beta-blockers also, appear to reduce mortality, an effect that may be greater even than that observed with ACE inhibitors. In contrast to metoprolol and bisoprolol, carvedilol is a nonselective beta-blocker that also has alpha-adrenoceptor blocking as well as antioxidant and anti-smooth-muscle-cell proliferative properties.[115] It is not clear how important the ancillary properties of carvedilol are to its effect on mortality, or whether the benefits of carvedilol can be extrapolated to other beta-blockers.

The investigators in the studies of beta-blockers selected relatively young patients, predominantly with dilated cardiomyopathy. Thus the study population is very different from the general population of patients with heart failure. Wider clinical experience is required before extrapolation of the data from the beta-blocker trials.

Beta-blocker Studies in Progress

Further placebo-controlled trials are underway with bisoprolol (CIBIS-II; $n = 2500$) and bucindolol (BEST; $n = 2800$).[87,116] Trials comparing metoprolol and carvedilol (COMET; $n = 3000$) are in the planning phase.[108]

Other Studies

There are several studies ongoing with other groups of agents. The WASH study[67] is comparing aspirin, warfarin, and a no antithrombotic treatment control arm in an open-label prospective randomized study. Patient entry criteria include evidence of major impairment of left ventricular systolic function and a requirement for diuretic therapy. Patients recruited will be mainly NYHA II–III. After ascertaining baseline characteristics, the patients are randomized by telephone. The primary endpoint is all-cause mortality. A subanalysis of the SOLVD data suggests that warfarin may improve prognosis,[117] although a similar analysis has suggested that antiplatelet agents may be effective.[65] Other sources of data and other interpretations of the SOLVD data highlight the potential for aspirin to exert a deleterious effect on prognosis in heart failure.[66,67]

Currently, losartan appears to be superior to placebo in terms of preventing worsening heart failure, but possibly not as good as an ACE inhibitor.[118] ELITE[128] ($n = 722$) compared losartan (50 mg daily), an angiotensin-II receptor antagonist, and captopril (50 mg three times daily) in patients with heart failure and ejection fraction $< 40\%$, two-thirds of whom were over 70 years of age.[128] The study was designed to assess the tolerability of each agent as well as the outcome in terms of worsening heart failure and death. Losartan was better tolerated than captopril but was not superior in terms of its effect on increasing serum creatinine. However, 32 deaths occurred on captopril versus 17 on losartan ($P < 0.05$). Whether the results reflect a greater efficacy of losartan over ACE inhibitors in general or were a consequence of fewer withdrawals from treatment remains to be determined.

RALES[87,119] ($n = 1400$) will compare a range of doses of spironolactone added to background ACE inhibition to assess any additional effect on mortality. Patients recruited into RALES are either in NYHA class IV or have a history of NYHA class IV heart failure in the last 6 months. Patients intolerant of ACE inhibitors are included.

No adequate randomized study of the benefits of coronary bypass surgery in heart failure exists as yet. Operative mortality ranges from under 5% to around 20%, depending on the patient-selection criteria (especially age, gender, the amount of viable but jeopardized myocardium, and the severity of ventricular dysfunction and heart failure) and the center where the surgery is performed.[120,121] Data from a recent report from Duke University are given in *Table 18.18*.[122] A total of 1088 patients with an EF $< 40\%$ and in NYHA class II–IV were included. The Duke University experience shows what is possible, but does not show if their experience is widely applicable.

With advances in medical therapy, it is obvious that a randomized, controlled trial of transplantation versus medical therapy is needed, although it is doubtful if one will be done. This is particularly the case when transplantation is being advised for improvement in prognosis rather than because of a failure of medical treatment to control symptoms.

Table 18.18 Mortality after coronary bypass surgery versus medical therapy[122]

Year	Medical therapy (%)	Coronary bypass surgery (%)	P-value
1	71	77	0.17
5	35	55	0.0001
10	15	35	0.0001

Summary

Although still in its infancy, the art and science of clinical trials is rapidly growing up. Below is a list of factors, by no means exhaustive, that will improve future trials.

(1) We need to know much more about the patients entering clinical trials. This includes:

- *Better diagnosis*. It has been suggested that drug therapy may generally improve the prognosis of patients without ischemic heart disease (IHD) to a greater extent than those with IHD. This is curious, as patients without IHD generally have a better prognosis. To what extent age plays a role in the better prognosis of non-IHD patients is unclear. Patients without IHD as the cause of heart failure could reflect a predominantly young population with dilated cardiomyopathy (DCM) or an old population with hypertensive heart disease. Patients without IHD as the cause of heart failure should not be assumed to have DCM. Epidemiological studies of DCM indicate that only about 50% of patients so diagnosed undergo coronary angiography, but 50% of patients with presumptive DCM turn out to have important coronary disease.[18] Sutton's use of a 'diagnosis uncertain' category[123] is better than being unable to distinguish guesswork from a proper diagnosis. A full diagnostic work-up, including a coronary arteriogram in all cases (unless the presence of coronary disease has already been declared by clinical, electrocardiographic and, perferably, enzyme diagnosis of myocardial infarction), is ideal but often impractical, especially in studies incorporating elderly patients. It is quite possible that the debate on the effects of etiology on response to therapy is spurious. It is sobering to recall that enalapril had a significantly greater effect ($P < 0.04$ for heterogeneity) in reducing myocardial infarction in patients without IHD at baseline than in patients with IHD.[58]
- *Detailed reporting of drug therapy*. It is important to know about concomitant therapy that may interact with the study treatment. The apparent negation of ACE inhibitor benefit with aspirin is a good example. The intensity of treatment, in particular the dose of diuretic, is probably a more important guide to prognosis than is the NYHA class. A patient in NYHA class I on frusemide 120 mg daily probably has a worse outcome than a patient in NYHA class III on no therapy. It is likely that the intensity of treatment biases the NYHA class to which the doctor ascribes the patient, although it should not. This may be why NYHA class seems better than quality-of-life scales in predicting outcome.

(2) It is not inappropriate for trials to select specific groups of patients for study, as lack of patient selection can mean dilution and loss of a real benefit. However, it is inappropriate to extrapolate the data from highly selected populations to the general community. For a drug to be truly sucessful requires it to demonstrate efficacy in a broad range of patients. The most notable group of patients absent from clinical trials of heart failure is the elderly, although this omission is being redressed.

(3) More thought needs to be put into endpoints.

- Health economists as well as statisticians should be consulted before planning large trials. Counting the number of hospitalizations is not enough. The duration and complexity of hospitalization needs to be assessed. Total hospitalization rather than cause-specific hospitalization is the only valid measure for health economic purposes, unless it can be shown that the reason for admission influences the duration and complexity of hospital stay.
- Too many endpoints are reported in a superficial manner. This prevents insight into the natural history of disease that might indicate better means of treatment. Superficial reporting also stops doctors thinking more deeply about the problem, as they feel they have been given the answer. A good example is 'hospitalization for worsening heart failure'. What does this mean? Does it include dehydration, hypotension, and renal dysfunction (consequences of treatment rather than disease)? Acute exacerbations of heart failure can be due to dietary indiscretion, infection, ischemia, or atrial fibrillation. We should know what led to the exacerbation.
- Transplantation or being scheduled for it is a lottery owing as much to the play of chance, age, body size, and blood group as the severity of heart failure. By all means record transplantation, but is should not be an endpoint. The data should be censored around the time of surgery. On the other hand, more patients die waiting for transplants than get them, so when studying severe heart failure there is no need to exclude such patients from trials.

(4) More clarity. Large clinical trials, regardless of their result, are likely to find a 'good home' in a 'respectable' journal. Doctors need to know about and learn from the result. It would be useful if a standard mode of reporting for large trials was developed that, for instance, laid emphasis on total hospitalization, the true marker of morbidity and economic cost, rather than hospitalization for just one cause that happened to be favorably influenced. The protocol and endpoint definition of all landmark trials should be published prior to the randomization code of the trial being broken. By placing the endpoints in the public domain arguments about endpoint definitions will be reduced or eliminated. Journals specifically for this purpose are now available.

(5) Trial duration.

- *Can mortality trials be too short?* The CONSENSUS and US carvedilol trials demonstrated a reduction in mortality with a mean follow-up of a little over 6 months. Trials that have a large enough number of endpoints can show a reduction in mortality in the short term. It is reassuring to see short-term data confirmed by long-term data, but if a treatment improves symptoms, morbidity, and mortality in the short-term, it seems churlish not to accept the balance of evidence. It has been said that short-term trials do not provide enough insight into the impact on the natural history of the disease. Patients are inevitably recruited into clinical trials at varying points in their clinical course, and thus a clinical trial will usually give information over a broad range of the course of the condition. On the other hand, a surprise result on mortality in one trial with a drug that has increased mortality at other doses and belongs to a class of drugs that have had deleterious effects needs to be viewed with caution.[90] The duration of the trial would be irrelevant.
- *Can trials be too long?* Despite the lack of strong evidence of long-term symptomatic benefit with ACE inhibitors,[124,125] intelligent, informed guesses can be made on the basis of circumstantial evidence influenced by known benefits on hospitalization and mortality. In general, longer term trials on symptoms and morbidity are to be

welcomed, although where the sample size is less than 50 patients studies of 3–6 months in duration are most likely to demonstrate the activity of an agent on symptoms.[124] More emphasis should be placed on collecting data on symptoms in long-term 'mortality' trials. Arguments about mortality benefit in short-term trials would be resolved by publishing in advance, before the randomization code is broken, the endpoints of the study.

(6) A more liberal attitude to study design. Undoubtedly, the randomized, controlled trial is clinical medicine's most important research tool. Blinding is advisable whenever possible, and should always be implemented when investigating new agents. However, comparative trials of clinical practice (e.g. surgery, hospital versus community management) are valid as long as patients are truly randomized and followed strictly on an intention-to-treat basis. Mortality is an important consideration when conducting trials in heart failure, but is often not of overriding clinical importance. Paradoxically, it is those patients with the highest mortality risk (i.e. those with severe symptomatic heart failure) in whom small improvements in survival are least important. Improvement in symptoms should be the primary goal of treatment for severe symtomatic heart failure. The tiny fraction of patients awaiting definitive therapy, such as transplantation, may be an exception to this rule. The prognosis of patients with 'mild' heart failure is generally better, although still poor compared to that of patients with many other diseases. In 'mild' heart failure, improving mortality is the primary goal. It is unfortunate that the quest for a positive mortality result is driving attention away from symptoms and towards prognosis in the group of patients with heart failure in whom this is least appropriate. It is also unfortunate that the cost and difficulty of mounting studies that are large and long enough to address the mortality issue in milder heart failure is driving attention away from this issue. The concept of large trials with substudies is well developed. The concept of multiple studies with a common trunk protocol (as with the US carvedilol studies) is an interesting development that should be pursued further.

References

1. Cohn JN, Archibald DG, Ziesche S, *et al*. Effect of vasodilator therapy on mortality in chronic congestive heart failure: results of a Veterans Administration Cooperative Study. *N Engl J Med* 1986; **314**: 1547–52.
2. Cleland JGF, Oakley CM. Vascular tone in heart failure: the neuroendocrine–therapeutic interface. *Br Heart J* 1991; **166**: 264–7.
3. Cannon PJ, Powers ER, Reison DS, *et al*. A placebo-controlled trial of captopril in refractory chronic congestive heart failure. *J Am Coll Cardiol* 1983; **2**: 755–63.
4. Doval HC, Nul DR, Grancelli HI, Perrone SV, Bortman GR, Curiel R. Randomised trial of low-dose amiodarone in severe congestive heart failure. *Lancet* 1994; **344**: 493–8.
5. Cleland JGF, Poole Wilson PA. ACE inhibitors for heart failure: a question of dose. *Br Heart J* 1994; **72**: S106–10.
6. Cohn JN, Johnson G, Ziesche S, *et al*. A comparison of enalapril with hydralazine-isosorbide dinitrate in the treatment of chronic congestive heart failure. *N Engl J Med* 1991; **325**: 303–10.
7. Captopril-Digoxin Multicentre Group. Comparative effects of therapy with captopril and digoxin in patients with mild to moderate heart failure. *JAMA* 1998; **259**: 539–44.
8. Just H, Drexler H, Taylor SH, Siegrist J, Schulgen G, Schumacher M. Captopril versus digoxin in patients with coronary artery disease and mild heart failure. A prospective, double-blind, placebo-controlled multicenter study. *Herz* 1993; **18**: 436–43.
9. Swedberg K, Idanpaan Heikkila U, *et al*. Effects of enalapril on mortality in severe congestive heart failure. Results of the Cooperative North Scandinavian Enalapril Survival Study (CONSENSUS). *N Engl J Med* 1987; **316**: 1429–35.
10. Yusuf S. Effect of enalapril on survival in patients with reduced left ventricular ejection fractions and congestive heart failure. *N Engl J Med* 1991; **325**: 293–302.
11. Yusuf S, Nichlas JM, Timmis G, *et al*. Effect of enalapril on mortality and the development of heart failure in asymptomatic patients with reduced left ventricular ejection fractions. *N Engl J Med* 1992; **327**: 685–91.

12. Eriksson SV, Kjekshus J, Offstad J. Swedberg K. Patient characteristics in cases of chronic severe heart failure with different degrees of left ventricular systolic dysfunction. *Cardiology* 1994; **85**: 137–44.

13. Bangdiwala SI, Weiner DH, Bourassa MG, *et al*. Studies of Left Ventricular Dysfunction (SOLVD) registry: rationale, design, methods and description of baseline characteristics. *Am J Cardiol* 1992; **70**: 347–53.

14. Carew BD, Ahn SA, Boichot HD, *et al*. Recruitment strategies in the studies of left ventricular dysfunction (SOLVD): strategies for screening and enrollment in two concurrent but separate trials. *Controlled Clin Trials* 1992; **13**: 325–38.

15. Johnstone D, Limacher M, Rousseau M, *et al*. Clinical characteristics of patients in studies of left ventricular dysfunction (SOLVD). *Am J Cardiol* 1992; **70**: 894–900.

16. Young JB. Clinical heart failure trials and the design rationale of studies of left ventricular dysfunction (SOLVD). *J Hypertens* 1991; **9**: S57–61.

17. Parameshwar J, Shackell MM, Richardson A, Poole Wilson PA, Sutton GC. Prevalence of heart failure in three general practices in north west London. *Br J Gen Pract* 1992; **42**: 287–9.

18. Brookes CIO, Hart P, Keogh BE, Cleland JGF. Angiography and the aetiology of heart failure. *Postgrad Med J* 1995; **71**: 480–2.

19. Parameshwar J, Poole Wilson PA, Sutton GC. Heart failure in a district general hospital. *J R Coll Physicians London* 1992; **26**: 139–42.

20. Sutton GC. Epidemiologic aspects of heart failure. *Am Heart J* 1990; **120**: 1538–40.

21. Narang R, Cleland JGF, Erhardt L, *et al*. Mode of death in chronic heart failure: a request for more accurate classification. *Eur Heart J* 1996; **17**: 1390–1403.

22. Ziesche S, Rector TS, Cohn JN. Inter-observer discordance in the classification of mechanisms of death in studies of heart failure. *J Cardiac Failure* 1995; **1**: 127–32.

23. Kjekshus J, Swedberg K, Snapinn S. Effects of enalapril on long-term mortality in severe congestive heart failure. *Am J Cardiol* 1992; **69** 103–7.

24. Kjekshus J, Swedberg K. Tolerability of enalapril in congestive heart failure. *Am J Cardiol* 1988; **62**: 67A–72A.

25. Ljungman S, Kjekshus J, Swedberg K. Renal function in severed congestive heart failure during treatment with Enalapril (the Cooperative North Scandinavian Enalapril Survival Study (CONCENSUS) trial). *Am J Cardiol* 1992; **70**: 479–87.

26. Swedberg K. Eneroth P, Kjekshus J. Wilhelmsen L. Hormones regulating cardiovascular function in patients with severe congestive heart failure and their relation to mortality. *Circulation* 1990; **82**: 1730–6.

27. Hughes CV, Wong M, Johnson G. Cohn JN. Influence of age on mechanisms and prognosis of heart failure. *Circulation* 1993; **87**: VI111–17.

28. Carson PE, Johnson GR, Dunkman WB, Fletcher RD, Farrell L, Cohn JN. The influence of atrial fibrillation on prognosis in mild to moderate heart failure: the V-HeFT studies. *Circulation* 1993; **87**: VI102–10.

29. Dunkman WB, Johnson GR, Carson PE, Bhat G, Farrell L, Cohn JN. Incidence of thromboembolic events in congestive heart failure. *Circulation* 1993; **87**: VI94–101.

30. Smith RF, Johnson, G, Ziesche S, Bhat G, Blankenship K, Cohn JN. Functional capacity in heart failure: comparison of methods for assessment and their relation to other indexes of heart failure. *Circulation* 1993; **87**: V188–93.

31. Loeb HS, Johnson G, Henrick A, *et al*. Effect of enalapril, hydralazine plus isosorbide dinitrate, and prazosin on hospitalization in patients with chronic congestive heart failure. *Circulation* 1993; **87**: V178–87.

32. Rector TS, Johnson G, Dunkman WB, *et al*. Evaluation by patients with heart failure of the effects of enalapril compared with hydralazine plus isosorbide dinitrate on quality of life V-HeFT II. *Circulation* 1993; **87**: V171–7.

33. Wong M, Johnson G, Shabetai R, *et al*. Echocardiographic variables as prognostic indicators and therapeutic monitors in chronic congestive heart failure: Veterans Affairs Cooperative Studies V-HeFT I and II. *Circulation* 1993; **87**: V165–70.

34. Ziesche S, Cobb FR, Cohn JN, Johnson G, Tristani F. Hydralazine and isosorbide dinitrate combination improves exercise tolerance in heart failure: results from V-HeFT I and V-HeFT II. *Circulation* 1993; **87**: V156–64.

35. Fletcher RD, Cintron GB, Johnson G, Orndorff J, Carson P, Cohn JN. Enalapril decreases prevalence of ventricular tachycardia in patients with chronic congestive heart failure. *Circulation* 1993; **87**: V149–55.

36. Francis GS, Cohn JN, Johnson G, Rector TS, Goldman S, Simon A. Plasma norepinephrine, plasma renin activity, and congestive heart failure: relations to survival and the effects of therapy in V-HeFT II. *Circulation* 1993; **87**: V140–8.

37. Johnson G, Carson P, Francis GS, Cohn JN. Influence of prerandomization (baseline) variables on mortality and on the reduction of mortality by enalapril: Veterans Affairs Cooperative Study on Vasodilator Therapy of Heart Failure (V-HeFT II). *Circulation* 1993; **87**: V132–9.

38. Goldman S, Johnson G, Cohn JN, Cintron G, Smith R, Francis G. Mechanism of death in heart failure: The Vasodilator–Heart Failure Trials. *Circulation* 1993; **87**: V124–31.

39. Cintron G, Johnson G, Francis G, Cobb F, Cohn JN. Prognostic significance of serial changes in left ventricular ejection fraction in patients with congestive heart failure. *Circulation* 1993; **87**: V117–23.

40. Cohn JN, Johnson GR, Shabetai R, *et al*. Ejection fraction, peak exercise oxygen consumption, cardiothoracic ratio, ventricular arrhythmias, and plasma norepinephrine as determinants of prognosis in heart failure. *Circulation* 1993; **87**: V15–16.

41. Cohn JN. The Vasodilator–Heart Failure Trials (V-HeFT) mechanistic data from the VA cooperative studies: introduction. *Circulation* 1993; **87**: VI1–4.

42. Kostis JB. The effect of enalapril on mortal and morbid events in patients with hypertension and left ventricular dysfunction. *Am J Hypertens* 1995; **8**: 909–14.

43. Pratt CM, Gardner M, Pepine C, *et al*. Lack of long-term ventricular arrhythmia reduction by enalapril in heart failure. *Am J Cardiol* 1995; **75**: 1244–9.

44. Benedict CR, Francis GS, Shelton B, *et al*. Effect of long-term enalapril therapy on neurohormones in patients with left ventricular dysfunction. *Am J Cardiol* 1995; **23**: 1151–7.

44. Greenberg B, Quinones MA, Koilpillai C, *et al*. Effects of long-term enalapril therapy on cardiac structure and function in patients with left ventricular dysfunction: results of the SOLVD echocardiography substudy. *Circulation* 1995; **91**: 2573–81.

46. Young JB, Weiner DH, Yusuf S, *et al*. Patterns of medication use in patients with heart failure: a report from the Registry of Studies of Left Ventricular Dysfunction (SOLVD). *South Med J* 1995; **88**: 514–23.

47. LeJemtel TH, Liang CS, Stewart DK, *et al*. Reduced peak aerobic capacity in asymptomatic left ventricular systolic dysfunction: A substudy of the studies of left ventricular dysfunction (SOLVD). *Circulation* 1994; **90**: 2757–60.

48. Henzlova MJ, Blackburn BH, Bradley EJ, Rogers WJ. Patient perception of a long-term clinical trial: experience using a close-out questionnaire in the Studies of Left Ventricular Dysfunction (SOLVD) trial. *Control Clin Trials* 1994; **15**: 284–93.

49. Benedict CR, Johnstone DE, Weiner DH, *et al*. Relation of neurohumoral activation to clinical variables and degree of ventricular dysfunction: A report from the registry of studies of left ventricular dysfunction. *J Am Coll Cardiol* 1994; **23**: 1410–20.

50. Rogers WJ, Johnstone DE, Yusuf S, *et al*. Quality of life among 5025 patients with left ventricular dysfunction randomized between placebo and enalapril: the studies of left ventricular dysfunction. *J Am Coll Cardiol* 1994; **23**: 393–400.

51. Hart W, Rhodes G, McMurray J. The cost effectiveness of enalapril in the treatment of chronic heart failure. *Br J Med Econ* 1993; **6**: 91–8.

52. Kostis JB, Shelton BJ, Yusuf S, *et al*. Tolerability of enalapril initiation by patients with left ventricular dysfunction: results of the medication challenge phase of the studies of left ventricular dysfunction. *Am Heart J* 1994; **128**: 358–64.

53. Konstam MA, Kroneberg MW, Rousseau MF, *et al*. Effects of the angiotensin converting enzyme inhibitor enalapril on the long-term progression of left ventricular dilatation in patients with asymptomatic systolic dysfunction. *Circulation* 1993; **88**: 2277–83.

54. Bittner V, Weiner DH, Yusuf S, *et al*. Prediction of mortality and morbidity with a 6-minute walk test in patients with left ventricular dysfunction. *J Am Med Assoc* 1993; **270**: 1702–7.

55. Benedict CR, Weiner DH, Johnstone DE, *et al*. Comparative neurohormonal responses in patients with preserved and impaired left ventricular ejection fraction: results of the studies of left ventricular dysfunction (SOLVD) registry. *J Am Coll Cardiol* 1993; **22**: 146A–53A.

56. Pouleur H, Rousseau MF, Van Eyll C, *et al*. Effects of long-term enalapril therapy on left ventricular diastolic properties in patients with depressed ejection fraction. *Circulation* 1993; **88**: 481–91.

57. Gorkin L, Norvell NK, Rosen RC, *et al*. Assessment of quality of life as observed from the baseline data of the Studies of Left Ventricular Dysfunction (SOLVD) trial quality-of-life substudy. *Am J Cardiol* 1993; **71**: 1069–73.

58. Yusuf S, Pepine CJ, Garces C, *et al*. Effect of enalapril on myocardial infarction and unstable angina in patients with low ejection fractions. *Lancet* 1992; **340**: 1173–8.

59. Konstam MA, Rousseau MF, Kroneberg MW, *et al*. Effects of the angiotensin converting enzyme inhibitor enalapril on the long-term progression of left ventricular dysfunction in patients with heart failure. *Circulation* 1992; **86**: 431–8.

60. Hood WB, Youngblood M, Ghali JK, *et al*. Initial blood pressure response to enalapril in hospitalized patients (studies of left ventricular dysfunction (SOLVD)). *Am J Cardiol* 1991; **68**: 1465–8.

61. Stewart DK, Liang CS, Kirlin PC, *et al*. Effect of enalapril on exercise response of SOLVD patients with left ventricular dysfunction and mild symptoms. *Heart Failure* 1995; **11**: 243–51.

62. Young JB, Gheorghiade M, Packer M, Uretsky B, Hull H, on behalf of the PROVED and RADIANCE investigators. Are low serum levels of digoxin effective in chronic heart failure? Evidence challenging the accepted guidelines for a therapeutic serum level of the drug. *J Am Coll Cardiol* 1993; **21**: 378A (abstract).

63. Benedict CR, Shelton B, Johnstone DE, *et al*. Prognostic significance of plasma norepinephrine in patients with asymptomatic left ventricular dysfunction. *Circulation* 1996; **94**: 690–7.

64. Shindler DM, Kostis JB, Yusuf S, *et al*. Diabetes mellitus, a predictor of morbidity and mortality in the Studies of Left Ventricular Dysfunction (SOLVD) trials and registry. *Am J Cardiol* 1996; **77**: 1017–20.

65. Al-Khadra AS, Salem DN, Rand WM, Udelson JE, Smith JJ, Konstam MA. Effect of antiplatelet agents on survival in patients with left ventricular systolic dysfunction. *Circulation* 1995; **92**(Suppl 1): I665–6 (abstract).

66. Cleland JGF, Poole-Wilson PA. Is aspirin safe in heart failure? More data. *Heart* 1996; **75**: 426–7.

67. Cleland JGF, Bulpitt CJ, Falk RH, *et al*. Is aspirin safe for patients with heart failure? *Br Heart J* 1995; **74**: 215–19.

68. Glick H, Cook J, Kinosian B, *et al*. Costs and effects of enalapril therapy in patients with symptomatic heart failure: an economic analysis of the studies of left ventricular dysfunction (SOLVD) treatment trial. *J Cardiac Failure* 1995; **1**: 371–80.

69. Cleland JGF. ACE inhibitors for the prevention and treatment of heart failure: Why are they 'under-used'? *J Human Hypertens* 1995; **9**: 435–42.

70. Cleland JGF. The clinical course of heart failure and its modification by ACE inhibitors: insights from recent clinical trials. *Eur Heart J* 1994; **15**: 125–30.

71. Rutherford JD, Pfeffer MA, Moye LA, *et al*. on behalf of the SAVE Investigators. Effects of captopril on ischemic events after myocardial infarction. Results of the Survival and Ventricular Enlargement trial. *Circulation* 1994; **90**: 1731–8.

72. Carson P, Johnson G, Fletcher R, Cohn J, for the V-HeFT Cooperative Study Group. Mild systolic dysfunction in heart failure (left ventricular ejection fraction (>35%): baseline characteristics, prognosis and response to therapy in the vasodilator in heart failure trials (V-HeFT). *J Am Coll Cardiol* 1996; **27**: 642–9.

73. Cohn JN, Johnson G. Heart failure with normal ejection fraction; the V-HeFT study. *Circulation* 1990; **81**: 48–53.

74. Francis GS, Benedict C, Johnstone DE, *et al*. Comparison of neuroendocrine activation in patients with left ventricular dysfunction with and without congestive heart failure. A substudy of the studies of left ventricular dysfunction (SOLVD). *Circulation* 1990; **82**: 1724–9.

75. Cleland JGF. ACE inhibitors for myocardial infarction: how should they be used? *Eur Heart J* 1995; **76**: 153–9.

76. Cleland JGF, Puri S. How do ACE inhibitors reduce mortality in patients with left ventricular dysfunction with and without heart failure: remodelling, resetting, or sudden death? *Br Heart J* 1994; **72**: S81–6.

77. Cleland JGF, Dargie HJ, East BW, *et al*. Total body and serum electrolyte composition in heart failure: The effects of captopril. *Eur Heart J* 1985; **6**: 681–8.

78. Cleland JGF, Dargie HJ, Balls SG, *et al*. Effects of enalapril in heart failure: a double blind study of effects on exercise performance, renal function, hormones, and metabolic state. *Br Heart J* 1985; **54**: 305–12.

79. Poole-Wilson PA, on behalf of the NETWORK Investigators. The NETWORK study. The effect of dose of an ACE-inhibitor on outcome in patients with heart failure. *J Am Coll Cardiol* 1996; **27**(Suppl A): 141A (abstract).

80. Haywood GA, Adams KF, Gheorghiade M, McKenna WJ. Is there a role for epoprostenol in the management of heart failure? *Am J Cardiol* 1995; **75**: 44A–50A.

81. Gogia H, Mehra A, Parikh S, *et al*. Prevention of tolerance to hemodynamic effects of nitrates with concomitant use of hydralazine in patients with chronic heart failure. *J Am Coll Cardiol* 1995; **26**: 1575–80.

82. Bayliss J, Norell MS, Canepa-Anson R, *et al*. Clinical importance of the renin-angiotensin system in chromic heart failure: double-blind comparison of captopril and prazosin. *Br Med J* 1985; **290**: 1861–5.

83. Cleland JGF. Dutka DP. Optimising heart failure pharmacotherapy: the ideal combination. *Br Heart J* 1994; **72**(Suppl): S73–9.

84. Packer M. Calcium channel blockers in chronic heart failure. The risks of 'physiologically rational' therapy. *Circulation* 1990; **82**: 2254–7.

85. Packer M. Second generation calcium channel blockers in the treatment of chronic heart failure: are they any better than their predecessors? *J Am Coll Cardiol* 1989; **14**: 1339–42.

86. O'Connor CM, Belkin RN, Carson PE, *et al*. Effect of amlodipine on mode of death in severe chronic heart failure: the PRAISE trial. *Circulation* 1995; **92**(Suppl 1): I143 (abstract).

87. McMurray J, Cleland JGF, Cowley A. Ongoing and planned clinical trials in chronic heart failure and left ventricular dysfunction. *Expert Opinion Invest Drugs* 1995; **4**: 1069–80.

88. Cohn JN, Ziesche SM, Loss LE, Anderson GF, and the V-HeFT Study Group. Effect of felodipine on short-term exercise and neurohormones and long-term mortality in heart failure: results of V-HeFt-III. *Circulation* 1995; **92**: I143 (abstract).

89. Cleland JGF, Dargie HJ, Ford I. Mortality in heart failure: clinical variables of prognostic value. *Br Heart J* 1987; **58**: 572–82.

90. The Digoxin Investigation Group: The effect of digoxin on mortality and morbidity in patients with heart failure. *N Engl J Med* 1997; **336**: 525–33.

91. Packer M, Gheorghiade M, Young JB, *et al*. Withdrawal of digoxin from patients with chronic heart failure treated with angiotensin-converting-enzyme inhibitors. *N Engl J Med* 1993; **329**: 1–7.

92. Packer M, Carver JR, Rodeheffer RJ, *et al*. Effect of oral milrinone on mortality in severe chronic heart failure. *N Engl J Med* 1991; **325**: 1468–75.

93. Feldman AM, Bristow MR, Parmley WW, *et al*. Effects of vesnarinone on morbidity and mortality in patients with heart failure. *N Engl J Med* 1993; **329**: 149–55.

94. Hampton J. Prime–II: hotline session at the American College of Cardiology. 1966.

95. Matsui S, Matsumori A, Matoba Y, Uchida A, Sasayama S. Treatment of virus-induced myocardial injury with a novel immunomodulating agent, vesnarinone. Suppression of natural killer cell activity and tumor necrosis factor-alpha production. *J Clin Invest* 1994; **94**: 1212–17.

96. Matsumori A, Shioi T, Yamada T, Matsui S, Sasayama S. Vesnarinone, a new inotropic agent, inhibits cytokine production by stimulated human blood from patients with heart failure. *Circulation* 1994; **89**: 955–8.

97. Rogers WJ, Epstein AE, Arciniegas JG, *et al*. Preliminary report: effect of encainide and flecainide on mortality in a randomized trial of arrhythmia suppression after myocardial infarction. *N Engl J Med* 1989; **321**: 406–12.

98. Rogers WJ, Epstein AE, Arciniegas JG, *et al*. Effect of the antiarrhythmic agent moricizine on survival after myocardial infarction. *N Engl J Med* 1992; **327**: 227–33.

99. Echt DS, Liebson PR, Mitchell LB, *et al*. Mortality and morbidity in patients receiving encainide, flecainide, or placebo – The Cardiac Arrhythmia Suppression Trial. *N Engl J Med* 1991; **324**: 781–8.

100. Anderson JL, Platia EV, Hallstrom A, *et al*. Interaction of baseline characteristics with the hazard of encainide, flecainide, and moricizine therapy in patients with myocardial infarction: a possible explanation for increased mortality in the Cardiac Arrhythmia Suppression Trial (CAST). *Circulation* 1994; **90**: 2843–52.

101. Peters RW, Mitchell LB, Brooks MM, *et al*. Circadian pattern of arrhythmic death in patients receiving encainide, flecainide or moricizine in the Cardiac Arrhythmia Suppression Trial (CAST). *J Am Coll Cardiol* 1994; **23**: 283–9.

102 Hallstrom AP, Anderson JL, Carlson M, *et al*. Time to arrhythmic, ischemic, and heart failure events: exploratory

analyses to elucidate mechanisms of adverse drug effects in the Cardiac Arrythmia Suppression Trial. *Am Heart J* 1995; **130**: 71–9.

103. Breithardt G. Amiodarone in patients with heart failure. *N Engl J Med* 1995; **333**: 121–2.

104. Singh SN, Fletcher RD, Fisher SG, *et al.* Amiodarone in patients with congestive heart failure and asymptomatic ventricular arrhythmia. *N Engl J Med* 1995; **333**: 77–82.

105. Gottlieb SS, Kukin ML, Medina N, Yushak M, Packer M. Comparative hemodynamic effects of procainamide, tocainide, and encainide in severe chronic heart failure. *Circulation* 1990; **81**: 860–4.

106. Gottlieb SS, Kukin ML, Yuskak M, Medina N, Packer M. Adverse hemodynamic and clinical effects of encainide in severe chronic heart failure. *Ann Intern Med* 1989; **110**: 505–9.

107. Massie BM, Fisher SG, Deedwania PC, *et al.* For the CHF-STAT Group. Effect of amiodarone on clinical status and left ventricular function in patients with congestive heart failure. *Circulation* 1996; **93**: 2128–34.

108. Cleland JGF, Swedberg K. Carvedilol for heart failure, with care. *Lancet* 1996; **347**: 1199–201.

109. Nicholas G, Oakley C, Pouleur H, *et al.* Xamoterol in severe heart failure. *Lancet* 1990; **336**: 1–6.

110. Waagstein F, Bristow MR, Swedberg K. *et al.* Beneficial effects of metoprolol in idiopathic dilated cardiomyopathy. *Lancet* 1993; **342**: 1441–6.

111. Lechat P, Jaillon P, Fontaine ML, *et al.* A randomized trial of beta-blockade in heart failure: The Cardiac Insufficiency Bisoprolol Study (CIBIS). *Circulation* 1994; **90**: 1765–73.

112. Krum H, Tonkin A, Trotter A, *et al.* Effects of carvedilol, a vasodilator- beta-blocker, in patients with congestive heart failure due to ischemic heart disease. *Circulation* 1995; **92**: 212–18.

113. Australia–New Zealand Heart Failure Research Collaborative Group. Randomised, placebo-controlled trial of carvedilol in patients with heart failure due to ischaemic heart disease. *Lancet* 1997; **349**: 375–80.

114. Packer M, Bristow MR, Cohn JN, *et al.* for the US Carvedilol Study Group. The effect of carvedilol on morbidity and mortality in patients with chronic heart failure. *N Engl J Med* 1996; **334**: 1349–55.

115. Feuerstein GZ, Ruffolo RR. Carvedilol, a novel multiple action antihypertensive agent with antioxidant activity and the potential for myocardial and vascular protection. *Eur Heart J* 1995; **16**: 38–42.

116. The BEST Steering Committee. Design of the beta-blocker evaluation survival trial (BEST). *Am J Cardiol* 1995; **75**: 1220–3.

117. Al-Khadra AS, Salem DN, Rand WM, Udelson JE, Smith JJ, Konstam MA. Effect of warfarin anti-coagulation on survival in patients with left ventricular systolic dysfunction. *J Am Coll Cardiol* 1996; **27**(Suppl A): 142A (abstract).

118. Cleland JGF. Angiotensin II receptor antagonists for heart failure: do we need them? In: McMurray JJV, Cleland JGF (eds), *Heart Failure in Clinical Practice*. London: Martin Dunitz, 1996: 271–90.

119. Pitt B. 'Escape' of aldosterone production in patients with left ventricular dysfunction treated with an angiotensin converting enzyme inhibitor: implications for therapy. *Cardiovasc Drug Ther* 1995; **9**: 145–9.

120. Milano CA, White WD, Smith LR, *et al.* Coronary artery bypass in patients with severely depressed ventricular function. *Ann Thorac Surg* 1993; **56**: 487–93.

121. Mickleborough LL, Maruyama H, Takagi Y, Mohamed S, Sun Z, Ebisuzaki E. Results of revascularisation in patients with severe left ventricular dysfunction. *Circulation* 1995; **92**(Suppl II): I73–9.

122. O'Connor CM, Puma JA, Gardner LH, Califf RC, Jones RH. A 25-year experience in patients (pts) with coronary artery disease (CAD) and chronic heart failure (CHF): outcomes with medical therapy and bypass surgery (CABG). *J Am Coll Cardiol* 1996; **27**(Suppl A): 142A (abstract).

123. Sutton GC. Epidemiologic aspects of heart failure. *Am Heart J* 1990; **120**(Suppl): 1538–40.

124. Narang R, Swedberg K. Cleland JGF. What is the ideal study design for evaluation of treatment for heart failure? Insights from trials assessing the effects of ACE inhibitors on exercise capacity. *Eur Heart J* 1996; **17**: 120–34.

125. Rogers WJ, Johnstone DE, Yusuf S, *et al.* Quality of life among 5025 patients with left ventricular dysfunction randomized between placebo and enalapril: The studies of left ventricular dysfunction. *J Am Coll Cardiol* 1994; **23**: 393–400.

126. Konstam V, Salem D, Pouleur H, *et al.* Baseline quality of life as a predictor of mortality and hospitalization in 5025 patients with congestive heart failure. *Am J Cardiol* 1996; **78**: 890–5.

127. Califf RC, Adams KF, Armstrong PW, *et al.* Flolan international randomised survival trial (FIRST): final results. *J Am Coll Cardiol* 1996; **27**(Suppl): 141A (abstract).

128. Pitt B, Segal R, Martinez FA, *et al.*, on behalf of the ELITE study group: Randomised trial of losartan versus captopril in patients over 65 with heart failure (Evaluation of losartan in the elderly study, ELITE). *The Lancet* 1997; **349**: 747–52.

19

Rehabilitation

Robert West

Introduction

Before undertaking a detailed examination of the trials of cardiac rehabilitation, it is useful to consider the definition of rehabilitation, outline its principal components, and review briefly its history. The definition most commonly cited for cardiac rehabilitation is: 'The sum of activity to ensure them the best possible physical, mental and social conditions so that they by their own efforts regain as normal as possible a place in the community and lead an active productive life' (WHO 1964).[1] This definition best suits myocardial infarction patients and places it as that activity which helps patients negotiate the transition between dependency on highly technical treatment and care during the acute phase in hospital and the loneliness of recuperation after discharge. The logical timing for rehabilitation to help patients manage this transition is as soon as practically possible after discharge: it then offers the patient a 'stepped discharge', a continuation of technical, specialist, and skilled help, and provides a 'lifeline' back to the hospital in case of need. The definition also helps to some degree in distinguishing between rehabilitation and treatment, opportunistic health promotion, and self-help.

Boundaries are necessarily somewhat arbitrary and activities are often perceived differently by the wide variety of doctors, nurses, and therapists who contribute to the totality of cardiac care. Nevertheless, to deliniate activities that might be considered in this chapter and those that are more obviously covered in other chapters, some outline of the boundaries is necessary. It seems logical to exclude medication by aspirin as 'treatment', although it may be part of long-term aftercare or risk reduction, and to include psychological therapy as rehabilitation, although it may be a treatment directed at reducing clinical anxiety, and in some centers may be initiated quite early in the patient's hospital stay. The dividing line between rehabilitation and opportunistic health promotion is less clear. Many clinicians, nurses, and therapists would feel that they were failing their patients if they did not provide clear encouragement in 'risk reduction', and many rehabilitation programs include significant elements of health promotion. However, others have argued that 'risk reduction' goes beyond the World Health Organization (WHO) definition of rehabilitation and returning patients to their pre-acute disease state. Be that as it may, one practical reason for separating health promotion from rehabilitation, when they can be separated, is that health-promotion trials fall more naturally into the lifestyle trials described in Chapter 7, and to minimize replication such trials are omitted from this review.

The principal components of rehabilitation are cardiac education, exercise training, psychological therapy, counseling, practical guidance, and opportunistic health education. Programs vary in their content, emphasis, and on their delivery, ranging from those that are almost entirely based on exercise training, with the implied assumption that if patients see their physical performance improve their other morbidities will follow in line, to those that concentrate almost entirely on psychological morbidities, with the implied assumption that patients without anxiety and depression will have confidence to get on with the rest of their lives. Many rehabilitators acknowledge the multifactorial nature of morbidity after acute myocardial infarction, the need for and relevance of a multifactorial approach, and the contribution of multidisciplinary therapy, and hence most established rehabilitation programs contain several of the principal components in their 'core' and refer on for further specialist therapies according to individual need.

The history of physical rehabilitation has its roots in the eighteenth century. In 1802, Heberden[2] advocated a routine half-hour of sawing wood for patients with angina, and some 50 years later Stokes prescribed a regulated course of exercise.[3] Despite these early antecedents, the consensus recommended treatment for myocardial infarction in the middle of this century was still 6 weeks of total bed rest. The origin of modern rehabilitation following myocardial infarction centers on the armchair treatment of Levine and Lown,[4] and since the 1960s there has been a progression towards earlier mobilization and shorter durations of hospital stay. A number of randomized controlled trials evaluated earlier mobilization during the 1970s,[5,6] but more recent further reductions in duration of hospital stay have not been formally evaluated, and early discharge is now often influenced by economic considerations. Armchair treatment, progressive mobilization, and early discharge led naturally to consideration of active measures to encourage physical rehabilitation.[7] The epidemiological studies of lifestyle and coronary heart disease mortality among London bus drivers and conductors and civil servants[8] suggested a cardioprotective effect of exercise in primary prevention. It was only a small step to consider the possibilities of a cardioprotective effect of exercise in secondary prevention. A number of physicians in North America and Israel began exercising patients after myocardial infarction.[9,10] These developments evaluated safety and monitored physical performance (maximum heart rate, oxygen uptake, double product or treadmill time), and a number of controlled trials sought to evaluate effectiveness relative to the untrained patient. Exercise-based rehabilitation was adopted in a very patchy fashion: several specialist centers were established, notably in parts of North America, while many hospitals continued to offer little or nothing in the way of formal rehabilitation.

The evolution of psychologically based rehabilitation following myocardial infarction paralleled that of exercise training. Adset and Bruhn[11] were perhaps the first to explore the effects of psychological therapy in these patients. Further observational studies demonstrated psychological morbidity in postinfarction patients and a number of (mostly small) randomized controlled trials followed, yet rehabilitation programs based on psychological therapy as a principal component remain rare. Psychological therapy has become more commonly accepted as a component of multidisciplinary or 'comprehensive' rehabilitation. The slower adoption of the psychological component than the physical training component may be attributed to weaker evidence of effectiveness and poorer understanding of a mechanism, or also to practical considerations such as the availability of suitable qualified and trained staff and their proximity to cardiologists and physicians.

The education component of 'comprehensive' rehabilitation probably has its origin in the time urgency of most hospital doctors and, perhaps to a lesser extent, of hospital nurses. As the technology of coronary care developed and as patients' stay in hospital shortened, there became less time to explain to patients what their disease was, what had happened to them, what had been done for them in hospital, and what to expect after discharge. Thus a need was perceived to reintroduce formally some doctor–patient or, more usually, nurse–patient time. A second important basis for the educational component in 'comprehensive' rehabilitation rests with health education. The principal risk factors for heart disease (hypertension, hypercholesterolemia, overweight, and cigarette smoking) have been recognized for many years, not only by the medical profession but also by the public at large. Nevertheless, individuals mostly accept to 'live with these risks' (perhaps because they do not have a feel for statistics, chance, or probability) until they are shocked into acceptance of their own latent mortality by the sudden manifestation of myocardial infarction or, less forcibly, by myocardial infarction or cerebrovascular accident in a near relative. Ex-patients are much more likely to change their lifetime habits than are age- and sex-matched controls,[12] and hence education aimed at secondary prevention is likely to be more effective than that aimed at primary prevention. Secondary prevention is arguably also more ethical, since the patients have disease and seek professional assistance.

The parallel developments of exercise training and psychological therapy and recognition of the need for more doctor–patient or nurse–patient time for cardiac education and of the opportunities for health education and risk reduction led naturally to 'comprehensive' rehabilitation. Many programs became established in parts of America and Canada and in several Northern European countries. However, developments in the UK lagged far behind,[13] until recent pump-priming grants by the Chest Heart and Stroke Association and the British Heart Foundation and the adoption of 'health gain targets' in the National Health Service (NHS) combined to effect a rapid increase in the number of programs offered.[14] The apparent reluctance to accept rehabilitation or conservatism among clinicians may have its foundation in the relative paucity of sound evidence of effectiveness, by comparison for example with the many large trials and statistical overviews in the other areas of cardiology. This chapter is directed towards reviewing the principal evidence.

While myocardial infarction is the main cardiac diagnosis considered for rehabilitation, and the one which the WHO definition fits best, there are two other important groups that are also eligible. These are cardiac surgery, for which rehabilitation purposes might include angioplasty, and chronic cardiac conditions, in particular chronic stable angina and hypertension. There are common needs for patients of all three main groups, but there are also important differences. Surgery (and angioplasty) is planned and perceived by most patients as a practical physical solution for a physical condition, unlike unexpected myocardial infarction and its accompanying psychological trauma. Physiotherapy and progressive physical exercise is regarded by most patients as a logical requirement following many operations. Cardiac surgery patients nevertheless have particular needs, some of which parallel those of myocardial infarction patients.[15] Several rehabilitation programs now include surgery patients, either separately or with myocardial infarct patients.[14]

The chronic stable angina and hypertension group has different requirements again, and the term 'rehabilitation' (as defined by WHO) may not exactly suit their needs, which are essentially for preventive therapy, to prevent myocardial infarction or cardiac surgery. Although the therapeutic activity may be similar, it is rather differently focused in the chronic condition on the principal presenting symptom or on risk reduction rather than on an 'event', as in myocardial infarction or surgery. Therefore, angina management[16,17] or hypertension management[18] probably have more in common with primary prevention than with rehabilitation following myocardial infaction or surgery and primary prevention is reviewed in Chapter 7.

Trials of Rehabilitation: Design and Interpretation

The requirements for trial design and for interpretation of trial results have been clearly set out in Chapters 1 and 3. Before applying these basic principles of trial design and of critical appraisal of individual trials, it seems appropriate to consider their application in general to evaluations of rehabilitation. This is because the ideal trial design is modeled on the 'double-blind', placebo-controlled trial, a design which is possible with pharmaceuticals. Many clinical trials in cardiology (of aspirin, beta-bockers, thrombolysis, etc.) are basically pharmaceutical trials, and can therefore be judged critically against ideal criteria. By contrast, rehabilitation trials are examples of health-service evaluations and cannot be equated with the 'pharmaceutical'. In a number of important respects experimental evaluations of health services in general and rehabilitation in particular cannot conform to the ideal. The most obvious principal difference is that these trials are necessarily doubly open or 'unblind', in that both patients and therapists know whether or not treatment is prescribed. Secondly, the methods of randomization in health-service evaluations may often be nonideal, usually for practical reasons (e.g. in rehabilitation employing some form of 'block randomization' in order to create rehabilitation groups or mini cohorts). Thirdly, compliance in health-service evaluations can fall far short of ideal, again often for practical reasons. While in acute therapy trials the drug (e.g. streptokinase) is 'administered' and in chronic medication trials the drug (e.g. aspirin or beta-blocker) is 'prescribed', in rehabilitation trials patients are 'invited'. In addition, patients may be required to make considerably greater commitment to partake in rehabilitation (with perhaps half a day off work and travel costs for each session) than to take prescribed medication (before dinner), and this means many may decline the invitation or default early in the program. Some plausible justification can be found for rehabilitation trials failing almost all the ideal trial criteria outlined in Chapter 3.

However, practical considerations in healthcare evaluation should not be used as an excuse for sloppy research. The principles of the 'double-blind', randomized, controlled trial should still apply, and health-service trials should attempt to be as rigorous as possible. In exercise rehabilitation trials, for example, while partaking in exercise training is necessarily 'doubly unblind', in that both patients and therapists know who are the study patients and who are controls, the exercise test used to compare outcomes could be undertaken 'single-blind' by a third party not involved in any way in the exercise training program, and the test could be different from any of the exercises employed in the training program, so that cases are no more familiar with the apparatus and procedure than are controls. A compromise needs to be struck between rigor and the limitations imposed by practical realities. A review of rehabilitation trials that demanded rigor comparable with modern acute therapy trials might eliminate as 'inadmissible' most reported to date, which would leave practitioners and managers without the evidence necessary to plan and supervise appropriate rehabilitation services. However, to drop the rigor demanded of trials in other areas of cardiology, as reviewed in other chapters, would have the effect of endorsing some poorly executed trials and misleading findings. Accordingly, the standards (see Chapter 3) have been lowered rather than dropped in order to include in this review the principal trials in the development of cardiac rehabilitation.

Many outcome measures have been employed in the evaluation of cardiac rehabilitation. There is some justification for using more than one 'endpoint', since rehabilitation has more than one aim or objective and may 'add life to years as well as years to life'. Furthermore, there are also several dimensions to rehabilitation, which may neither add nor equate. Benefits in one dimension (e.g. physical-work capacity) may be accompanied by benefits in another (e.g. reduced anxiety state) for some patients and not for others, and again may not be appreciated as benefits at all by others. Despite using these arguments to justify more than one outcome measure in the evaluation of rehabilitation programs, readers will be aware of the potential misuse of 'multiple measurements': if enough are studied one may show benefit through chance alone.

Survival (or mortality) is generally seen by clinicians, epidemiologists, and patients as the 'hard statistic' and, when mortality statistics are available, they tend to dominate comparisons in many fields of healthcare evaluation. A well-known example in cardiology is of coronary artery bypass graft surgery, which was introduced for relief of intractable long-standing angina but, after three randomized controlled trials, is now widely regarded as life saving (although survival benefits have been extrapolated beyond the range of experimental evidence on left main stem or three-vessel disease). Many rehabilitation trials have reported mortality and cardiac mortality, but it should be appreciated that the latter contributes 80–90% of the former.

A number of clinical measures used to compare outcome following rehabilitation, common to other cardiology trials, have included further (confirmed) myocardial infarction, stroke, or coronary surgery or, in some trials, hospitalization for cardiovascular disease as proxy. Clinical examinations have included angina, dyspnea, arrhythmia, and heart failure.

Measurement of the quality of life is much more ambiguous than mortality – few pathologists disagree over death, although they may over the cause. Many quality-of-life measures have been developed over the years, but few measure directly patients' perceptions of improvement in their level of performance or their satisfaction with their level of health, although it is these that largely determine whether patients consider themselves to be recovered or in need of further care or treatment.[19] Different scales measure different aspects of health, including for example functional ability, psychological well-being, social support, and life satisfaction. These different scales may be relevant to patients' total health status, and contribute to patients' perceived quality of life and hence to whether patients see themselves as recovered, but it should be appreciated that these scales measure different features of health and that patients may be recovered and well on one scale and at the same time sick and in need of further treatment on another.

One pragmatic outcome measure, which may be regarded as the summation of a variety of health-status factors, is 'return to work'. This is a measurable factor, indeed almost a 'hard statistic', and perhaps removes some of the perceived subjectivity of health-status scales. However, it is limited in its applicability to younger men in areas of generally high employment. Since half of myocardial infarction patients are over retirement age, a quarter are women, and unemployment is nowadays by no means unusual, this simple measure of 'regaining a normal place in the community' has become barely relevant as a measure of effectiveness of rehabilitation.

Measurements of physical function are easier to obtain, standardize, and compare between case and control groups. These include, for example, resting heart rate, blood pressure, exercise time, maximum heart rate, oxygen intake, and rate–pressure product. Most exercise training trials have reported a number of these measures, but quite a diverse variety have been reported, which makes for difficulty in comparing trials. Fairly clearly, these measures of physical function have a direct relevance to monitoring physical training and fitness, but clinicians and therapists should be cautious against overreliance on such measures or overinterpreting change in these measures. First, they may reflect a short-term training effect. More fundamentally, although they may be very direct measures of physical functions, the physical functions themselves may not necessarily indicate successful rehabilitation.

Trial size is important, but it is also important to consider trial size in the context of the state of knowledge at the time when the trial was designed. With the wisdom of hindsight and with the results of large trials and of statistical overviews, many forget the importance of early 'phase I' and even 'phase 0' trials. The statistical calculation of trial size, to have sufficient power to seek a difference (between intervention and control) of a certain size and to find the difference statistically significant, requires a 'prior'. Where there is no prior knowledge of the effect of a proposed new therapy or intervention, the first ($n = 1$) experiment is highly significant. Although $n = 1$ experiments and 'uncontrolled' experiments on small numbers have an important role in the early evolution of a scientific theory, larger 'uncontrolled' observational studies have little power to demonstrate effectiveness of new therapies in practice. In rehabilitation, several 'uncontrolled' observations continue to make unjustifiable claims and, without fairly matched comparison groups, they probably reflect nothing more than the natural resolution of morbidity following myocardial infarction. The case for properly designed, randomized, controlled trials need not be emphasized in this book, but it might not be out of place to remind readers that there is a 'natural history' in trials (as part of the 'natural history' of evaluation) that follows the 'natural history' of adopting a new therapy. With the wisdom of hindsight (when, for example, it is discovered that the benefit of aspirin is to reduce 1-year mortality from 11% to 10%) it is all too easy to criticise early trials for being too small. It is necessary to consider trials in the context of existing knowledge at the time when they were designed, and appreciate that benefits might be larger than subsequently found or, more seriously, that risks or side-effects might be more significant or serious than they turned out to be. Therefore, the important trials of rehabilitation are reviewed here in order of publication, and it will be seen that the criteria for the ideal trial (Chapter 3) are applied more rigorously in the more recent trials.

Since practising clinicians and health-service managers are often too busy to appraise critically the primary scientific and medical literature, in the context of this book the original reports of individual cardiology trials, there is a clear role for the review or overview. An awareness of both the uses and the limitations of the review or overview is relevant to any assessment of the totality of available evidence.[20] There have been many changes recently in the practice of overviewing. In the past, reviews tended to appear (anonymously) as editorials, usually by senior authorities, and consensus permeated practice from the centers of excellence via those anonymous editorials. In many journals editorials have become much more numerous, so that one accompanies each new trial (or original paper) to help place the trial in context. However, they often do little more than rearrange the words of the original paper's discussion, and it is not uncommon for journals to carry contradictory editorials only a year or so apart. Thus editorials generally no longer perform the function of the review. The statistical overview (or meta-analysis) has largely replaced the editorial in summarizing the state of knowledge in many developing research areas. Following the explosion of scientific activity, literature and journals, reviewing has moved some way from being an art to being a science, with statisticians formalizing the review process. While a role for the statistical overview is clearly established, it needs to be undertaken properly and its findings still need to be interpreted, in an 'editorial of editorials'.

A few cautions on the use of statistical overview may be considered under five headings: representativeness, homogeneity, statistics, publication bias, and *post hoc* enquiry bias or inevitable prejudice.[21] The usual recommendations of the critical appraisal of the scientific (medical) literature are relevant in assessing the 'truth' behind any paper.[22,23] Readers must appreciate that in an overview, just as in a typical research paper, they are not told what really happened, they only have the author's word and often a very abbreviated word. It is important that the trials included in overviews are representative and homogeneous. There are clear examples of the effect of publication bias in fields where trial registration is practised; where the pooled effect of published trials may be significant and at the same time the pooled effect of registered trials not significant.[24] Homogeneity considerations include for example: Were the patient populations similar (e.g. did all subjects have a confirmed myocardial infarction, or did some trials include patients after cardiac surgery)? Were the interventions similar (e.g. have all trials compared formal exercise with no exercise or have some compared a lot of exercise with a little, or have some included significant amounts of risk factor reduction advice or counseling? Were end-points comparable (e.g. 2-year total mortality, or have some trials compared 6-month or 5-year mortality, or some compared fatal and nonfatal cardiac events together)?

Publication bias is popularly attributed to journal editors, behaving to some degree as purveyors of scientific news or interesting stories, and preferring papers with results to those without. Many besides editors may contribute to 'nonpublication' one way or another: for example, it has been reported that more negative studies are withdrawn by their authors than are rejected by editors.[25] In addition, publication bias is not 'black and white' (publish or reject): papers may be accepted after editor and referee feedback, which is often directed towards helping to mould the 'unacceptable' into the prevailing consensus.

The most fundamental criticism of statistical overviews is that they contravene one of the hallowed principles of science, 'first the hypothesis, then the test'.[26] By its very nature, the statistical overview is *post hoc*; the reviewer starts with a set of results (e.g. trials that compare mortality of exercise-trained patients after myocardial infarction with the mortality of untrained patients) and then selects from these results those that suit his or her purpose. The reviewer should be, and may attempt to be, as detached and as dispassionate as possible, and select trials on the basis of methodology, size, duration of intervention, etc. However, it is rare for the reviewer to be truly blind as to the result and the effect of its inclusion (or exclusion) on the pooled overall estimate. It is much more common that he or she starts with the answer (in the abstract or even in the title) and learns about the methodology, problems encountered, or errors committed on closer reading or by further interrogation of the authors.

Some statistical overviews have described a 'scientific' process of selecting and includ-ing trials, which requires a team: (a) to read articles and transcribe them into a results-free format, (b) to judge eligibility criteria and weighting of papers selected for inclusion, (c) to pool the findings of the selected papers, and (d) to interpret the pooled findings in the light of other relevant knowledge. To do all this properly requires several people, at least one of whom should be well informed methodologically and yet virtually ignorant of the subject of study, a very unlikely combination, and doing it properly requires considerable time. One statistical overview of exercise-based rehabilitation found considerable interrater differences in what the programs actually included (e.g. the number of weeks of exercise, the number of sessions per week) and what outcome measure the trials compared (e.g. comparing deaths after discharge, randomization, or start of rehabilitation).[27] Comparison of statistical overviews reveals that different reviewers interpreted and reported results, even the main results, of common papers differently.[21,22,28]

Exercise-based Rehabilitation Trials

Introduction of 'armchair treatment' by Levine and Lown[4] led to (gentle) exercising in bed, shorter bedrest, and earlier mobilization, and subsequently some physicians began exercis-ing selected myocardial infarction patients 6 weeks to 6 months after discharge.[9,10,29–31]

Several of these programs ran for years and enrolled hundreds of patients. These uncontrolled studies of exercise programs reported improved cardiac performance, typically 10–20% in rate–pressure product (heart rate $\times$ blood pressure) among compliant volunteer patients after a period of (re)training, but these improvements were not directly compared with comparable patients not offered rehabilitation, whose performance might have improved comparably with the passage of time after myocardial infarction or with familiarity with the testing procedure. Several reported mortality in their rehabilitation patients as lower than 'the average for the hospital' or the 'average for the country', but without satisfactory discussion of case selection for such novel and aggressive therapy the comparisons are of little value. The first direct comparison was by Rechnitzer et al.,[30] who compared eight exercised cardiac patients with eight cardiac controls (average of 3 years after myocardial infarction) and also eight exercised normals with eight nonexercised normals. Even with such small numbers they reported a statistically significant improvement ($P < 0.01$) in six items of a 5-minute muscular endurance test in cardiac exercises and in none in controls.

The early controlled trials of exercise rehabilitation programs were conducted in Scandinavia and were more fully described than many subsequent trials: each was reported as a whole journal supplement (see Table 19.1).[32–34] The Helsinki trial randomized nearly 300 consecutive male patients aged <65 years by year of birth on admission.[32] Exclusions for hospital death, living outside the area, unconfirmed diagnosis, coexisting severe disease, and incomplete information whittled numbers down to 77 in the rehabilitation group and 81 in the control group by the time of referral (6–8 weeks after myocardial infarction). The author undertook detailed examinations before, during, and after rehabilitation in both cases and controls, and the rehabilitation itself was conducted twice weekly by a physiotherapist in another department. The case and control groups were similar on a very extensive list of characteristics (anthropometric, cardiovascular disease history, clinical, radiological and biochemical findings, physical function, and risk factor profiles). Follow-up was thorough. The important findings at 12 months were that mortality was the same (11/77 and 11/81, respectively), that physical work capacity improved (significantly) almost identically in cases and controls (maximum workload 675 ± 360 SD and 650 ± 360 SD kpm min^{-1}, and similarly in virtually all the symptomatological, clinical, radiological, and biochemical findings. The outcomes of cases and controls were so similar that the results were pooled in a subsequent analysis of 'predictors' of maximal working capacity among more than 40 variables measured at baseline. The negative result could be attributed in part to self-training by controls, their working capacity showed improvement over time, and interviews recorded that nearly as many maintained physical activity at 'full training level'.

In a similar trial in Gothenburg, patients aged <57 years were randomized at discharge to form two groups of 158 cases and 157 controls, including 15 and 20 women, respectively.[33,35] Anthropometric measurements, cardiovascular disease, and risk-factor history and clinical findings were recorded before discharge, and baseline physical function was measured at 3 months, after which cases were referred to three half-hour exercise sessions per week for 9 months led by a physiotherapist. The risk profile of controls was slightly poorer than that for cases at 1 year, 14 cases and 15 controls had died, and at 4 years 28 and 35 had died, respectively. This nonsignificant difference ($P \simeq 0.4$) may be mostly explained by the poorer risk scores of controls at entry (risk-adjusted 4-year death rates 0.19 and 0.21, respectively). An average improvement in physical capacity (210 kpm min^{-1}) is reported as significant for cases ($P < 0.001$) but not for controls (80 kpm min^{-1}), but baseline measures were reported for only 129/157 cases and 95/158 controls and, since the further analysis is mostly not by intention to treat but by symptom

Table 19.1 Exercise-based rehabilitation trials

Author	Age (years)/sex	Sample size Rehabilitation	Sample size Controls	Time from MI to program (weeks)	Exercise duration (min), No. of sessions, program duration (months)	Follow-up (months)	No. of deaths Rehabilitation	No. of deaths Controls	No. of nonfatal reinfarctions		Physical fitness outcome measures
Kentala 1972[32]	<65 M	77	81	6–8	30 min supervised training, 2–3 per week, 10 months	24	11	11	6	4	Work capacity (NS)
Sanne 1973[33]	<57	158	157	12	30 min supervised training, 3 per week, 9 months	48	28	35	25	28	Work capacity ($P < 0.05$)
Palatsi 1976[34]	<65	180	200	10	30 min daily at home, supervised training once a month, 24 months	29	19	33	27	33	Work capacity (controls better)
Shaw 1981[38]	<65 M	323	328	8–128	60 min, 3 per week, laboratory for 2 months, gym for 34 months	36	15	24	15	11	Work capacity ($P < 0.001$)
Carson et al. 1982[40]	<70 M	151	152	6	Supervised exercise, 2 per week, 3 months	36	12	21	11	10	Mean cycling time ($P < 0.001$)
Rechnitzer et al. 1983[41]	<57 M	379	354	8–78	60 min, 2 per week supervised, 4 per week unsupervised, 48 months (Control: 1 per week supervised, 2 months)	48	(CHD only)		39	33	Heart-rate reduction ($P < 0.01$)
Roman et al. 1983[42]	<72	93	100	8	30 min supervised training, 3 per week, 40 months	56	16	27	9	8	Work capacity ($P < 0.01$)
Marra et al. 1985[43]	<65 M	81	80	8	90 min supervised training, 3 per week, 2 months	55	6	5	5	9	Work capacity ($P < 0.001$)
Bethell and Mullee 1990[44]	<66 M	99	101	4–6	20–45 min supervised training, 3 per week, 3 months	36	9	7	6	10	Maximum oxygen uptake ($P < 0.001$)

CHD, coronary heart disease; MI, myocardial infarction.

limitation, it is not clear how many follow-up measurements were averaged (possibly 82 male cases and 60 controls). Rather more than half of surviving cases (77/144) stopped training within 1 year. A small trial comparing 6 weeks of physical training among 29 men aged <65 years with 26 controls reported comparable improvement in maximal working capacity (from 570 to 750 $\pm$ 200 SD kpm min^{-1} among exercisers and from 510 to 610 $\pm$ 210 SD among controls) as significant for both cases and controls.[36]

The third trial was undertaken in Oulu in Northern Finland, within the Arctic Circle.[34] A total of 380 patients aged <65 years were recruited to the trial 6 weeks after myocardial infarction; it is said without exclusion. They were allocated to treatment or control in three blocks of 100, 50, and 50, which is not ideal. The block allocation resulted in 180 (including 37 women) in the treatment group and 200 (including 34 women) in the control group. The report compares a wide range of patient characteristics and potential confounders. Treatment and control groups appeared to be similar in most respects, although fewer women in the rehabilitation group had suffered a previous infarction (4/37 versus 7/34). Rehabilitation comprised only one 30-minute physiotherapist-supervised session in a gym per month to teach techniques that could be continued at home for 1 year. This may have been partly because of the very low outdoor temperature experienced in the area (parking meters are wired up with heater sockets in order to prevent cars freezing). The principal exercise was walking/running on the spot, and three-quarters of the treatment group exercised 6 or 7 days per week. All patients were recalled as outpatients for examination and exercise test at 3-month intervals, and exercise-test data were reported for nearly 85% at baseline, but for only about 67% of estimated survivors at the final 12 month follow-up.

Physical working capacity of all subjects improved between baseline (1 month) and the final test (1 year), but cases scored lower than controls both before (440 ± 170 SD, $n = 156$ versus 500 ± 200 SD, $n = 169$; $P < 0.01$) and after (500 ± 200 SD, $n = 110$ versus 590 ± 200 SD, $n = 130$; $P < 0.001$). Other objective measures were in the same direction, while subjective and clinical measures showed no differences. Mortality and reinfarction, on the other hand, point towards benefit in the training group: 17/143 men and 2/37 women cases versus 27/166 men and 6/34 women controls died after an average follow-up of 31 and 26 months, respectively, which suggests an (unadjusted) relative risk of 0.64 with a 95% confidence interval (CI) of 0.38–1.08. There were also 21 (12%) reinfarctions among cases and 28 (14%) among controls. These results should be interpreted with caution, since they are at variance with the principal performance measures, and allocation to case and control groups was not ideal and may have introduced a seasonal effect (a series of 100 patients would have taken nearly 7 months to recruit) and the control group may have been at greater initial risk.

Following the three Scandinavian trials one could reasonably expect some power calculations in the design of the next trial. This was done in the 'national exercise and heart disease project', which sought 4300 patients.[37] In practice, the trial enrolled 651 men aged <64 years 2 months to 3 years after myocardial infarction in five centers.[38] Patients were entered into a low-level exercise programme for 6 weeks prior to randomization in order to eliminate probable noncompliers. Patients were given exercise tests and clinical examinations before the exercise program and subsequently at 6-month intervals for 3 years. Baseline characteristics (history, clinical picture, and risk factors) of rehabilitation patients (323) and controls (328) were very similar. The exercise program started in an exercise laboratory with three 1-hour sessions per week with electrocardiogram (ECG) monitoring for 8 weeks and continued (3 sessions per week) in a gymnasium for nearly 3 years. Total mortality at 3 years was 15 (4.6%) in the rehabilitation group and 24 (7.3%) in controls, which suggests a relative risk of 0.63 (95% CI 0.33–1.21). Adjustments for cardiovascular status at baseline made little difference, since the two groups were very comparable. This apparent benefit was not seen in comparison of morbidity, nonfatal reinfarction (18 exercisers versus 13 controls), or hospitalizations (92 exercisers and 90 controls). The attrition rate was reported as low (7% among exercisers and 6% among controls), which may be attributed to the unusual pre-entry 'training' period. This trial is probably one of the most robust demonstrations of mortality reduction in a preselected 'compliant' group of patients (men aged <64 years) but, as numbers fell some way short of the pretrial target, even this result is nonsignificant. A separate paper reported comparison of postprogram work capacity and psychological measures.[39] Among those measured at the 1-year follow-up, exercisers increased work capacity by 0.5 METs (from 7.9 mean, $n = 241$) while controls decreased by 0.1 METs (from 8.0 mean, $n = 225$) ($P < 0.001$). There were no significant differences between exercisers and controls in a battery of psychological measures.

The first British trial of exercise-based rehabilitation was undertaken in Stoke on Trent.[40] Of 1029 men who attended the outpatient clinic 6 weeks after myocardial infarction, 303 were entered into the trial. The mean age of 151 exercisers (50.3 ± 0.6 SE years) was marginally younger than that of 152 controls (52.8 ± 0.7 SE years), and marginally more exercisers suffered anterior (or anterolateral) infarction (76 versus 70). The program compared patients offered twice-weekly exercise sessions in a hospital gym under medical supervision for 12 weeks against controls: 69% completed the course. Work capacity was recorded at baseline (6 weeks) and in reducing numbers at 3 months, and 1, 2, and 3 years: the results were reported as mean ($\pm$ SE) cycling time. At baseline a small advantage to exercisers (approximately 12.5 versus 11.5 minutes) was not significant ($t = 1.25$), while at the 1-year follow-up a significant difference was seen (approximately 16.2 versus 13.2 minutes; $t = 4.18$). However, work capacity was reported for only 175 (58%) and there were more dropouts in the exercising group: work capacity appears to have been measured only for those who completed the training program. Mortality was compared by the log-rank method over 3 years (average follow-up 2.1 years): 12 exercisers and 21 controls died, which suggests a relative risk of 0.58 (95% CI 0.29–1.13). The difference was not apparent in patients with inferior infarction. There were also 11 nonfatal further infarctions among exercisers and 10 among controls.

A multicenter trial in Eastern Canada compared high exercise with low exercise levels.[41] The power calculation was rather optimistically based on halving the rate of myocardial infarction recurrence (22 to 11%), but rather realistically on a 35% dropout rate. Male patients aged <56 years were recruited 2–17 months (mean 6 months) after myocardial infarction. Randomization was stratified by hypertension, social class, and type A/B personality. Detailed clinical examination on entry showed the two groups (379 high exercisers and 354 low exercisers) to be highly comparable. Exercise capacity was measured at baseline and every 6 months. The high-exercise program comprised two physician-supervised sessions per week plus a recommended further four sessions every week at home for up to 4 years. The low-exercise group met once weekly for recreational exercise. There was considerable attrition: overall, 45% dropped out before the end of the program. The principal trial endpoint (obtained for 92%) showed 54 reinfarctions among high exercisers compared with 46 in low exercisers: a relative risk of 1.09 (95% CI 0.61–1.96). A subset analysis, excluding dropouts in order to investigate 'treatment effect', gave a higher relative risk of 1.22. All-cause mortality was not reported (Rechnitzer, personal communication, 1995). A significant difference was reported in heart-rate reduction (at $1.25 \, l \, min^{-1}$) of 10 ± 13 SD (beats per min) among high exercisers compared with 4 ± 13 SD among low exercisers.

A single-center trial in Chile took 8 years to recruit 193 patients (men and women aged $\leqslant 71$ years).[42] The exercise group, randomized 2 days after admission, exercised 3 times a week for 6 months to 9 years. Follow-up reported significantly improved physical working capacity at 12 months (520 ± 80 SD versus 320 ± 60 SD kg min^{-1}), reduced angina prevalence (27/93 versus 47/100; $P < 0.05$), and possibly reduced total mortality (16/93 versus 27/100; RR = 0.6, 95% CI 0.4–1.1). A single-center Italian trial was too small to seek any realistic mortality reduction, but recruited patients (men aged <65 years) without contraindications after an exercise test sooner after myocardial infarction (6 ± 2 weeks) than in the American and Canadian trials.[43] Eighty-four men were entered into the supervised rehabilitation program, which comprised 4 sessions per week for 30 sessions, and 83 controls were advised to exercise at home. The two groups were similar at baseline with respect to clinical history and biochemical measures. Working capacity measured before and after the 8–9 week program showed improvement among cases (670 ± 140 SD versus 880 ± 170 SD kg min^{-1}), but not among controls (630 ± 170 SD versus 670 ± 170 SD kg min^{-1}), and there were no measures to demonstrate whether or not the training effect was maintained over the 4 years or more of follow-up. The exercising group showed slightly higher rates of return to work (nonsignificant, since the numbers were small) and a higher proportion were symptom free, but no benefit was seen in total mortality over 55 months (6/84 exercisers versus 5/83 controls; relative risk 1.2).

Another single-center trial was unusual in that the program was based at a sports center and run by a general practitioner, although it recruited nearly all its patients from one neighboring hospital.[44] Men aged <65 years without medical or orthopedic contra-indications living within 25 miles of the health center and not on the investigator's own practice list were randomized while in hospital. Baseline measures were taken at 4–5 weeks and 99 exercise patients and 101 controls were deemed similar. The program comprised an eight-station exercise circuit and patients attended 3 times a week for 12 weeks. The outcome assessment at the end of the program was conducted by the therapists. Predicted maximum oxygen uptake increased significantly among both exercised patients (22.2 ± 5.0 SD at baseline and 27.3 ml min^{-1} kg^{-1} at follow-up) and controls (23.4 ± 4.5 SD and 26.2, respectively), but fewer exercisers reported angina at follow-up (19 versus 32 controls). However, mortality at 3 months (2 versus 1) and 3 years recorded marginally more deaths among exercisers (9 versus 7; relative risk 1.3, 95% CI 0.5–3.4).[45] This might in part be attributable to an imbalance in the number of previous myocardial infarctions at baseline (17 versus 9). One important criticism of the trial, that baseline measures and outcome assessments were all undertaken by the therapist, was discussed. In defense, it might be borne in mind that such practice possibly occurred in other trials, but without comment.

Three other trials that contribute to the evaluation of exercise-based rehabilitation deserve brief mention. Sivarajan et al.[46] compared exercise ($n = 88$) and exercise plus education ($n = 86$) starting while in bed in hospital with controls ($n = 84$). Exercisers continued under supervision once per week and, on advice, at home twice daily for 3 months. Exercise tests at baseline and at 3 and 6 months showed no significant differences between groups, although the exercisers reported walking further (among 12 activities of daily living). However, at 6 months 6/174 of the exercisers died compared with 2/84 of the controls (relative risk 1.5). Miller et al.[47] described a trial of supervised gym training ($n = 61$) versus home exercise ($n = 65$) and a control group ($n = 71$), which further investigated duration of training. Their findings suggest little difference in functional capacity between gym and home and between brief (8 week) and extended (23 week) training. Goble et al.[48] compared heavy and light exercise (156 high versus 144 low) to see whether comparable effects were achievable with less intensive unsupervised training. The results suggested that those exercising at home fared as well as those who were supervised.

The pattern that emerges, through considerable intertrial heterogeneity, is that exercise training may improve physical working capacity in programs of quite short duration more than 'natural' rehabilitation, but that the relative improvement can be lost over time, through loss of training opportunity or through progressive exercise by controls. A pooled estimate of a standardized effect size on physical working capacity (variously measured) suggests improvement over controls at 3–6 months (at the end of most training programs) ($Z = 2.3$, $P < 0.05$ on 7 trials) but not at 12 months ($Z = 1.7$, NS). Some of this improved physical work capacity (relative to controls) may be attributable to 'measurement training' rather than 'exercise training', since many trials employed test machines that were similar to training machines (treadmills or cycle ergometers) and rehabilitation patients may become familiar with the surroundings, machine, routine, and possibly also operator, while controls do not develop the same familiarity.

Mortality in individual trials mostly 2–4 years after infarction shows considerable variation, from a relative risk of 0.58 (95% CI 0.29–1.13)[40] to 1.10 (95% CI 0.38–3.74).[43] The only two larger trials in America and Canada show nearly as much variation, from 0.63 (95% CI 0.33–1.21)[38] to 1.08 (0.52–2.23) in cardiac mortality.[41] In estimating an overall effect in these trials, all but two of which included fewer than 400 patients, one should bear in mind that the national study called for 4300 patients at its design stage.[37] Two statistical overviews[27,28] have been widely quoted as indicative of an overall mortality reduction. The two overviews included six exercise-based trials in common and both increased numbers by including also, as 'exercise-plus trials', selected centers of the WHO European collaborative trial of comprehensive rehabilitation (reviewed later). Two overviews arrived at similar pooled relative risks for total mortality of 0.75 (95% CI 0.62–0.93) and 0.80 (95% CI 0.66–0.96), respectively. Two trials[33,42] were included by Oldridge but not by O'Connor, and these lowered the former's point estimate. Inclusion of selected centers from the WHO collaborative trial added to the overall heterogeneity, since that trial was of comprehensive rehabilitation. Without inclusion of the WHO data, neither overview would be significant. Mortality in individual trials or WHO centers ranged from 3% (cardiac only) and 6% in the two larger trials[38,41] to over 25% in some WHO centers (which included typically 50–200 patients per center), so that small 'trials' (or centers) contributed disproportionately to the pooled relative risk. The effect of including or excluding the largest single trial[41] is very small. Oldridge excluded it from the estimate of total mortality, since the trial did not report total mortality, while O'Connor included cardiac mortality in place of total mortality. It is important also to appreciate that both overviews found increased odds ratios for nonfatal reinfarction (1.15, 95% CI 0.93–1.42, and 1.09, 95% CI 0.88–1.34, respectively). While these increases in incidence of nonfatal reinfarction are not statistically significant, the observations mitigate against the apparent reduction in mortality.

These findings of an overall effect on mortality, that is greater than that associated with aspirin or beta-blocker and comparable with that for thrombolysis, and no accompanying reduction in nonfatal reinfarction, raises questions about possible completion, reporting, and publication bias and needs cautious interpretation since no single trial has identified a significant reduction and no single trial of sufficient power has been undertaken.

Psychology-based Rehabilitation Trials

After the small pioneering trial by Adset and Bruhn,[11] Ibrahim *et al.*[49] reported a trial of 188 men aged 65 years following discharge after myocardial infarction (see *Table 19.2*). Patients were allocated to therapy or control as consecutive groups of nearly 12, a method that is not ideal when investigators have some choice about the order of discharge and

Table 19.2 Psychology-based rehabilitation trials

Study	Age (years)/sex	Sample size Rehabilitation	Sample size Controls	Time to program start	Counseling/therapy duration, No. of sessions, program duration	Follow-up (months)	No. of deaths Rehabilitation	No. of deaths Controls	No. of nonfatal reinfarcts Rehabilitation	No. of nonfatal reinfarcts Controls	Psychological outcome measures
Ibrahim et al. 1974[49]	<65 M	58	60	After discharge	90 min therapy sessions, weekly, 50 weeks	18	5	9	–	–	Social functioning (NS)
Rahe et al. 1979[50]	<60 M	22	22	Before discharge	Six group-therapy sessions, one every other week	48	0	3	0	4	Clinical judgement (NS)
Naismith et al. 1979[51]	<60 M	76	77	Before discharge	Counseling given when necessary	12	8	4	–	–	Eysenck personality inventry (NS)
Stern et al. 1983[53]	<70 M	35	29	6–52 weeks	75 min group sessions, weekly, 12 weeks	12	0	1	3	1	Taylor anxiety ($P < 0.03$), Zung depression ($P < 0.05$)
Horlick et al. 1984[54]	<65	83	33	<3 weeks after discharge	90 min discussions/education, weekly, 6 weeks	6	6	1	–	–	Spielberger MMPI (NS) locus of control (NS)
Friedman et al. 1984[55]	<65 M	592	265	>26 weeks	90 min sessions, 24 over 3-year period	36	21	11	24	28	Type 'A' measures ($P < 0.001$)
Frasure-Smith and Prince 1985[56]	<86 M	232	229	Before discharge	Monthly. GHQ by telephone, led to score ≥5 intervention	12	12	22	11	11	GHQ ($P < 0.05$)
Burgess et al. 1987[58]	<63	89	91	Before discharge	Home visits, 6 over 3 months	13	5	5	–	–	Taylor anxiety (NS), Zung depression (NS)
P re Cor 1991[59]	<66 M	61	61	4–9 weeks	Therapy sessions, weekly, 6 weeks	24	5	4	4	6	Lifestyle factors (NS)

GHQ, general health questionnaire.

assessment of eligibility. The 58 treatment patients were generally comparable with 60 controls, although the former included more patients aged 60–65 years and possibly had a slightly poorer (Peel) prognostic index. Group-therapy sessions led by a clinical phychologist of 1.5 hours weekly for 1 year explored emotions and attitudes of cardiac patients and stress reduction and avoided medication, diet, and exercise prescription. Psychological and social functioning were assessed by questionnaire at baseline and at 6, 12, and 18 months, and showed improvement with time in both treated patients and controls (natural history), with no difference between the groups. However, the treatment group experienced slightly better survival; 91% (SE 4%) compared with controls 85% (SE 5%), a difference which was more pronounced among patients with a poor prognostic index. The finding was not significant, since the numbers involved were small, and should be treated with caution in view of the admission procedures and the lack of effect on the psychosocial measures.

A smaller trial compared brief group therapy by a psychiatrist/physician in 22 men aged <60 years following myocardial infarction and 22 controls.[50] Group therapy involved only six fortnightly sessions of 1.5 hours in groups of 7 or 8 patients, and covered stress and myocardial infarction, physiological and psychological risk factors in heart disease, social problems, and concerns over return to work. A 4-year follow-up conducted by the therapy team revealed no deaths among therapy patients but 3 among controls. There were no reinfarctions (4 in controls) and one bypass operation (4 in controls) in the therapy group, plus hints in the same favorable direction in prevalence of depression, time urgency, and life dissatisfaction. After only 44 patients the trial was discontinued in favor of elective referral.

Two trials in the UK done at about the same time yielded rather different results. In a Glasgow trial, 153 men aged <60 years were randomized while in hospital to rehabilitation ($n = 76$) and control ($n = 77$).[51] Repeat assessment was made of physical and psychological states, and psychological counseling was provided, as necessary, by a nurse counsellor. Rehabilitation patients and controls were assessed psychologically (Eysenk personality inventory) at baseline and physically at 6 weeks and 6 months. No complete intention-to-treat analyses were presented, but of 59 rehabilitation patients and 66 controls fit for work, rehabilitation patients scored better on 'social independence' and returned to work 2 weeks earlier. However, it seems that 8 rehabilitation patients died within 6 months of discharge compared with 2 controls (Johnson, personal communication, 1994).

A trial in Oxford compared advice with exercise training with controls in 121 men aged <60 years.[52] Advice by a psychiatrist over three or four fortnightly visits included review of symptoms, activities, plans, and risk factor modification, and was 'such as might be given by a cardiac nurse'. At 3 months of follow-up, 5 deaths and 1 serious cerebrovascular accident (CVA) were observed, but it is not known to which of the three groups they should be attributed. Patients were less satisfied with advice than with exercise training, but at 18 months the advice group fared better on hours worked and sexual intercourse (data not presented).

Another three-way trial compared group counseling with exercise training with controls among patients aged <70 years, 6 weeks to 1 year after myocardial infarction.[53] A total of 106 patients with an exercise capacity <7 METs and with clinical anxiety (Taylor) or depression (Zung) were recruited from a potential pool of 450 patients: 31 men and 4 women were assigned to counseling and 22 men and 7 women served as controls. Group counseling led by psychiatrist, social worker, and nurse was given over 12 weekly 1-hour sessions. Detailed measurements prior to randomization and at 3, 6, and 12 months were summarized, and at 6 months the counseled patients showed less anxiety and depression than controls. Three counseled patients experienced further myocardial infarction; one control died and one experienced a CVA within 12 months. Although small, the trial suggested that targeted counseling can reduce anxiety and depression.

A Canadian trial included men and a few women aged <65 years who were employed before their index myocardial infarction; 83 were included in an education (counseling) group led by a nurse or clinical psychologist for 1.5 hours per week for 6 weeks, and 33 served as controls.[54] The sessions were mostly educational (heart, heart disease, recovery, and risk factors), with little evidence of psychological therapy. Several psychological questionnaires were administered at baseline and at 3 and 6 months. Comparisons at baseline show the groups to be similar in all important aspects. No significant differences at 6 months were reported other than a later return to work and a possibly higher mortality (6/83 versus 1/33; relative risk = 2.4) among the counseled group.

The first major trial of psychological rehabilitation was undertaken by Friedman *et al.*[55] in California. An extensive recruitment campaign, including use of the media, sought men aged <65 years, nonsmokers or exsmokers, who had experienced a myocardial infarction 6 months or more previously. The investigators' work on type A personality and heart disease was well known. Of the 862 volunteers 592 were randomly assigned to psychological counseling and cardiac education and 270 to cardiac education only. The psychological or type A behavior counseling patients were offered 44 group sessions over 3 years, which comprised progressive muscle relaxation training, behavioral learning (including self-assessment) and cognitive affective learning (including self-management). The control patients were offered 24 1.5-hour sessions over 3 years by cardiologists, designed to enhance compliance with medication, diet, and exercise prescriptions.

Full clinical examinations were undertaken prior to entry and at 18 months and 3 years. Type A behavior was assessed by questionnaires (Framingham, Jenkins) and taped interview, all of which intercorrelated. Type A behavior reduced from 2.7 ± 0.4 SD (n = 592) at baseline to 2.1 ± 0.4 SD (n = 328) among patients in the active treatment group, and less strongly from 2.7 ± 0.4 SD (n = 270) to 2.4 ± 0.4 SD (n = 139) among active controls. Total mortality and nonfatal infarctions at 3 years were 21 and 24/584 in the treatment group compared with 11 and 28/265 in the control group. The relative risk for mortality was 0.87 (95% CI 0.42–1.77). Further analyses comparing type A score reducers with nonreducers suggested a link between type A behavior and reinfarction.

The second largest trial was undertaken in Canada. Men discharged following an uncomplicated myocardial infarction with no other medical or psychological condition and, unusually, without an upper age cut-off were considered eligible and randomized to a monthly telephone follow-up (n = 281) or normal discharge (n = 258).[56] Baseline measures of demographic, clinical, and psychological characteristics revealed some differences between participants (n = 229) and controls (n = 224) in cardiac enzymes and medication. The 'treatment' program entailed monthly administration of the 20-item GHQ by telephone over 1 year and home visits by a cardiology-trained nurse if the GHQ score was above 5: nearly half the treatment group were visited (average 5 visits of 1 hour each) for counseling, discussion of problems, advice (after a case conference), and referral to specialist services as appropriate. At 1 year of follow-up the 'treatment' group experienced lower mortality (12 versus 22; relative risk 0.53, 95% CI 0.27–1.05). A long-term follow-up found that the difference continued for several years, and total mortality became comparable again only at about 6 years.[57]

Another trial of nurse counseling compared 89 patients (76 men, 13 women) aged <62 years with 91 controls.[58] The nurse provided psychosocial counseling and assistance with return to work over an average of six home visits in the first 3 months after discharge, but patients in both groups may or may not have received exercise training or cardiac education. There was a significant reduction in distress score (but not anxiety or depression) in counseled patients at 3 months (16 ± 14 SD versus 20 ± 15 SD; among 77 and 75 patients, respectively; $P < 0.05$), but there were no differences in return to work or mortality (5 versus 5) at the 13-month follow-up.

A three-way comparison done in Italy randomized men aged <65 years 4–8 weeks after uncomplicated myocardial infarction and an exercise test to exercise training ($n = 60$), psychological counseling ($n = 61$), or control ($n = 61$).[59] Group counseling sessions, one session per week for 6 weeks, were led by a cardiologist, psychiatrist, nutritionist, and physiotherapist. No results were presented for psychological morbidity over a 2-year follow-up, but comparable rates of return to work and all-cause mortality were observed for counseled patients and controls (5 and 4, respectively). This trial estimated the proportion of myocardial infarction patients enrolled in the trial to be 14%.

The only multicenter trial of psychological rehabilitation evaluated outpatient programs for men and women (no age restriction) with minimal exclusion in 2300 patients.[60] Psychological morbidity was measured on standard scales (Bedford, Spielberger) both before and after a 7-week program led by a clinical psychologist and health visitor. The program comprised 2 hours of progressive muscle relaxation, stress awareness and management, cardiac advice, and counseling. The trial remains reported only as an abstract and thus it is perhaps premature to include its findings in a review.

Some further studies that have contributed to the evaluation of psychological rehabilitation include small trials of bedside nurse counseling during the earliest stages of recovery. Gruen[61] reported a trial of 38 patients and 37 controls in which patients were offered 30 minutes of counseling a day and psychological support from day 2 until discharge. A significantly reduced score on the Multiple Anxiety Adjective Check List (Zucherman) was recorded on day 11. However, no such reduction was seen on several other standard scales, and subjective follow-up at 4 months was conducted by the therapist. Thompson and Meddis[62] described a similar trial, in which 30 patients received four 0.5-hour sessions of cardiac education and counseling by a cardiac nurse. Evaluation by a third party showed significantly reduced anxiety and depression on the HAD scale 5 days after infarction compared with 30 controls, but not at 6 months. Langosch et al.[63] compared stress-management training ($n = 28$) with relaxation training ($n = 30$) and with controls ($n = 30$), while patients were still in hospital and suggested that although the methods differed the outcomes were similar. Van Dixhoorn et al.[64] evaluated relaxation therapy superimposed on an exercise training program ($n = 76$) compared with exercise training alone ($n = 80$). The 6-week psychologist-led program of active–passive respiratory relaxation increased physical work capacity and reduced anxiety.[65]

The trials of psychology-based rehabilitation suffer some methodological problems similar to those associated with the trials of exercise-based rehabilitation. For example, the measurement of psychological state, even using questionnaires or standardized interviews, interrogates areas that are covered in therapy sessions: thus improvement on a scale may reflect 'learning' rather than 'health'. This may be accentuated when the programs use similar questionnaires (or base questions) to monitor therapy and thereby 'train' patients how to answer questions. There may also have been more confusion over monitoring and evaluation, particularly in smaller trials, when the therapist and researcher were one and the same. While many exercise-training trials were directed by a physician, who referred patients to a physiotherapist for training and called upon a registrar to undertake baseline and outcome measurements, the organization of clinical psychological services seems to have led several of the psychology-based rehabilitation trials to be undertaken by one enthusiast, with little separation of the roles of therapist, assessor, and author.

The overall pattern in psychological rehabilitation trials is more heterogeneous than the exercise trials in terms of program content, trial design, primary endpoint measures, and duration of follow-up. The heterogeneity in the program content may indicate differences in opinion between experts as to the needs of these patients and as to the appropriate therapy for addressing these needs. Although the primary objective was generally to reduce psychological morbidity, particularly anxiety and depression associated with the trauma of severe unexpected illness, few trials have presented clear comparisons of anxiety and depression on validated scales at the end of a program or over the longer term. The two larger trials (in the USA and Canada) reported a reduction in reinfarction and mortality rates comparable with trials of exercise based programs, but the late recruitment and volunteer factor in the Friedman trial and the very modest therapeutic input of the Frasure-Smith trial make the interpretation of these findings somewhat problematic. A 'mechanism' would be helped by clear improvements in clinical anxiety and depression, particularly in those patients most affected at discharge.

Comprehensive Rehabilitation Trials

The WHO definition of rehabilitation includes 'the sum of activity', which is almost synonymous with 'comprehensive'. For the purposes of this review, the WHO European collaborative trial and a few subsequent trials are regarded as comprehensive. The WHO European collaborative trial was, in many respects, exemplary for a trial of the period. There was a clear appreciation at the design stage that the patient numbers required would necessitate pooling the findings of many centers, with each center providing approximately the same number of patients as in the three Scandinavian exercise-training trials of the same period.[66,67] Altogether, 26 centers joined from many Northern and some Eastern European countries, with the common objective of evaluating rehabilitation for men aged <65 years hospitalized for myocardial infarction by provision of exercise training, cardiac education, health education, counseling, assistance with social security, and occupational retraining. Programs were designed to run for 2 years and evaluations to be undertaken at 3 and 6 months, and at 1, 2, and 3 years. The preferred allocation to rehabilitation or control was by randomization on discharge, but not all centers achieved this. Six groups of outcome measures were chosen: physical work capacity, cardiac risk factors, psychological morbidity, return to work, cardiac recurrences, and mortality. A power calculation suggested a trial size of 2200 patients followed for 3 years.

In practice, there was variation between centers in program content and trial management. Before comparing this multicenter trial critically against recent practice in multinational trials of pharmacological preparations, one should bear in mind the state of development of rehabilitation at the time and the practical considerations inherent in health-service evaluations outlined previously. The trial is perhaps more appropriately described as 'cooperative' rather than 'multicenter'. The report summarizes the findings of those 17 centers that best conformed to the intended trial design and program content. Therefore, the results may be regarded as a 'pooling' of the findings of 17 rehabilitation trials in 11 countries, but with the major differences from *post hoc* statistical overviews that the pooling was intended from the outset and the constituent trials set out to follow a common protocol, even if somewhat loosely defined. Some centers have reported their findings separately.[68] Comparisons between rehabilitation and control groups at baseline are presented, and reveal a number of differences in several centers. For example: age distributions that favored the rehabilitation group in Moscow and Erfurt; 23 versus 40 previous myocardial infarctions in Bucharest; and intermittent claudication (7% versus 9%), arterial claudication (21% versus 25%), NYHA class III and IV (3% versus 5%), and smoking (65% versus 68%) in the pooled 17 centers all favoring the rehabilitation group.

The report presents results at 3 and 6 months and at 1, 2, and 3 years for all principal outcome variables. Physical work capacity at 3 years was significantly improved in three centers, but overall the benefit was seen to reduce with age (<50 years, 700 versus 620 kpm min^{-1}; 50–59 years, 590 versus 530 kpm min^{-1}; 60–65 years, 500 versus 490 kpm min^{-1}). Anxiety and depression prevalence at follow-up were not presented for individual centers, but there were intercenter differences during phase 1. Rehabilitation patients fared worse on anxiety in one center and better in one other, and fared worse on depression in one center and better in two. Rehabilitation patients fared rather better in terms of return to work, significantly so in five centers, and overall 74% of rehabilitation patients compared with 67% of controls of those aged <60 years returned to work within 3 years. Total mortality was reported as significantly lower in one center (6% versus 16%) and higher in another (18% versus 4%), and as almost significantly lower and higher in another two centers. A pooling of 3-year mortality data suggests an overall relative risk of all-cause mortality of 0.86 (95% CI 0.72–1.03). However, the overall incidence of nonfatal myocardial infarction within 3 years was higher in the rehabilitation group (10.0% versus 8.7%), almost balancing the benefit in fatal myocardial infarction. The report drew attention to a lower than expected overall mortality and concluded that endpoint data were robust enough to compare outcomes only on reinfarction and mortality, and that these differences were inconclusive. While this major international collaboration suggested possible, and less than expected, benefits in mortality and return to work, it raised far more questions than it answered.

Three further trials of comprehensive rehabilitation have been reported since the WHO European collaborative. Vermeulen *et al.*[69] reported 2/49 deaths in 5 years among rehabilitation patients (men aged <55 years) compared with 5/51 among controls, and a similar reduction in nonfatal reinfarctions. Bengtsson[70] reported rather different death rates (10/62 at 1 year compared with 6/64 among controls) for men and women aged <65 years, but significant, although modest, reductions in blood pressure at rest and under exercise at 14 months of follow-up. Oldridge *et al.*[71] reported 3/99 deaths compared with 4/102 at 1 year among patients (men and women aged <65 years) who were clinically anxious (Spielberger) or depressed (Beck) while in hospital and who were offered 8 weeks of exercise training, progressive muscle relaxation, and cognitive behavior therapy. No differences were observed in exercise tolerance, anxiety, or depression. Finally, one trial[72] has evaluated comprehensive rehabilitation in the form of a self-help manual and audio-tape, designed to encourage home exercise, cardiac and risk factor education, and self-treatment for anxiety and depression. Patients ($n = 88$) were given information leaflets on cardiac disease, risk, and rehabilitation and compared with controls ($n = 88$). Significant improvements in anxiety and depression scores were recorded at 6 weeks, particularly among those anxious or depressed at baseline. Except for the self-help trial, these trials add relatively little to the WHO trial, and thus the evaluation of comprehensive rehabilitation rests strongly on the WHO European collaborative study. Although the WHO international collaborative study is undoubtedly the most thorough attempt to evaluate rehabilitation to date, the findings remain somewhat inconclusive. The trial failed to demonstrate a statistically significant reduction in total mortality, although target numbers were achieved and morbidity findings were generally less significant.

Interpretation and External Validity of Trials

Overall heterogeneity in terms of the content of rehabilitation programs, the design of randomized trials to evaluate programs, and in endpoints or outcome measures by which trials are judged, even within the three broad classifications, makes for difficulties when undertaking a statistical overview. As recorded in the report of the WHO European collaborative trial, endpoint data were only sufficiently robust to make meaningful judgements on mortality and nonfatal infarction. Subject to possible completion, reporting, and publication bias, overviews of trials suggest a possible mortality reduction of borderline statistical significance in exercise-based, psychology-based, and comprehensive programs.

The variety of measures of morbidity, particularly psychological morbidity, reported in trials make for greater difficulties in pooling data to determine any general treatment effect. While most trials offer one or two statistically significant measures of benefit, few indicate how many outcome measures were planned for and hence how many were not indicative of benefit. Exercise-based trials generally showed some (short-term) improvement in physical performance. However, the measures that showed benefit were often measures of 'training' rather than independent measures of quality of life. This allows the advocate of rehabilitation to select favorable results from trials and create estimates of 'treatment effect' and, perhaps, add different outcome measures in different trials. However, it also allows the critic to question the objectivity of reports and question the ability of treatment to produce meaningful clinical benefit. There were few independent outcome measures with comparable data between the majority of trials. The common measures reported in most trials were further nonfatal myocardial infarction and return to work. Pooling further nonfatal myocardal infarction, to avoid double counting, with total mortality, which is mostly from further myocardial infarction, shows a possible overall benefit only in psychology-based trials (relative risk 0.54, 95% CI 0.36–0.80), largely due to the Friedman trial. Neither exercise-based nor comprehensive trials showed any benefit in nonfatal infarction (relative risk 0.99 and 1.15, respectively).

In general, only a modest benefit was seen in the 'return to work' measure. For example, the WHO European collaborative study reported return to work among men aged <60 years at 3 years averaging 74% for rehabilitation patients and 67% for controls. As a measure of the success of rehabilitation, 'return to work' remains less than ideally objective, since many comprehensive programs facilitated 'return to work' as part of the rehabilitation package. In more recent years, this measure has become less relevant as a measure of effectiveness of rehabilitation, not only because rehabilitation has been extended to include older patients, but also because this outcome is more influenced by the state of the economy.

The external validity of most trials reported over the past 20 years in a number of countries is, in general, poor, particularly with respect to rehabilitation programs as now offered in the UK.[73] Most trials included only men (e.g. the WHO study[67]), and those few trials that did include women contained only very modest numbers (e.g. 35/315[33]), yet approximately 30% of myocardial infarction patients are women. Secondly, most trials included only patients aged <65 years, yet more than 40% of myocardial infarction patients are >65 years. Thirdly, many programs employed further exclusion criteria (e.g. concomitant disease, second infarcts, residence too far from base hospital) so that possibly as few as 15% of the total patient population was studied and reported on.[59] Some trials noted the effects of such 'nonrepresentativeness'; for example, Shaw[38] found the total mortality to be only one-third of that expected. Therefore, considerable caution should be exercised in extrapolating results reported in trials of selected younger men to the total patient population. The rehabilitation needs of women or older patients may be different, and hence it may be necessary to adjust the goals in future evaluations.[74] Appropriate rehabilitation may be as effective in older patients with concomitant disease as in younger men with uncomplicated myocardial infarction, but objective benefits may be fewer (e.g. work capacity did not show any improvement among 60–65 year olds in the WHO collaborative study). If, as is quite possible, the selection criteria employed in trial programs were 'appropriate', or if (informal) patient selection by experienced therapists in clinical situations identifies those patients most amenable to treatment, it might be unrealistic to expect comparable benefits in other patients. The effectiveness of rehabilitation for all potentially eligible myocardial infarction patients is largely untested. Overviews that have pooled the findings of selected, mostly small, trials of often highly selected patients, or volunteers in specialist centers in a number of countries, over the past 25 years provide only rather weak guidance regarding the overall effectiveness of rehabilitation generally. These points should be borne in mind during the expansion phase of rehabilitation from selected patients in specialist centers treated by enthusiastic experts to the broad service commitment of providing a basic program for all (or most) in every acute general hospital.

Finally, brief mention should be made of the evaluation of rehabilitation following cardiac surgery. Coronary artery bypass graft (CABG) and percutaneous transluminal coronary angioplasty (PTCA) patients are being referred to rehabilitation programs, in a few instances to dedicated programs in surgical centers but more often to join myocardial infarction patients in more local programs.[14,75] There is very little in the literature on the effectiveness of rehabilitation following surgery. One or two dedicated trials are in progress at regional surgical centers (Caine, personal communication, 1995),[76] but to date there are only reports of very small numbers of surgical patients who were included with myocardial infarction (and angina) patients in general programs. For example, Froelicher *et al.*[77] described a trial of 72 patients with 74 controls, that showed improved aerobic capacity, but the trial included patients with history of myocardial infarction, GABG surgery, or symptoms of stable angina, and subgroups were not distinguished. The nature of the hospitalization experience for planned surgery is not the same as for unexpected myocardial infarction, and it is unlikely that the rehabilitation needs and responses will be the same in the two types of patient.[15] Although the number of surgical (and PTCA) patients is somewhat smaller than the number of myocardial infarction patients, these operations have been common for many years and there is a clear need for more formal evaluation of rehabilitation in these patients.

In conclusion, trials in cardiac rehabilitation have not kept abreast of pharmocological trials in cardiology. There have been no large multicenter and international trials that are comparable with those for aspirin or thrombolysis, although rehabilitation is relevant to the same patient population. Consequently, several important questions remain unanswered, or only partly answered. The principal explanations for the absence of large multicenter trials of healthcare practice were outlined earlier in this chapter. The practical difficulties make it somewhat doubtful whether trials of healthcare delivery will ever grow to resemble the recent international pharmacological trials. That notwithstanding, since trials provide the most valid answers, researchers should strive to follow, as far as possible, the examples given in other chapters. The goals of rehabilitation are long term by comparison with, for example, the objective of thrombolytic therapy and, therefore, long-term follow-up is important. The goals of rehabilitation include quality of life and, therefore, trials should look at this factor and not only at mortality. Even if in the future the suggested mortality benefit vanishes in large trials, rehabilitation might be justified on grounds of quality of life. The important challenge for future research lies in the development and choice of suitable valid measures of quality of life.

References

1. World Health Organization. Rehabilitation of patients with cardiovascular disease: report of WHO expert committee. *WHO Technical Report Series* 1964; **270**.
2. Heberden W. *Commentaries on the History and Cure of Disease.* In: Willins FA, Keys TW (eds), *Classics in Cardiology,* Vol. 1. New York: Dover, 1961.
3. Stokes W. *Diseases of the Heart and Aorta.* Dublin, 1854.
4. Levine SA, Lown B. Armchair treatment of acute coronary thrombosis. *JAMA* 1952; **148**: 1365–9.
5. Glasgow Royal Infirmary. Early mobilisation after uncomplicated myocardial infarction: prospective study of 538 patients. *Lancet* 1973; **ii**: 346–9.
6. West RR, Henderson AH. Randomised multi-centre trial of early mobilisation after uncomplicated myocardial infarction. *Br Heart J* 1979; **42**: 381–5.
7. Cain HD, Frasher WG, Stivelman R. Graded activity program for safe return to self-care after myocardial infarction. *JAMA* 1961; **177**: 111–15.
8. Morris JN, Chave SPW, Adam C, *et al.* Vigorous exercise in leisure time and incidence of coronary heart disease. *Lancet* 1973; **i**: 333–9.
9. Kellerman JJ, Levy M, Feldman S, Kariv I. Rehabilitation of coronary patients. *J Chron Dis* 1967; **20**: 815–21.
10. Gottheiner V. Long range strenuous sports training for cardiac rehabilitation. *Am J Cardiol* 1968; **22**: 426–35.
11. Adset CA, Bruhn JG. Short-term group psychotherapy for post myocardial infarction patients and their carers. *Can Med Assoc J* 1968; **99**: 577–84.
12. West RR, Evans DA. Lifestyle changes in long-term survivors of acute myocardial infarction. *J Epidemiol Commun Health* 1986; **40**: 103–9.
13. Horgan J, Bethell H, Carson P, *et al.* Working party report on cardiac rehabilitation. *Br Heart J* 1992; **67**: 412–18.
14. British Cardiac Society. Report of a working group: cardiac rehabilitation services in the United Kingdom 1992. *Br Heart J* 1995; **73**: 201–2.
15. Broustet JP, Douard H. Rehabilitation after cardiac surgery. In: Jones D, West R (eds), *Cardiac Rehabilitation.* London: BMJ Books, 1995: 128–43.
16. Todd IC, Bradnam MS, Cooke MBD, *et al.* Effects of daily high-intensity exercise on myocardial perfusion in angina pectoris. *Am J Cardiol* 1991; **68**: 1593–9.
17. Lewin B, Cay EL, Tod I, *et al.* The angina management programme: a rehabilitation treatment. *Br J Cardiol* 1995; September: 221–6.
18. Patel C, Marmot MG, Terry DJ, *et al.* Trial of relaxation in reducing coronary risk: four year follow up. *Br Med J* 1985; **290**: 1103–6.
19. Bowling A. *Measuring Health: Review of Quality of Life Measurement Scales.* Milton Keynes: Open University Press, 1992.
20. Spector ID, Thompson SG. Potential and limitations of meta-analysis. *J Epidemiol Commun Health* 1991; **45**: 89–92.
21. West RR. A look at the statistical overview (or meta-analysis). *J R Coll Phys* 1993; **27**: 111–15.
22. Gehlbach SH. *Interpreting the Medical Literature: A Clinician's Guide.* Lexington, MA: Collamore Press, 1982.
23. Elwood JM. *Causal Relation Steps in Medicine: A Practical System for Critical Appraisal.* Oxford: Oxford University Press, 1988.
24. Begg CB, Berlin JA. Publication bias: a problem in interpreting medical data. *J R Stat Soc* 1988; **151**: 419–63.
25. Dickersin K, Min YI, Meinert CL. Factors influencing publication of research results. *JAMA* 1992; **267**: 374–8.
26. West RR. Assessment of evidence versus consensus or prejudice. *J Epidemiol Commun Health* 1992; **46**: 321–2.
27. Oldridge NB, Guyatt GH, Fischer MD, Rimm AA. Cardiac rehabilitation after myocardial infarction: combined experience of randomised clinical trials. *JAMA* 1988; **260**: 945–50.
28. O'Connor GT, Buring JE, Jusuf E, *et al.* Overview of randomised trials of rehabilitation after myocardial infarction. *Circulation* 1989; **80**: 234–44.
29. Hellerstein HK. Exercise therapy in coronary heart disease. *Bull NY Acad Med* 1968; **44**: 1208–47.
30. Rechnitzer PA, Yuhasz MS, Paivio A, *et al.* Effects of 24 weeks exercise programme on normal adults and patients with previous myocardial infarction. *Br Med J* 1967; **ii**: 734–5.
31. Wenger NK, Gilbert CA, Siegel W. Symposium: the use of physical activity in the rehabilitation of patients after myocardial infarction. *Southern Med J* 1979; **63**: 891–7.
32. Kentala E. Physical fitness and feasibility of physical rehabilitation after myocardial infarction in men of working age. *Ann Clin Res* 1972; **4**(Suppl 9): 1–84.
33. Sanne H. Exercise tolerance and physical training of non-selected patients after myocardial infarction. *Acta Med Scand* 1973; Suppl 551: 1–124.
34. Palatsi I. Feasibility of physical training after myocardial infarction and its effect on return to work, morbidity and mortality. *Acta Med Scand* 1976; Suppl 599: 4–84.
35. Wilhelmsen L, Sanne H, Elmfeldt D, *et al.* A controlled trial of physical training after myocardial infarction: effects on risk factors, nonfatal reinfarction, and death. *Prev Med* 1975; **4**: 491–508.
36. de Backer G, Depoorter A, Willens P, Varewijck E. The influence of rehabilitation on the physical performance after myocardial infarction: a controlled trial. *Acta Cardiol* 1974; **6**: 427–40.
37. Naughton J. National exercise and heart disease project. *Cardiology* 1978; **63**: 352–67.
38. Shaw LW. Effects of a prescribed supervised exercise program on mortality and cardiovascular morbidity in patients after a myocardial infarction. The National Exercise and Heart Disease Project. *Am J Cardiol* 1981; **48**: 39–461.

39. Stern MJ, Cleary P. The National Exercise and Heart Disease Project: long-term psychosocial outcome. *Arch Int Med* 1982; **142**: 1093–7.
40. Carson P, Phillips R, Lloyd M, *et al.* Exercise after myocardial infarction: a controlled trial. *J R Coll Phys* 1982; **16**: 147–51.
41. Rechnitzer P, Cunningham DA, Andrew GM, *et al.* Relation of exercise to the recurrence rate of myocardial infarction in men. Ontario exercise–heart collaborative study. *Am J Cardiol* 1983; **51**: 65–9.
42. Roman O, Guitierrez M, Luksie I, *et al.* Cardiac rehabilitation after myocardial infarction: nine year controlled follow-up study. *Cardiology* 1983; **70**: 223–31.
43. Marra S, Paolillo V, Spadaccini F, *et al.* Long-term follow-up after a controlled randomized post-myocardial infarction rehabilitation programme: effects on morbidity and mortality. *Eur Heart J* 1985; 656–63.
44. Bethell HJN, Mullee MA. Controlled trial of community-based coronary rehabilitation. *Br Heart J* 1990; **64**: 370–5.
45. Bethell HJN. Rehabilitation in the community of patients recovering from acute myocardial infarction: a randomised control trial. MD thesis, Cambridge University, UK, 1995.
46. Sivarajan E, Bruce R, Bronwen D, *et al.* Treadmill test responses to an early exercise program after myocardial infarction: a randomized study. *Circulation* 1982; **65**: 1420–8.
47. Miller NH, Haskell WL, Berra K, De Busk RF. Home versus group exercise training for increasing functional capacity after myocardial infarction. *Circulation* 1984; **70**: 645–9.
48. Goble AJ, Hare DL, Macdonald PS, *et al.* Effect of early programmes of high and low intensity exercise on physical performance after transmural acute myocardial infarction. *Br Heart J* 1991; **54**: 126–31.
49. Ibrahim MA, Feldman JG, Sultz HA, *et al.* Management after myocardial infarction: a controlled trial of the effect of group psychotherapy. *Int J Psychiatry Med* 1974; **5**: 253–68.
50. Rahe RH, Ward HW, Hayes V. Brief group therapy in myocardial infarction rehabilitation: three-to-four-year follow-up of a controlled trial. *Psychosom Med* 1979; **41**: 229–41.
51. Naismith LD, Robinson JF, Shaw GB, MacIntyre MMJ. Psychosocial rehabilitation after myocardial infarction. *Br Med J* 1979; **1**: 439–46.
52. Mayou R, Macmahon D, Sleight P. Florencio MJ. Early rehabilitation after myocardial infarction. *Lancet* 1981; **ii**: 1399–401.
53. Stern MJ, Gorman PA, Kaslow L. The group counselling vs. exercise therapy study: a controlled intervention with subjects following myocardial infarction. *Arch Intern Med* 1983; **143**: 1719–25.
54. Horlick L, Cameron R, Firor W, *et al.* Effects of education and group discussion in post myocardial infarction patients. *J Psychosom Res* 1984; **28**: 485–92.
55. Friedman M, Thorenson CE, Gill JJ, *et al.* Alteration of type A behaviour and reduction in cardiac recurrences in post-myocardial infarction patients. *Am Heart J* 1984; **108**: 237–48.
56. Frasure-Smith N, Prince R. The ischemic heart disease life stress monitoring program: impact on mortality. *Psychol Med* 1985; **47**: 431–45.
57. Frasure-Smith N, Prince R. Long-term follow-up of the Ischaemic Heart Disease Life Stress Monitoring Program. *Psychosom Med* 1989; **51**: 485–513.
58. Burgess A, Lerner D, D'Agostino, *et al.* A randomised control trial of cardiac rehabilitation. *Soc Sci Med* 1987; **24**: 359–70.
59. P re Cor. Comparison of rehabilitation programme, counselling programme and usual care after acute myocardial infarction: results of a long-term randomized trial. *Eur Heart J* 1991; **12**: 612–16.
60. Jones DA, West RR. Multicentre randomised controlled trial of rehabilitation following myocardial infarction. *Br Heart J* 1993; **69**(Suppl 5): 37 (abstract).
61. Gruen W. Effects of brief psychotherapy during hospitalisation period on the recovery process in heart attacks. *J Consult Clin Psychol* 1975; **43**: 223–32.
62. Thompson DL, Meddis R. Prospective evaluation of in-hospital counselling for first time myocardial infarction. *J Psychosom Res* 1990; **34**: 237–48.
63. Langosch W, Seer P, Brodner G, *et al.* Behaviour therapy with coronary heart disease patients: results of a comparative study. *J Psychol Res* 1982; **26**: 475–84.
64. Dixhoorn J van, Duivenvoorden HJ, Stahl HA, *et al.* Physical training and relaxation therapy in cardiac rehabilitation assessed through a composite criterion for training outcome. *Am Heart J* 1989; **118**: 545–52.
65. Dixhoorn J van, Duivenvoorden HJ, Pool J, *et al.* Psychic effects of physical training and relaxation therapy after myocardial infarction. *J Psychol Res* 1990; **34**: 327–37.
66. World Health Organization. Evaluation of comprehensive rehabilitate and preventive programmes for patients after acute myocardial infarction: report on two working groups. *EURO 8206(8)*. Copenhagen: WHO, 1973.
67. World Health Organisation. Rehabilitation and comprehensive secondary prevention after acute myocardial infarction. *EURO Report 84*. Copenhagen: WHO, 1983.
68. Kallio V, Hamalainen H, Hakkila J, Luturila OJ. Reduction in sudden death by a multifactorial intervention programme after acute myocardial infarction. *Lancet* 1979; **ii**: 1091–4.
69. Vermeulen A, Liew KI, Durrer D. Effects of cardiac rehabilitation after myocardial infarction: changes in coronary risk factors and long-term prognosis. *Am Heart J* 1983; **105**: 798–801.
70. Bengtsson K. Rehabilitation after myocardial infarction, a controlled study. *Scand J Rehab Med* 1983; **15**: 1–9.
71. Oldridge N, Guyatt G, Jones N, *et al.* Effects on quality of life with comprehensive rehabilitation after acute myocardial infarction. *Am J Cardiol* 1991; **67**: 1084–9.

72. Lewin B, Robertson I, Cay E, *et al*. Effects of self-help post-myocardial infarction rehabilitation on psychological adjustment and use of health services. *Lancet* 1992; **339**: 1036–40.
73. Davidson C. Cardiac rehabilitation in the district hospital. In: Jones D, West R (eds), *Cardiac Rehabilitation*. London: BMJ Books, 1995: 144–66.
74. Cay EL. Goals of rehabilitation. In: Jones D, West R (eds), *Cardiac Rehabilitation*. London: BMJ Books, 1995: 31–53.
75. Kavanagh T. The role of exercise training in cardiac rehabilitation. In: Jones D, West R (eds), *Cardiac Rehabilitation*. London: BMJ Books, 1995: 54–82.
76. Worsornu D, Allardyce W, Ballantyne D, *et al*. Influence of power and aerobic exercise training on haemostatic factors after coronary artery surgery. *Br Heart J* 1992; **68**: 181–6.
77. Froelicher V, Jensen J, Genter F, *et al*. A randomised trial of exercise training in patients with coronary disease. *JAMA* 1984; **252**: 1291–7.

Index